RADIOISOTOPE STUDIES IN CARDIOLOGY

DEVELOPMENTS IN NUCLEAR MEDICINE
Series editor Peter H. Cox

Cox, P.H. (ed.): Cholescintigraphy. 1981. ISBN 90-247-2524-0

Cox, P.H. (ed.): Progress in radiopharmacology 3. Selected Topics. 1982. ISBN 90-247-2768-5

Jonckheer, M.H. and Deconinck, F. (eds.): X-ray fluorescent scanning of the thyroid. 1983. ISBN 0-89838-561-X

Kristensen, K. and Nørbygaard, E. (eds.): Safety and efficacy of radiopharmaceuticals. 1984. ISBN 0-89838-609-8

Bossuyt, A. and Deconinck, F.: Amplitude/phase patterns in dynamic scintigraphic imaging. 1984. ISBN 0-89838-641-1

Hardeman, M.R. and Najean, Y. (eds.): Blood cells in nuclear medicine I. Cell kinetics and bio-distribution. 1984. ISBN 0-89838-653-5

Fueger, G.F. (ed.): Blood cells in nuclear medicine II. Migratory blood cells. 1984. ISBN 0-89838-654-3

Biersack, H.J. and Cox, P.H. (eds.): Radioisotope studies in cardiology. 1985. ISBN 0-89838-733-7

Radioisotope studies in cardiology

edited by

H.J. BIERSACK

Institute of Clinical and Experimental Nuclear Medicine
University of Bonn
Federal Republic of Germany

P.H. COX

Department of Nuclear Medicine
Rotterdam Radio-Therapeutic Institute
Rotterdam, The Netherlands

1985 **MARTINUS NIJHOFF PUBLISHERS**
a member of the KLUWER ACADEMIC PUBLISHERS GROUP
DORDRECHT / BOSTON / LANCASTER

Distributors

for the United States and Canada: Kluwer Academic Publishers, 190 Old Derby Street, Hingham, MA 02043, USA
for the UK and Ireland: Kluwer Academic Publishers, MTP Press Limited, Falcon House, Queen Square, Lancaster LA1 1RN, UK
for all other countries: Kluwer Academic Publishers Group, Distribution Center, P.O. Box 322, 3300 AH Dordrecht, The Netherlands

Library of Congress Cataloging in Publication Data

```
Main entry under title:

Radioisotope studies in cardiology.

   (Developments in nuclear medicine)
   Includes index.
   1. Radioisotope scanning.  2. Radioisotopes in
cardiology.  3. Heart--Diseases--Diagnosis.  4. Diagnosis,
Noninvasive.  I. Biersack, H. J.  II. Cox, Peter H.
III. Series.  [DNLM: 1. Cardiology--methods.  2. Heart--
radionuclide imaging.  3. Radioisotopes--diagnostic
use.  W1 DE998KF / WG 141.5.R2 R129]
RC683.5.R33R33  1985      616.1'207575      85-8859
```

ISBN-13: 978-94-010-8724-7   e-ISBN-13: 978-94-009-5022-1
DOI: 10.1007/978-94-009-5022-1

Copyright

CONTENTS

FOREWORD

During the last decade many significant advances have been made in the in vivo diagnosis of disease. An area of particular success has been the application of nuclear medical procedures to the detection of cardiac disease.

Not only is it possible to detect infarction or ischemia by scintigraphic techniques but by the use of labelled metabolites and analogues of potassium the viability of myocardial tissue can be evaluated. The efficiency of the heart pump can be calculated and wall motility observed in one simple procedure. The use of ultra short life radionuclides has made the evaluation of rapid changes in myocardial function feasible. Altogether a broad and impressive diagnostic package.

In this volume up-to-date reviews of all of the available techniques have been collected including methods which are still in the development phase. There is an inherent emphasis on European experience in Nuclear Cardiology which is then placed in context with world wide experience in the field.

This volume will be of interest to all concerned with cardiac diseases and we hope that it will serve to stimulate further developments in the future.

H.J. Biersack, Bonn
P.H. Cox, Rotterdam

CONTRIBUTORS

Bauer, R. — Nuklearmedizinische Klinik und Poliklinik rechts der Isar der Technischen Universität München, FRG.

Biersack, H.J. — Institut für klinische und experimentelle Nuklearmedizin der Universität Bonn, FRG.

Breuel, H.P. — Degussa Pharma Homburg, Frankfurt 1, FRG.

Cox, P.H. — Department of Nuclear Medicine, Rotterdamsch Radio-Therapeutisch Instituut, Rotterdam, The Netherlands.

Dressler, J. — Abteilung Allgemeine Nuklearmedizin, Zentrum der Radiologie, Klinikum der Universität, Frankfurt/Main, FRG.

Dudczak, R. — Department of Nuclear Medicine, I. Medizinische Universitätsklinik, Vienna, Austria.

Klepzig jr., H. — Abteilung Kardiologie- ZIM Universitätskliniken, Frankfurt/Main, FRG.

Knopp, R. — Institut für klinische und experimentelle Nuklearmedizin der Universität Bonn, FRG.

Pachinger, O. — Kardiologische Universitäts-Klinik, Wien, Austria.

Remme, W.J. — Department of Cardiology, Zuiderziekenhuis, Rotterdam, The Netherlands.

Reske, S.N. — Institut für klinische und experimentelle Nuklearmedizin der Universität Bonn, FRG.

Schmoliner, R. — First medical department University of Vienna, Austria.

Schümichen, C. — Department of Nuclear Medicine Albert-Ludwigs-University of Freiburg i. Br., FRG.

Vyska, K. — Institut für Medizin der Kernforschungsanlage Jülich, FRG.

Wackers, F.J.Th. — Cardiology Section, Yale University School of Medicine, New Haven, Connecticut, USA.

I. BASIC SCIENCE

MYOCARDIAL ISCHEMIA: A PROFILE OF ITS PATHOPHYSIOLOGICAL
BASIS AND ITS DETECTION BY NUCLEAR CARDIOLOGY

W.J. REMME

INTRODUCTION

As a muscular pump with the specific task of ensuring the
optimal circulation of blood under the most variable conditions,
the heart continuously consumes energy at a very high rate. A
large quantity of high energy phosphates are produced continuously to meet its specific requirements which makes a normal
oxygen and substrate delivery, removal of wastage and an undisturbed cellular metabolism essential. During myocardial
ischemia however, myocardial blood-flow and hence the oxygen
and substrate supply is reduced. Due to diminished venous
efflux from the ischemic area metabolic endproducts accumulate
and myocardial metabolism and function quickly deteriorates.

By means of nuclear medical techniques coronary blood-
flow and myocardial function can be monitored and metabolic
and hemodynamic changes registered. In this chapter the normal
physiology of myocardial perfusion, metabolism and cardiac
function, the pathophysiological changes which occur during
myocardial ischemia and possible approaches to a better understanding of its inherent problems via nuclear medical procedures will be discussed.

Coronary circulation

The coronary arterial system can be subdivided into the
large epicardial arteries (the conductance vessels), from which
smaller arteries branch off to penetrate the myocardial wall
at an approximate 90° angle and eventually form the arterioles
and capillary bed. Resistance to coronary flow is determined
mainly by the arterioles, the resistance vessels, which under
maximal pharmacological vasodilation have the capacity to increase

coronary blood-blow by a factor 4 to 5. In the wide conductance vessels the resistance to flow under normal conditions will be low. The compressive forces of walltension exerted on intra-myocardial vessels also creates a certain resistance to flow, which will be especially noticeable in the subendocardial region where the walltension is highest (fig 1a). In the normal situation this already results in vasodilatation of the sub-endocardial resistance vessels to ensure sufficient coronary flow. This is particularly important in view of the higher oxygen consumption of the subendocardial cells which are subjected to higher loading conditions than the subepicardial cells. This, however, implies that during progressive proximal coronary artery narrowing and hence increase in conductance vessel resistance the possibility of further dilation of the coronary reserve, will be exhausted earlier in the subendo-cardial region compared with the subepicardial region. Thus, myocardial ischemia always begins in the subendocardium, and only progresses in a subepicardial and lateral direction during more severe and prolonged periods of reduced coronary blood-flow (fig 1b and 1c).

The regulation of coronary blood-flow
With equal myocardial performance, coronary blood-flow will be constant in spite of varying perfusion pressures. The continuous adjustment of coronary resistance and flow to meet the instantaneous oxygen need of the muscle exists strictly on the basis of local mechanisms which are mainly metabolic. This is known as autoregulation. The most important and instantaneous regulator of flow is the nucleoside adenosine, the first catabolite of the high energy phosphates, which can diffuse across the intact cell membrane. This is formed as a result of cleavage of a phosphate group from 5'-adenosine monophosphate (5'-AMP) by the enzyme 5'-nucleotidase located at the cell membrane, which facilitates the release of adenosine into the surrounding interstitial fluid (1-3). It then presumably combines with specific adenosine receptors on the perivascular myocytes and directly influences arteriolar

5

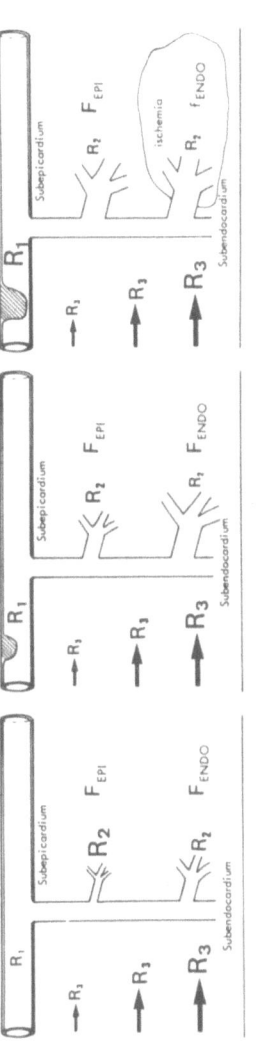

Fig. 1. Schematic representation of the various resistances in the coronary arterial bed and their effect on flow (F) in a normal coronary artery (fig 1a) and in the situation of a moderate and severe stenosis (fig 1b and fig 1c, resp). Due to higher walltension and compressive forces (R3) in the subendocardial region vasodilatation with decreased arteriolar resistance (R2) is already present in the normal situation (fig 1a). During progressive coronary stenosis and hence increase in conductance vessel resistance (R1), a compensating vasodilatation and decreased arteriolar resistance is found, which in moderate lesions results in unchanged regional flow (fig 1b). However, with a severe stenosis subendocardial arterioles eventually cannot further dilate and local coronary flow will diminish resulting in ischemic, even at rest (fig 1c).

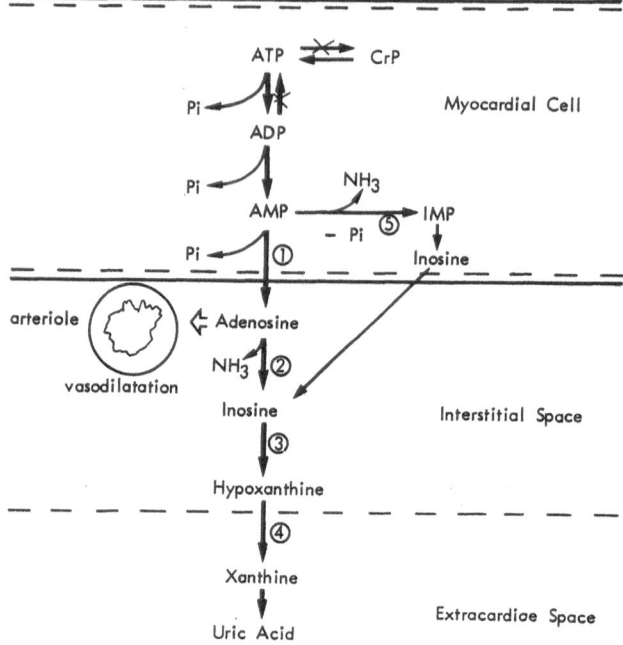

Fig. 2. Adenine nucleotide breakdown during myocardial ischemia. In the absence of oxydative phosphorylation resynthesis of ATP from ADP is inhibited which results in the accumulation of AMP and P_1. AMP can either be dephosphorylated to adenosine or deaminated to IMP. The latter reaction however will be inhibited by the accumulating P_1, resulting in an increase of adenosine which is the first ATP catabolyte able to pass the cellmembrane into the interstitial space. It then presumably combines with specific adenosine receptors on the arterioles and induces vasodilatation. Adenosine is easily and quickly deaminated to inosine and is only found in very small amounts in the venous effluent. Its breakdown products inosine and especially hypoxanthine can be detected more easily and may be used as biochemical markers of myocardial ischemia.
1. 5'-nucleotidase
2. adenosine deaminase
3. nucleoside phosphorylase
4. xanthine oxidase
5. adenylic acid deaminase.

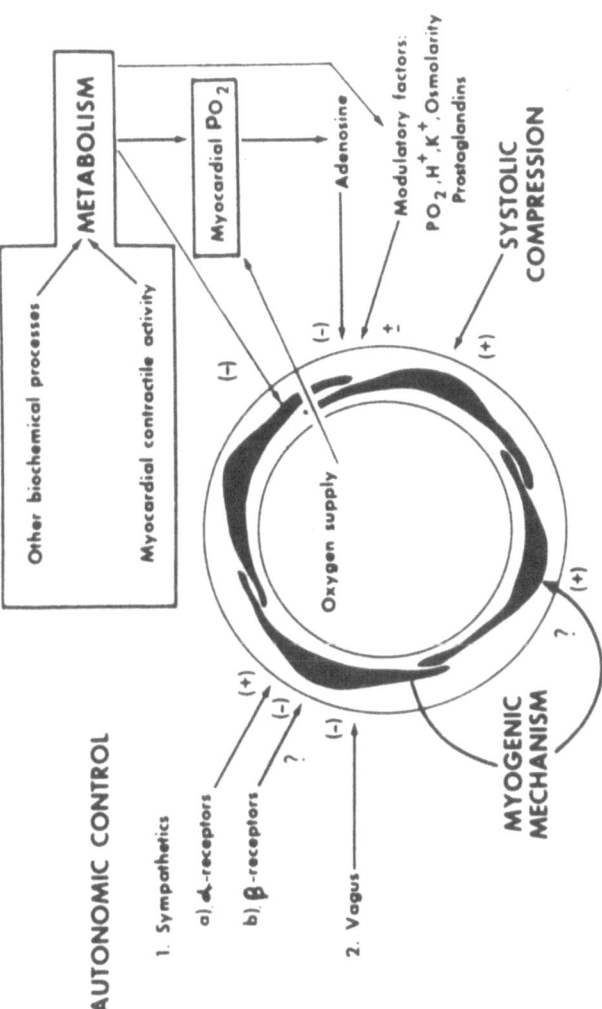

Fig. 3. Schematic representation of the various mechanisms influencing coronary blood-flow. (+) = Factors that reduce arteriolar lumen by vasoconstriction or compression. (-) = Factors that relax vascular smooth muscle tone. Force exerted by blood-pressure to stretch the vessel is not shown (from Berne RM Rubio R, Coronary Circulation. In: Handbook of Physiology, Sect. 2, The Cardiovascular System. Berne RM, Sperelakis N, Geiger SR, Bethesda MD (eds), Amer. Physiol. Soc. p 897 (1979) with permission.

vascular tone (4). This provides an immediate metabolic link
between energy production and oxygen delivery. During ischemia
adenosinetriphosphate (ATP) is not resynthesized from adenosine diphosphate (ADP) and 5'-AMP accumulates. Although 5'-AMP
may be converted into 5'-IMP, by the enzyme adenylic acid
deaminase, this is inhibited by the reduction of ATP and
accumulation of inorganic phosphate (p_i), which results in
the formation of adenosine (1) (fig 2). An increase of adenosine or its breakdown products inosine and hypoxanthine in
the venous effluent during ischemia has been demonstrated in
both animal and human studies (5-10) and the release of these
nucleosides by the heart are used as an indicator of myocardial
ischemia. Hypoxanthine especially seems to be a promising
metabolic indicator of myocardial ischemia in man (8,9). Work
induced vasodilatation however is more difficult to explain.
It is possible that relative decreases in pO_2 are sensed by
chemoreceptors on specific pericyte type cells, which then
increase local activity of the enzyme 5-nucleotidase and thus
stimulate adenosine production (11). Other metabolic factors
which influence coronary vascular tone without direct autoregulatory effects are pH, pCO_2, osmolarity changes and the
prostaglandins (fig 3). Although a direct autoregulatory
effect of pH and pCO_2 is unlikely on quantitative grounds,
i.e. nonphysiological large changes are needed to adapt the
coronary flow to instantaneous O_2 demand, changes in pH and
pCO_2 presumably modulate the sensitivity of the autoregulatory
(adenosine?) receptors.

Metabolic acidosis will enhance coronary blood-flow while,
on the other hand, alkalosis induces vasoconstriction with
small decreases in flow, i.e. during hyperventilation. A
continuous neural regulation of coronary vascular resistance
exists; vasoconstriction being induced by sympathetic impulses
and vasodilatation by parasymphathetic stimulation. A constant
degree of neurally induced vasoconstriction normally exists
which is continuously reflex modulated. However, these changes
in coronary resistance are low (30-40%) when compared to the
alterations caused by metabolic stimulation which can be 5-6
fold (12). Furthermore, autonomic nerve stimulation is mainly

confined to the resistance vessels. Excessive sympathetic vasoconstriction which results in coronary artery spasm of the large epicardial vessels seems an unlikely event because of their sparse sympathetic innervation.

Coronary insufficiency and myocardial ischemia

Coronary insufficiency is a pathophysiological disturbance in coronary perfusion and therefore of oxygen and substrate supply to the myocardial cell in relation to demand. In nearly all cases coronary insufficiency is the result of a local stenosis in one or more of the greater epicardial coronary arteries. This stenosis can be fixed (the arteriosclerotic lesion) or dynamic (the coronary artery spasm). As a result of this local stenosis a regional disturbance of coronary artery flow occurs with a subsequent relative or absolute shortage of oxygen and substrates which results in regional myocardial ischemia.

Although exercise-induced myocardial ischemia is nearly always caused by arteriosclerotic coronary artery lesions a clinical syndrome of myocardial ischemia in patients with normal coronary arteries without obvious spasm (syndrome X) has been described (13). In these patients a diminished coronary dilatory reserve was found without histologic abnormalities of the small intramyocardial vessels. Degenerative changes of the myocardial cell with mitochondrial alterations were, however, often present.

The vasodilatory reserve of the coronary vasculature prevents flow reduction in a moderate coronary artery diameter narrowing of 40-50% or less. A progressive reduction of normal resting coronary artery flow was found with acute diameter reductions of 85% or more with minimal or absent vasodilatory reserve (14) (fig 4). With stenoses of more than 50% of diameter, the blood-supply can either be improved by peripheral arteriolar dilatation or will remain unchanged in the event of an exhausted coronary vasodilatory reserve.

Whether coronary flow will be sufficient to prevent ischemia in lesions of 50 to 85%, depends both on the remaining vasodilatory reserve as well as on instantaneous myocardial

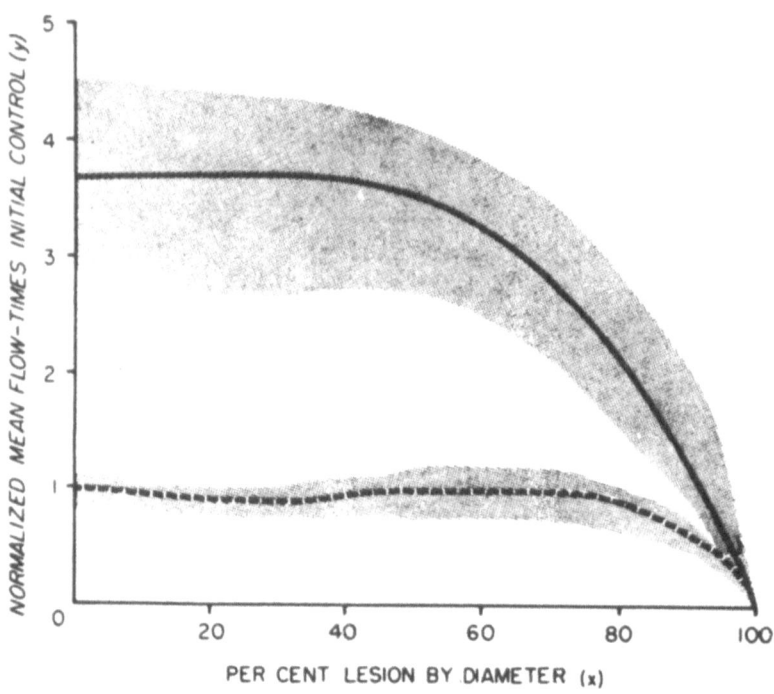

Fig. 4. Coronary artery flow and vasodilatory reserve. The relation
between percentual coronary artery diameter constriction to resting
mean flow (------------) and the hyperemic response (───────)
to intracoronary contrast injections in dogs is shown. Flows are
expressed as ratios to control resting mean values at the beginning
of each experiment. The shaded area indicates the limits of the
relation plotted for individual dogs. (From Gould KL et al, Amer. J.
Cardiol. 33:89 (1974) with permission.

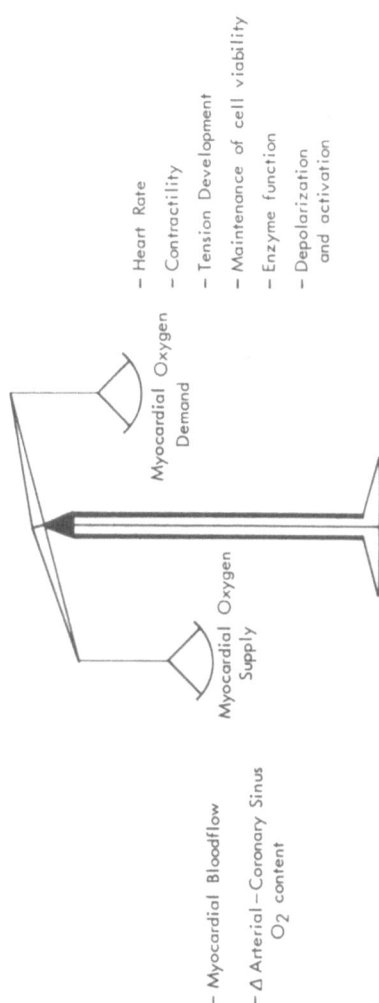

- Myocardial Bloodflow

- Δ Arterial–Coronary Sinus O₂ content

Myocardial Oxygen Supply

Myocardial Oxygen Demand

- Heart Rate
- Contractility
- Tension Development
- Maintenance of cell viability
- Enzyme function
- Depolarization and activation

Fig. 5. Factors influencing the instantaneous myocardial oxygen supply/demand ratio. The major determinants of myocardial oxygen demand are heartrate, contractility and walltension. The basic processes needed for normal enzyme and membrane function and cell viability consume far less oxygen.

oxygen demand. The occurence of myocardial ischemia has now become critically dependent on the extent to which myocardial energy consumption, and therefore oxygen need, is raised and will be determined by the direct supply/demand ratio (fig 5). Recent studies in animals suggest an actual decrease in flow over a critical coronary lesion during maximal peripheral vasodilatation (15). A decrease in peripheral perfusion pressure and increase in stenotic resistance has been suggested. Also, the occurrence of a steal phenomenon, during coronary vasodilatation, of blood from areas with a reduced coronary reserve i.e. supplied by collaterals to low resistance areas has been described (16,17).

The myocardial oxygen demand depends only to a small extent on the basic cellular functions needed for cell viability. Whilst the beating canine heart consumes 8-15 ml/min/100 gr oxygen only 2 ml/min/100 gr is needed in the quiescent non-beating heart (18).

Walltension, especially in the enlarged heart, contractility and heart rate are the major determinants of myocardial oxygen consumption. The occurence of ischemia in the event of a critical coronary lesion largely depends on these hemodynamic variables.

Coronary spasm

The concept of the supply-demand ratio for the development of ischemia is of less importance when spasm occurs in one of the epicardial vessels. Although originally described in patients with normal coronary arteries (19), pharmacologically induced spasm has been shown to occur predominantly in existing arteriosclerotic lesions (20). Furthermore, even relative small luminal reductions due merely to increased vasotone rather than frank spasm can alter a moderate lesion into a critical stenosis with diminished coronary flow reserve (fig 6). Depending on the severity of the constriction, clinical signs of only subendocardial or complete transmural ischemia will be found. In the same patient, exercise-induced angina pectoris due to a fixed arteriosclerotic lesion and angina at rest, presumably of vasopastic origin, may be found.

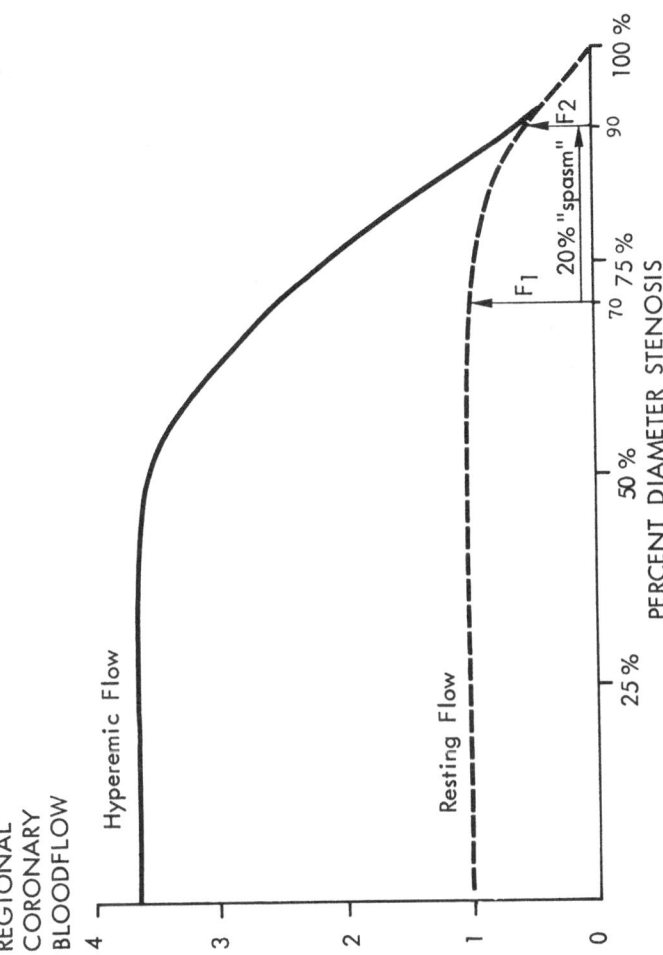

Fig. 6. Theoretical example of the effect of a relatively small reduction in diameter by increased vasomotor tone on the severity of an underlying coronary artery lesion. A 20% narrowing due to vasoconstriction can change a moderate lesion with sufficient coronary reserve into a critical stenosis without any reserve left or with even a decrease in resting coronary flow.

14

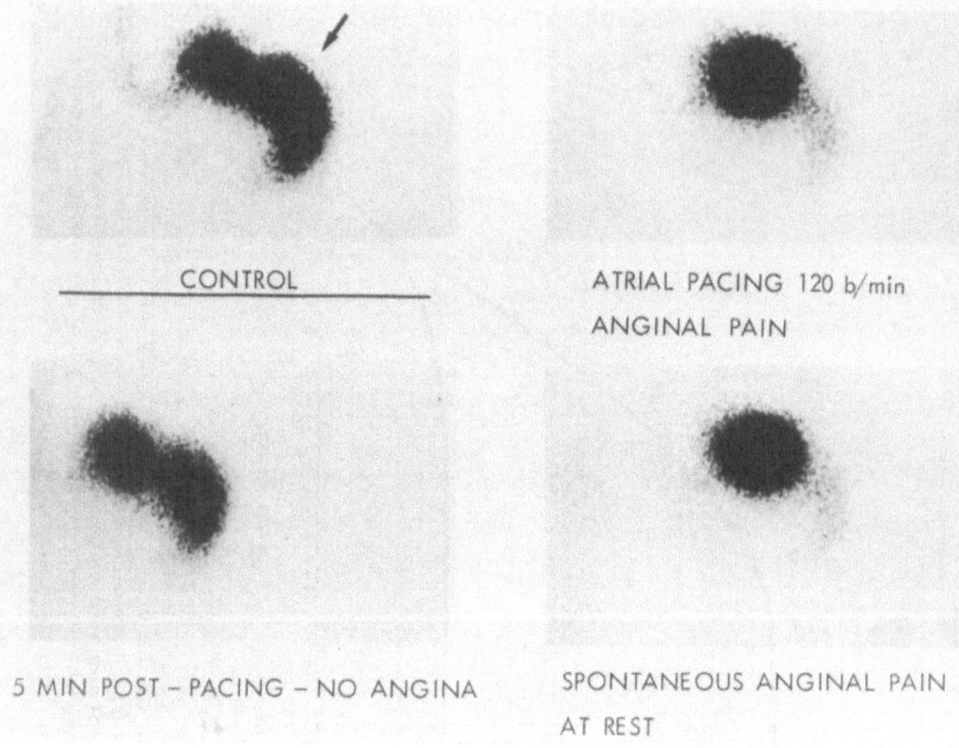

CONTROL

ATRIAL PACING 120 b/min

ANGINAL PAIN

5 MIN POST – PACING – NO ANGINA

SPONTANEOUS ANGINAL PAIN

AT REST

Fig. 7. Reduction of regional coronary flow during spontaneous angina pectoris at rest in the same area as during atrial pacing induced ischemia. In this patient Kr81m is continuously infused into the left circumflex artery which has a 70-90% stenosis (arrow). During pacing-induced anginal pain Kr81m distribution is decreased over the post-stenotic area with an increase over the normal area. 5 min after pacing the Kr81m changes have nearly returned to the control situation after angina has subsided for several minutes. However, thereafter, during spontaneous anginal pain Kr81m again disappears in the same area with an increase over the normal region suggesting a reduction in coronary flow due to spasm of the artery at the site of the stenosis.

During our studies using intracoronary Kr^{81m} (see later
in this volume), several patients developed angina at rest
with similar reductions in coronary blood-flow as were observed
during atrial pacing induced ischemia (fig 7). Various
mechanisms have been proposed to explain the occurrence of
spasm, including the effects of α-adrenergic and serotonergic
stimulation (21). The opposing effects of arachidonic acid
metabolites thromboxane A$_2$ and the prostanoid PGI$_2$ (prosta-
cyclin) on blood-platelets and vascular smooth muscle are
believed to be relevant to the pathophysiology of vasospasm
and intravascular platelet aggregation (22,23). The strong
vasospastic properties of thromboxane A$_2$, released from plate-
lets adhering to the rough surface of an arteriosclerotic
plaque, could be of importance in the absence of locally
produced prostacycline (24).

This prostaglandin which is formed in the normal, undamaged
vessel wall has strong counteracting vasodilating properties
at low doses. A vicious circle may be envisaged with continuous
platelet adherence during spasm producing small thrombusforma-
tions and thromboxane release, which in turn prolong arterial
spasm and induce myocardial ischemia with the final outcome
of an occluding thrombus and myocardial infarction (20,25).

Myocardial metabolism

In contrast to other types of muscle, the heart with its
ever continuing sequence of contraction and relaxation, is
not allowed an oxygen debt. It is in constant need of large
quantities of energy which are generated and kept as ATP with
a small reserve of creatinine phosphate (CrP). Under normal
conditions this ATP is formed exclusively by oxidative metabolism with only 1% production via anaerobic pathways. Under
normal circumstances oxygen extraction from the blood is already maximal (± 75% compared to only 25% in other types of
muscle) and any extra supply of oxygen has to be met by
augmentation of the coronary flow. The energy eventually
generated will be used for contraction/relaxation of the cell,
biosynthesis and membrane transport.

The substrates used by the heart for its ATP-production

in declining order of importance are: free fatty acids (FFA),
glucose, lactic acid and ketone bodies. Their rate of incorporation and utilization will depend on plasmaconcentration, hormonal activity (i.e. insuline, catecholamines) and the immediate
metabolic rate.

FFA metabolism

Free fatty acids provide up to 60-70% of the total substrate during oxydative metabolism (26). Uptake by the cell
depends on blood-concentration, the ratio of total FFA to
high-binding sites on albumen and the chain length and degree
of unsaturation. During the first passage 40-50% of labelled
FFA is extracted by the myocyte (27). Membrane passage is
both by diffusion as well as by carrier. Intra-cellulary FFA
are mainly esterified to lipids and stored as glycerol (90%)
or transformed to phospholipids to partake in membranefunction
(10%) (28,29). A small portion remains soluble and another
small, but rapidly replenished portion, is metabolized (fig 8).
Before metabolism in the β-oxidation pathway can take place
FFA must be transformed into the mitochondria by way of Acyl-
CoA and carnitine. During β-oxydation Acyl-CoA is degraded
stepwise to form Acetyl-CoA fragments, which then can enter
into the tricarboxylic acid (Krebs) cycle.

Glucose metabolism

The normale rate of glucose utilization is low (10-30%) at
a normal workload. When the only available substrate glyto-
lytically derived acetyl-CoA can rise to 70% during extreme
workloads, aerobic conditions and high glucose uptake, while
at the same tome a slight increase (7%) of the anaerobic
production of ATP is found (30). This, however, is insufficient
for normal contractility. FFA will therefore always be required
for optimal contractile function.

Glucose is transported over the sarcolemma carrier-bound
with increased uptake stimulation by insulin, adrenaline and
intracellular hypoxia (fig 9). It is then transformed to
glucose-6-phosphate by hexokinase and either follows the
glycolytic pathway to pyruvate entering the Krebs cycle via

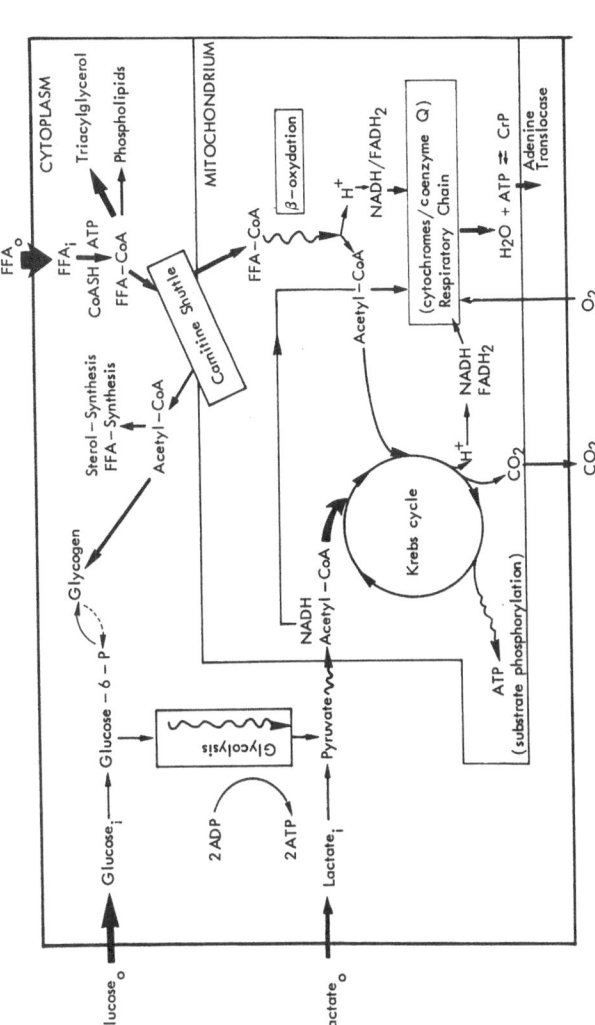

Fig. 8. Myocardial substrate metabolism under normal, aerobic conditions. In declining order of prevalence FFA, glucose and lactate are taken up by the cell and metabolized, eventually to form Acetyl-CoA, which enters the Krebs cycle. During the latter process 1 mole ATP is generated directly (substrate phosphorylation) however more important is the formation of the reduced co-enzymes NADH and FADH2, which subsequently are oxidized in the respiratory chain, eventually to form 33 mole of ATP. FFA enters the cell by diffusion or carrier-bound, where the majority is stored as glycerol. Only a small portion is metabolized in the β-oxidation pathway after binding to Acetyl-CoA and entering the mitochondria via the carnitine shuttle system. During β-oxidation Acetyl-CoA fragments are formed as well as the reduced co-enzymes NADH and FADH2, which are then oxidized in the respiratory chain. For a more detailed description of glucose metabolism see fig 9.

18

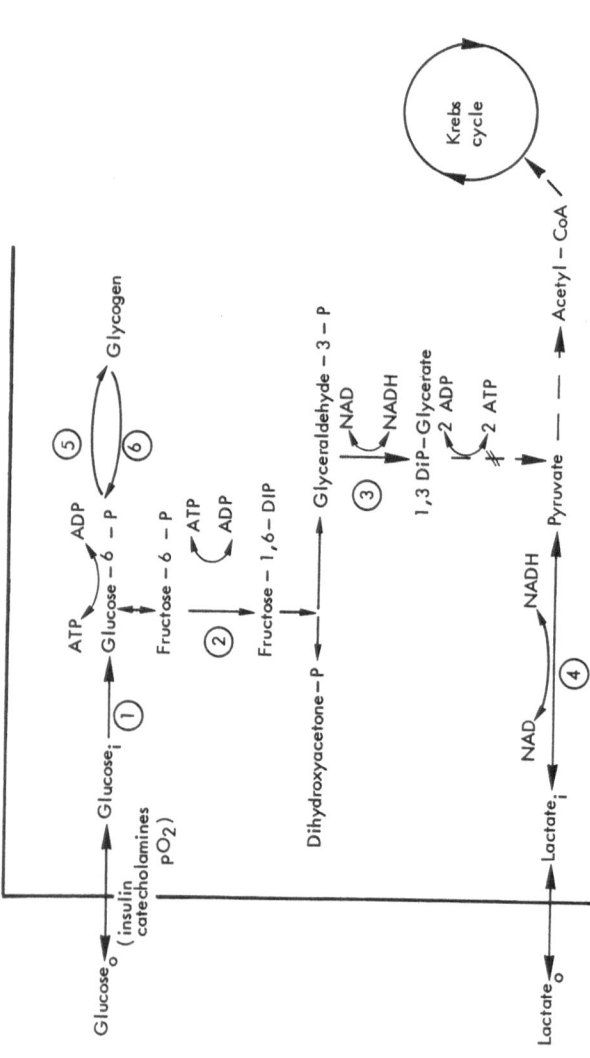

Fig. 9. Glucose and lactate metabolism under normal aerobic conditions. Glucose uptake by the cell is carrier-bound and dependent on insulin and adrenalin stimulation. Once inside it is phosphorylated by hexokinase (1) to glucose-6-P. It then enters the glycolytic pathway or is transformed to glycogen by the enzyme glycogensynthe-tase (5). The glycolytic flux is mainly governed by the enzymes phosphofructokinase (2) and glyceraldehyde-3-P-dehydrogenase (4). When there is sufficient O_2 supply glycolysis is regulated mainly by instantaneous ATP content at the phosphofructokinase level. Although ATP is utilized at 2 steps a net gain of 2 mole ATP per mole of glucose is achieved at the end of glycolysis. Pyruvate, formed both by the glycolytic pathway as well as from lactate thereupon is converted to Acetyl-CoA and enters the Krebs cycle.

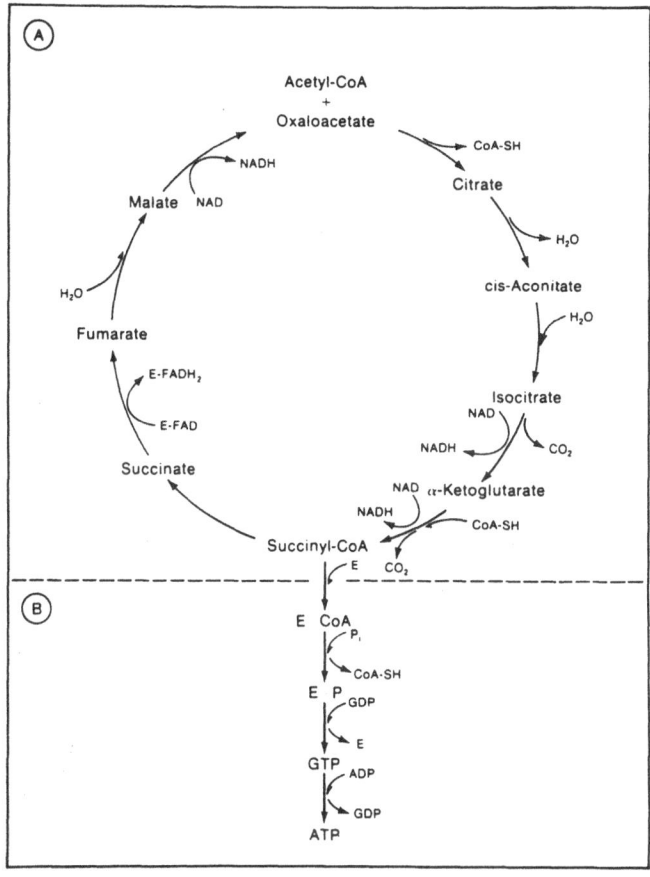

Fig. 10. Pathways of Acetyl-CoA oxydation. a. Tricarboxylic acid cycle or Krebs cycle. Citrate is formed after condensation of acetyl-CoA with oxaloacetate and eventually transformed in the Krebs cycle to oxaloacetate, during a process of oxydation and decarboxylation, where a number of reduced co-enzymes are formed. b. Substrate level phosphorylation. Each mole of enzyme-bound CoA released from succinyl-CoA provides for the generation of a single mole of ATP. From Katz AM, Physiology of the heart, Raven Press, New York, p 57 (1977) with permission.

acetyl-CoA or is stored as glycogen. During its passage
through the glycolytic pathway a net yield of 2 moles of ATP
per mole of glucose is produced.

Lactate

Under normal conditions lactate is never produced by the
myocardium. The net extraction pattern varies between 0-35%;
largely depending on arterial lactate level, catecholamine
stimulation and substrate competition (FFA). It enters the
Krebs cycle via transformation to pyruvate and acetyl-CoA.

Energy generation by phosphorylation

After condensation with oxaloacetate to citrate, acetyl-
CoA is oxidized and decarboxylated in the Krebs cycle, during
which process substrate phosphorylation at the succinyl-CoA
level yields 1 mole ATP (fig 10).

More important is the formation of the reduced co-enzymes
NADH and $FADH_2$, which also occurs during β-oxidation. NADH
and $FADH_2$ are then oxidized during the respiratory chain
phosphorylation, where under the influence of the mitochondrial
membrane-bound enzymes (cytochromes and co-enzyme Q) the
electrons initially carried by the reduced co-enzymes NADH
and $FADH_2$ are transferred to molecular oxygen, producing O^{2-},
which combines with $2H^+$ to H_2O. During this process chemical
energy in the form of ATP is generated. Energy, that can be
stored as ATP or CrP, or used for a great variety of chemical
processes, including enzymeregulation, membranefunction,
contractility and relaxation. To this purpose ATP has to be
transported from the mitochondria into the cytoplasm, a process
which is carried out by the adenine nucleotide translocase
system.

Although ATP is in part formed by substrate phosphorylation, virtually all of the aerobic generated ATP is obtained
by the respiratory chain linked phosphorylation with a total
yield of 36 moles of ATP per mole of glucose.

Myocardial metabolism during ischemia

During myocardial ischemia oxidative phosphorylation will soon be halted when no oxygen is available. Secondary to the diminished electrontransport and subsequent rise in NADH/NAD and $FADH_2$/FAD ratios in the mitochondria, an inhibition of β-oxidation occurs (31). This leads to accumulation of intracellular acetyl-CoA bound FFA, followed by a rapid decline of FFA cellular uptake, diminished transport into the mitochondria and an increased formation of triacyl-glycerol ("fat droplets") (32,33). The increased intracellular FFA levels are thought to induce various deleterious effects, including an inhibition of adenine nucleotide translocase, possibly also of the enzymes Na/K ATP-ase of the sarcolemma and Mg/Ca ATP-fase of the sarcoplasmatic reticulum with inhibition of the calcium pumping system into the sarcoplasmatic reticulum (34-36). At the mitochondrial level uncoupling of the electrontransport has been described (37). Elevated FFA levels could also lead to a detergent effect on the cellmembrane by disruption of enzyme binding function, resulting in an altered permeability with electrolyte loss and cell swelling (38).

When FFA-utilization is reduced during ischemia, glycolysis will be activated mainly by the increased activity of the enzymes, phosphofructokinase (PFK) and glyceraldehyde-dehydrogenase (G3PDH) due to accumulation of the ATP-catabolites (ADP, AMP and P_i (32) (fig 11). Uptake of glucose by the cell will be maximal (insulin), as well as the formation of glucose-6-P by hexokinase. However, this supply of substrate is critically dependent on the level of myocardial ischemia and the possibility of blood reaching the ischemic cells.

Glycogenolysis will also be increased to supply as much substrate for glycolysis and anaerobic ATP-production as possible. However, these reserves are limited and during severe anoxia will be exhausted within minutes (39). The pyruvate formed during glycolysis cannot enter the Krebs cycle, but will be transformed to lactate. Myocardial lactate production rather than the normal extraction pattern is found very early during the ischemic process and serves as a sensit-

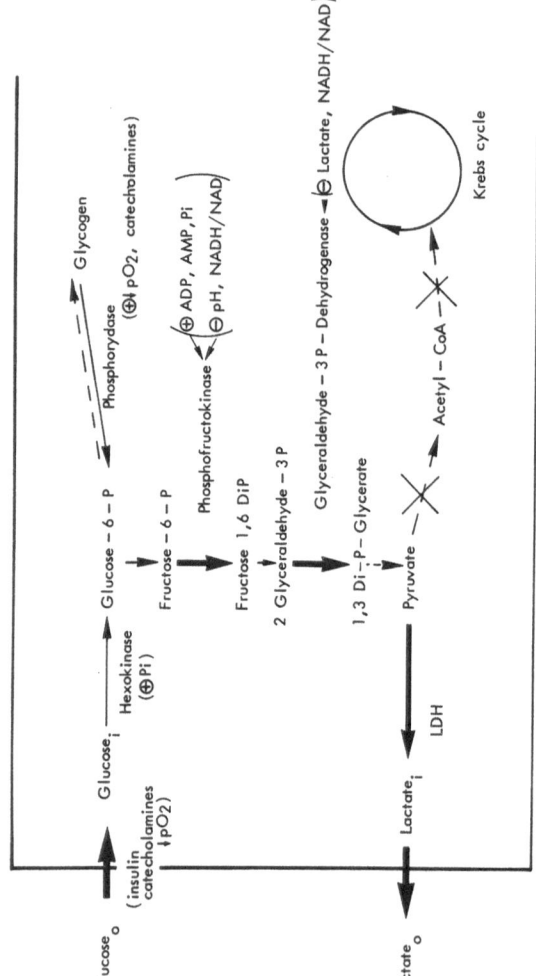

ive marker of myocardial ischemia (40). In our experience
lactate production during pacing-induced ischemia was observed
in 92% of patients with left coronary artery disease, as
compared to ECG-changes and anginal pain in only 72% and 78%
respectively (41). However, although being a good indicator
of short lasting periods of ischemia, lactate production will
again decline during longer episodes of coronary flow reduction,
due to inhibition of glycolysis, especially at the G3PDH level
(42,43). This is mainly caused by accumulation of H^+-ions and
lactate due to reduced venous efflux from the ischemic area,
which results in pH changes and a rise in the NADH/NAD ratio.
The ensuing inhibition of glycolytic flux leads to a decrease
in (anaerobic) ATP production.

Hemodynamic and electrophysiological changes during
ischemia

Contraction of the myocardial myofilaments occurs as a
sliding movement of the thin filaments (actin) over the thick
filaments (myosin) under the influence of regulatory proteins
(troponins, tropomyosin) and in the presence of a critical
amount of Ca-ions.

During this movement the actin filaments attached to
either end of the sarcomere, the fundamental unit of myocardial
muscle, shift to the centre of the sarcomere causing it to
shorten; an energy (ATP) consuming process.

ATP, which is bound to the myosin cross-bridges is hydro-
lyzed by myosin ATP-ase stimulated by actin and forms an
actin-myosin (+ADP+P_i) active complex in which release of phosphate bound energy results in a shift in position of the
myosin cross-bridges and sliding of the filaments. This interaction of actin with the myosin cross-bridges inhibited by the
troponin-tropomyosin complex, attached to actin and being more
or less "in the way" of the reaction at low free calcium
levels in the cytoplasm (fig 12). The increase in cytoplasmatic
free calcium as it occurs during excitation allows for binding
of Ca^{2+} to troponin C, which then results in a re-arrangement
of the troponin-tropomyosin complex and de-inhibition of the
interaction between actin and myosin (44). The very complex

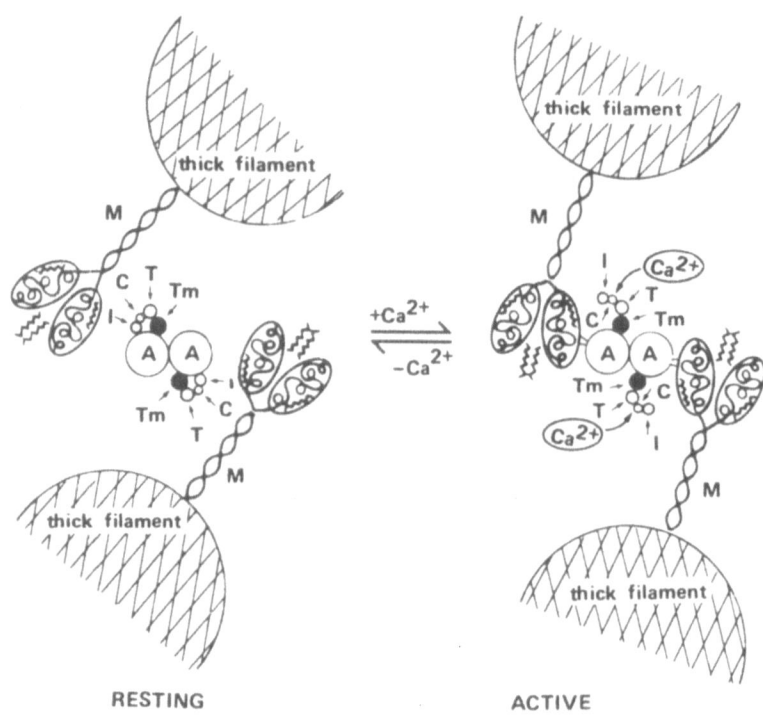

RESTING   ACTIVE

Fig. 12. Possible mechanism by which calcium binding troponin iniates contraction. In resting muscle the troponin/tropomyosin complex prevents interaction between actin (A) and myosin (M). Release of calcium upon excitation in the cytoplasm enables binding of Ca^{2+} to troponin C (C) (right), thereby reducing the affinity of troponin I (I) to actin and a shift of the position of tropomyosin (Tm), which allows actin to inter-act with the myosin crossbridges and thereby to initiate muscular activity. (From Katz AM, Physiology of the heart, Raven Press, New York, p 110 (1977), with permission.

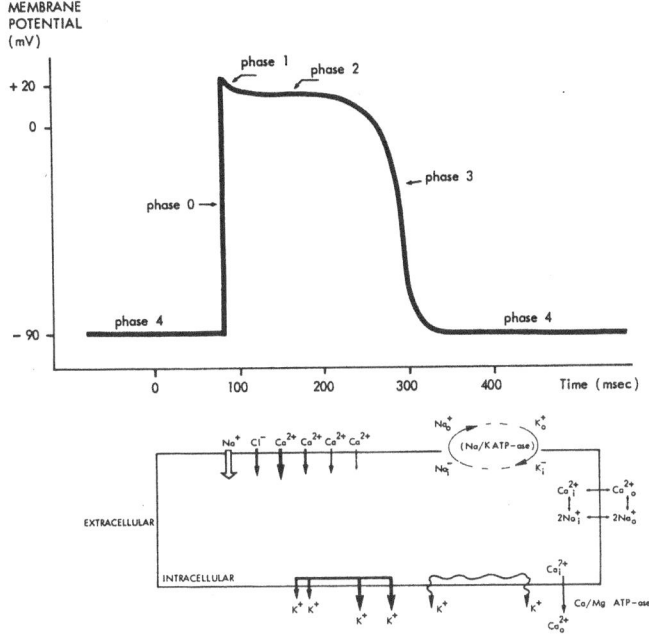

Fig. 13. Transsarcolemmal ionic fluxes during the various phases of the
action potential. After an initial depolarization from the resting membrane potential (phase 4) to threshold level a fast inward current carried
by Na+ions depolarizes the cellmembrane to a positive value (phase 0).
This is immediately followed by a small repolarization (phase 1) due to
ongoing Cl⁻-ions and a voltage dependent inhibition of the fast inward
current to the plateauphase (phase 2), maintained by a voltage-dependent
slow inward current (mainly Ca2+ and Na+/Ca2+-ions) and the gradual onset
of K+ movement out of the cell. After termination of the slow inward
current this K+-ion efflux repolarizes the membrane (phase 3) until phase
4 is reached. During this phase active Na/K exchange (Na/K pump) Na/K-
ATP-ase or sodium potassium pump takes place to reinstitute their respective original intercellular levels. A different, voltage dependent K+
efflux is present during phase 4 which may result in a gradual depolarization of the diastolic membrane potential. Apart from the slow channels
transsarcolemmal Ca2+ transport also depends on a 2Na+(Ca2+ exchange
system and an active Ca2+ pump (Ca/Na-ATP-ase), which removes Ca2+ from
the cell.

series of processes beginning with depolarization of the sarcolemma to calcium-binding of troponin C is called the excitation-contraction coupling. Mainly because of the relatively slow diffusion of Ca^{2+} over the cellmembrane to the contractile proteins other mechanisms for Ca^{2+} delivery and removal are utilized, including various subcellular storage systems such as the sarcoplasmatic reticulum.

Sarcolemmal permeability for ions is governed by the action-potential (fig 13). During diastole the sarcolemma is highly permeable for K^+; however not for Na^+ and Ca^{2+} ions.

At phase O the rapid upstroke of the action potential is caused by a fast inward current, carried by Na^+ ions.

Sodium ion conductance through the fast sodium channels in the sarcolemma is a voltage dependent process starting after an initial partial depolarization of the cellmembrane to its threshold potential and terminating abruptly after complete depolarization (45,46). Full recovery of these channels takes place only after complete repolarization to the resting membrane potential, so similar ingoing Na^+ fluxes can not be found until this period (phase 4).

A brief period of rapid repolarization (phase 1) occurs immediately after the initial upstroke due to a transient increased chloride conductance into the cell. The ensuing plateau (phase 2) is caused by the slow inward current carried mainly Ca^{2+} ions, however, in part also by slow Na^+/Ca^{2+} currents

K^+ ions efflux starts during this phase and together with an impermeability for Ca^{2+} during phase 3 results in repolarization of the action potential to its original resting diastolic level. During this diastolic period (phase 4) intra- and extracellular Na^+ and K^+ ion levels have to be rearranged to anable the next depolarization. In order to achieve this against their gradients energy is required and a specific enzyme in the sarcolemma Na-K-ATP-ase, or the so-called sodium-potassium pump. Prerequisites for proper functioning of this sodium-potassium pump is the availability of sufficient ATP and Mg^{2+} ions. Digitalis glycosides are known to specifically inhibit Na/K-ATP-ase (47), depending on the extracellular

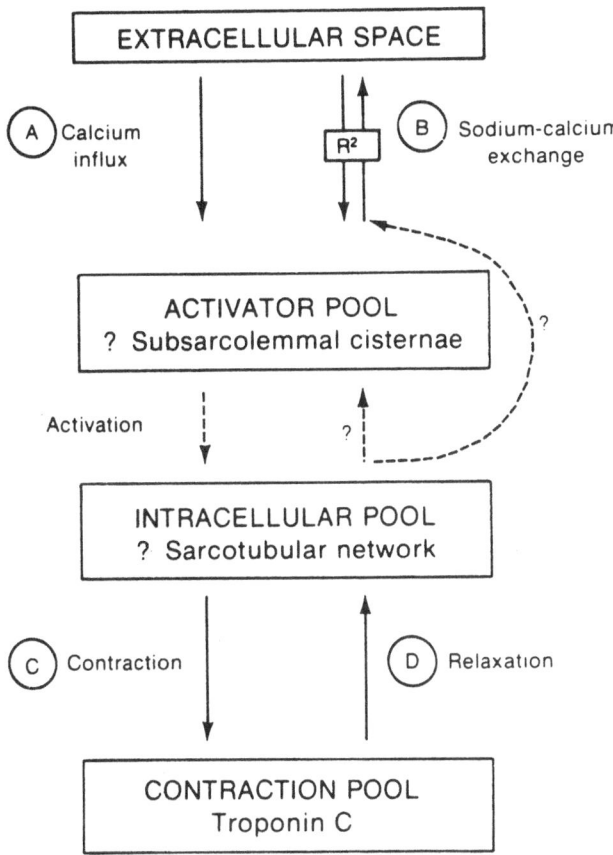

Fig. 14. Calcium fluxes during excitation-contraction coupling. Calcium influx (A) is a "downhill" flux over the sarcolemma largely by the slow channels to the "activator pool", presumably the subsarcolemma cisternae. This Ca^{2+}, entering the cell during each cycle, is in itself quantitatively insufficient to occupy all binding sites on troponin C. A relatively small Ca^{2+} flux from the activator pool may trigger the release of a larger amount of calcium from an intracellular pool, most likely the sarcoplasmatic reticulum (activation) to enable contraction (C). Relaxation (D) occurs by a cyclic-AMP dependent Ca^{2+}-ATP-ase, which pumps Ca^{2+} back into the sarcoplasmatic reticulum. The resulting fall in cytosolic Ca^{2+} concentration causes calcium to become dissociated from its binding site on troponin C. The sodium-calcium exchange system (B) can transport calcium in both directions, however is mainly involved in a nonelectrogenic exchange of Ca^{2+} for Na^+, removing it out of the cell against its gradient. (From Karz AM, Physiology of the heart, Raven Press, New York, p 144 (1977) with permission.

K^+ level and it is of interest that Thallium transport over
the sarcolemma is partly inhibited both by ouabain and increasing extracellular K^+ levels (48). Apart from the potassium
fluxes mentioned above several other voltage dependent out-
going K^+ movements have been described, particularly in connection with spontaneous phase 4 depolarization (49). Calcium
fluxes within the myocardial cell are quite complex and at
least 3 separate calcium pools are involved: the subsarcolemmal
cisternae, the sarcoplasmatic reticulum and the calcium-binding
sites on troponin C (50) (fig 14). Calcium entering the myocardial cell via the slow channels is apparently retained in
the subsarcolemmal cisternae. This calcium, which in itself
is quantitatively insufficient for binding with troponin C
might serve as an activator for calcium release from the more
important calcium pool: the sarcoplasmatic reticulum. While
this process is non-energy consuming the successive removal
of calcium from troponin C against its concentration gradient
into the sarcoplasmatic reticulum however is carried out by
hydrolysis of ATP by a cyclic-AMP dependent Ca^{2+}-ATP-ase.

Impaired relaxation will be an early event during myocardial ischemia and can be found seconds after coronary artery
occlusion. Depending on the severity and size of the area with
impaired relaxation, a reduced compliance of the left ventricle
develops with elevated enddiastolic pressures, which may
account for the dyspnoe the anginal patients so often experience.

The elevated enddiastolic and pulmonary wedge pressures
may be the reason for increased Tl^{201} uptake in the lung
during myocardial ischemia (51). Both impaired relaxation and
reduced contractility can be attributed to derangements in
intracellular Ca^{2+} metabolism. Shortage of ATP will effect
both myosin-ATP-ase activity which results in diminished
contractility and wallmotion disturbances as well as the Ca^{2+}-
ATP-ase of the sarcoplasmatic reticulum leading to impaired
relaxation. Contractility will further be effected by the
development of acidosis during ischemia, when H^+ ions tend to
replace Ca^{2+} ions from its binding sites on troponin C (52).

Ischemia also results in dysfunction of the sodium-potassium

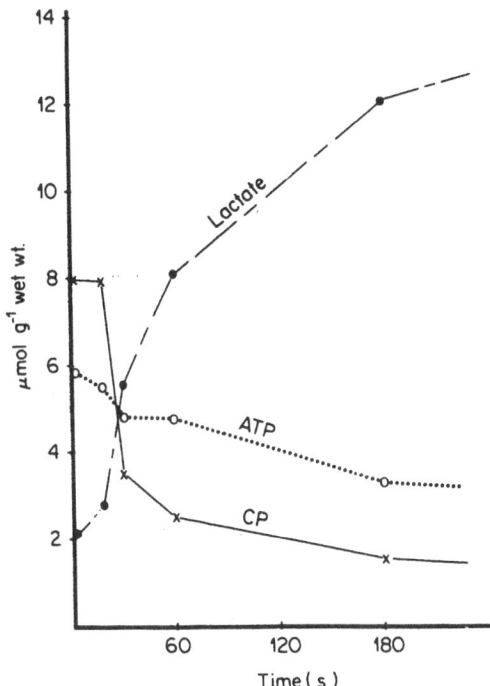

Fig. 15. Immediate changes of intracellular high energy phosphate and lactate content after complete coronary occlusion in dogs. During the first 15 sec there is little change. However, a marked increase in lactate and decrease in CrP occurs during the following 15 sec, indicating both the appearance of anaerobic glycolysis and the immediate effect of depression of aerobic metabolism on high energy phosphate metabolism. Note that ATP content decreases relatively little during the first 3 min. (From Jenning RB, Reimer KA, Biology of experimental acute myocardial ischemia and infarction. In: Enzymes in Cardiology, Diagnosis and Research. Hearse DJ, De Leiris J, (eds), John Wiley & Sons, Chichester, p 30 (1979) with permission.

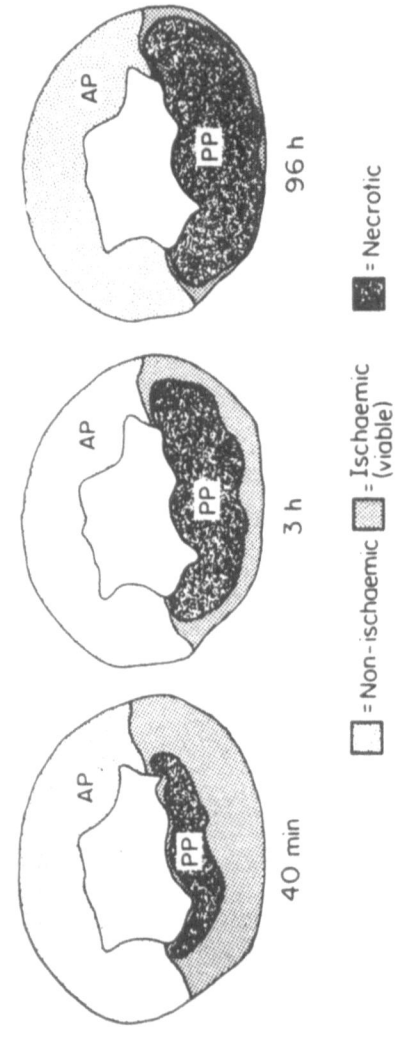

PROGRESSION OF CELL DEATH VS TIME
AFTER LEFT CIRCUMFLEX CORONARY OCCLUSION

AP   AP   AP

PP   PP   PP

40 min   3 h   96 h

☐ = Non-ischaemic   ▨ = Ischaemic (viable)   ▦ = Necrotic

Fig. 16. Diagrammatic summary of cross-sections through the left ventricle of the dog heart to show the progression of ischemic myocardial cell death in relation to the duration of coronary artery occlusion. Necrosis is observed first in the subendocardium but extends in lateral and epicardial direction during longer periods of ischemia. The lateral border of the infarct is sharp and in the dog there is still a significant amount of viable subepicardial tissue present, as late as 3 hours after coronary occlusion, which can be salvaged by reperfusion. (From Reimer KA, Jenning RB, Laboratory Investigation 40:633 (1979) with permission.

pump of the sarcolemma (Na/K-ATP-ase) with K^+ loss and Na^+
gain of the cell (53). Accompanied by accumulation of H_2O this
eventually will lead to cell swelling and oedema (54).

Progression to infarction

All metabolic, hemodynamic and electrophysiological changes
are completely reversible when the ischemic period is of short
duration. With continuing coronary blood-flow reduction and
ischemia, irreversible alterations develop. In animal experiments
total occlusion of a coronary artery leads to complete utilization of oxygen dissolved in the cytoplasm during the first
seconds. Anaerobic glycolysis increases with a quadrupling of
lactate in 1 min (55) (fig 15). The CrP content will be
exhausted to 20% within 3 min, while total ATP decreases at a
slower rate. This does not mean that compartmentalized ATP
pools (i.e. near the sarcoplasmatic reticulum) could not be
deplenished at a faster rate, which is suggested by the
immediate decrease in contractile force. Within 15 min total
ATP will be diminished by 65% and by 85% in 30 min (56). Ultrastructural changes with swelling of the mitochondria can be
seen after 20 min and small patches of subendocardial necrosis
are observed. Disruption of lysosomes and leakage of lysosomal
enzymes is found after 30 min with extension of the region of
cell death, so that after 40 min an area of confluent subendocardial necrosis is present, which tends to spread in a
lateral and transmural way. With continuing coronary obstruc-
tion, 50-60% of the transmural wall will be necrotic after 3
hours and 75% after 6 hours (57). Throughout this process of
progressive necrosis, the infarct area always is surrounded by
an area of ischemic, but still viable tissue (58) (fig 16).

The application of nuclear techniques for the evaluation
of myocardial ischemia

The great majority of current nuclear cardiological investigations are applied in the detection of myocardial ischemic
events. Functionally they can be divided in the study of:

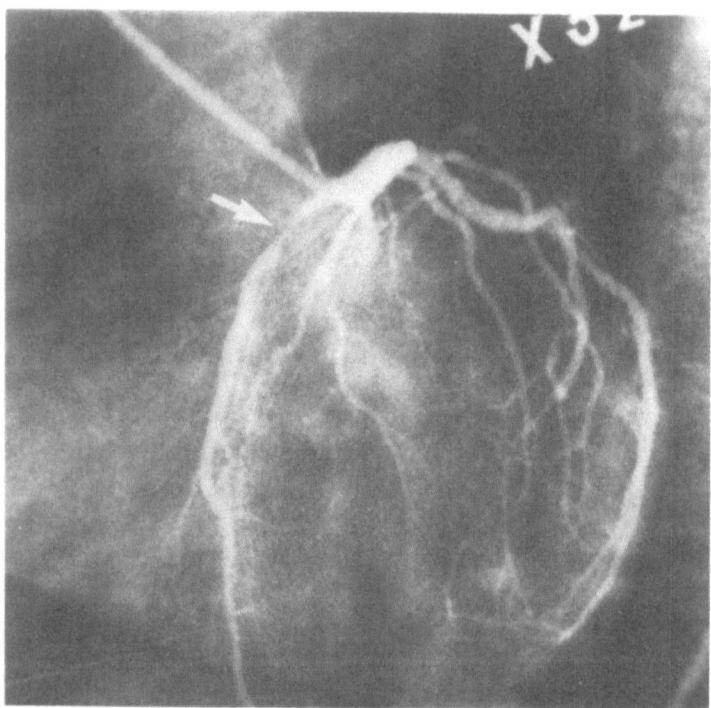

Fig. 17a. Kr^{81m} distribution changes during atrial pacing induced myocardial ischemia in a patient with an 80% proximal stenosis of the left
anterior descending (arrow), and normal circumflex artery. $Kr^{81}m$ is
continuously infused in the left coronary artery and images taken during
succesive 15 sec intervals (fig 7b). At rest there is normal, equal
distribution. During pacing induced anginal pain $Kr^{81}m$ distribution
decreases over the poststenotic area with an increase over the normal
area, signifying the functional significance of this lesion.
(b/min = beats/min; P-P = post pacing).

a. myocardial blood-flow

b. myocardial cell perfusion

c. myocardial metabolism

d. hemodynamics or myocardial function

e. myocardial cell necrosis.

Myocardial blood-flow

The application of microspheres, labelled with various

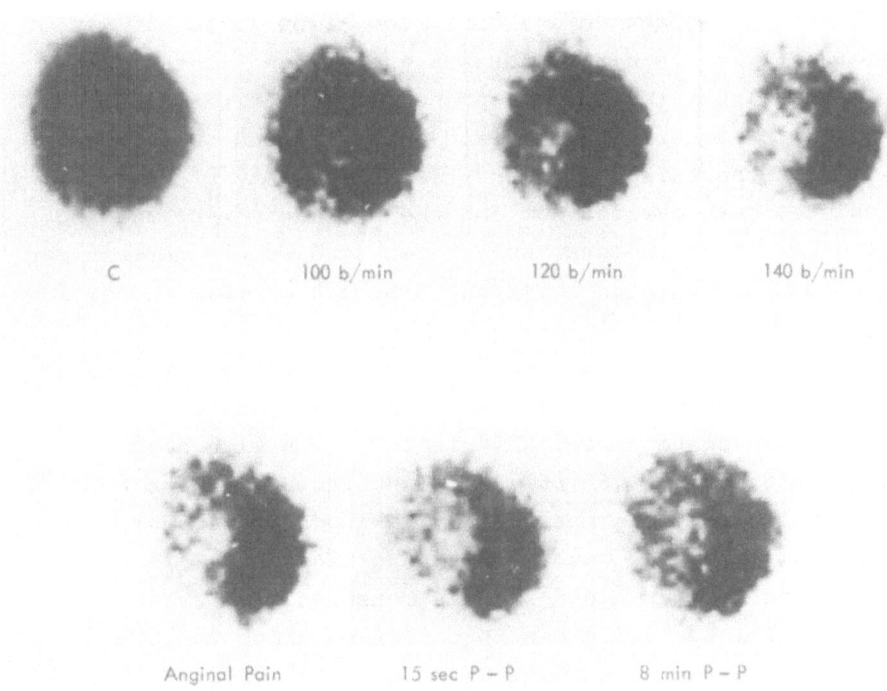

C   100 b/min   120 b/min   140 b/min

Anginal Pain   15 sec P – P   8 min P – P

Fig. 17b.

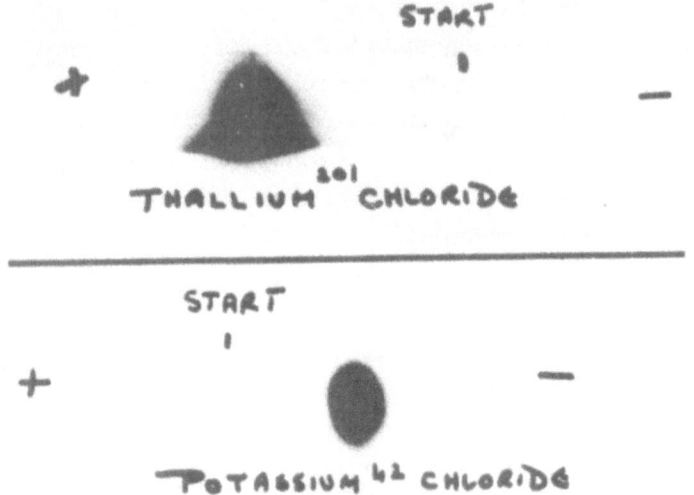

Fig. 18. Electrophoresis of $K^{43}Cl$ and $Tl^{201}Cl$ solutions demonstrating the negative charge on the Thallium ion.

nuclides, is presently the most accurate technique for the
measurement of regional myocardial blood-flow (59). However,
precise and multiple determinations are limited to the animal
experimental laboratory, where proper mixing of the microspheres in the arterial system and accurate counting after
sacrifice of the animal is guaranteed. A variety of human
studies have been carried out and the procedure reported to be
safe (60-63). Nevertheless, only a few studies per patient can
be performed which is an important drawback of this method in
man.

The inert gas technique for the measurement of myocardial
blood-flow has been used for many years (64). Argon in particular was shown to be a realiable tracer, even with high
coronary artery flows (65,66). One disadvantage is its poor
resolution in time; one measurement taking approximately 4-5
min. The main drawback with this kind of technique, is that
only left ventricular blood-flow is measured.

Regional flow studies can be performed using the precordial mapping technique with Xe^{133} or Kr^{81m} as diffusable
tracers (fig 17. Xe^{133} has been applied for many years and its
potentials and disadvantages are well recognized (67-71).
Kr^{81m} has only recently been used in man and seems not to
share some of the disadvantages of Xe^{133} (72-75). The most
important advantage is its very short half-life (13,3 sec),
which together with its biological and chemical inertness
makes it an ideal tracer for regional coronary flow studies
when administered directly into the coronary artery system
(76-79). The main drawback of both techniques however, is the
invasive nature of the procedure.

Myocardial perfusion

Myocardial blood-flow studies as described above should be
distinguished from the myocardial perfusion studies using
radiopharmaceutical agents like radio-potassium (K^{43}) or
radioisotopes of its cationic analogues, rubidium and Thallium.
Of these, Tl^{201} has gained widespread use for the detection of
myocardial ischemia (80-84). The principal difference with the

inert gas or microsphere method for the determination of myo-cardial flow is that myocardial perfusion images with cationic tracers will not only depend on regional myocardial blood-flow, but also on their biological properties which affect uptake and release by the myocyte. Although the ionic radii of potassium and Thallium are close, their biological properties now seem not to be so identical as originally believed. Tl^{201} uptake by the myocyte is dose-dependent and of a greater magnitude that K^{43}. Also, there is doubt about its dependence of the Na/K-ATP-ase system of the sarcolemma (85). It has been suggested that Thallium complexes in the presence of NaCl form $TlCl^{4-}$ complexes, which in contrast with K^{43} chloride are negatively charged (86,87) (fig 18). Although precise knowledge about the cellular mechanism of Thallium uptake is lacking, widespread clinical practice has demonstrated its value in the visualization of ischemic areas and distinction between reversible vs irreversible myocardial injury.

Application of quantitative measurements of uptake and redistribution and tomographic devices have improved its diagnostic potential (88,89). Yet, its relatively low energy profile (95% mercury K X-rays of 60-83 KeV) and long half-life of 73 hours calls for the search of other, better markers of myocardial (cell) perfusion. Promising results have been published with Rb^{82} (half-life 78 sec) (90) and N^{13} (half-life 9.9 min) (91,92). These radionuclides however are positron emitters, narrowing down their application to a limited field of investigators. Also it has to be realized that these compounds do not behave as pure perfusion agents, but are dependent on cellular extraction as well. The intracellular behaviour of NH^{13}_3, which circulates in the blood as an NH^{13}_3/ $NH^{13}_4^+$ complex, is complicated (93). Incorporation in glutamine and carbamylphosphate is believed to occur, so that its clearance from the myocardium depends on a variety of metabolic processes, including the Na^+/K^+-ATP-ase and glutamine synthetase activity, as well as the possibility of carbamylphosphate to enter the urea cycle (94-96).

Myocardial metabolism

Free fatty acids, the most important substrates for oxydative metabolism have been used increasingly for the detection of myocardial ischemia and infarction. Studies with C^{11}-palmitate have demonstrated its usefulness in the detection and quantification of ischemic areas and infarcted regions of the heart (93,97-99). For this, positron emitting computer tomography (PECT) and an in-house cyclotron are required. Labelling of medium-chain FFA with I^{123} in the omega-position does not alter their normal biological behaviour significantly (100,101). Studies with labelled phenylpenta-, hexa- and heptadecanoic acid have been conducted measuring its half-life of disappearance from the myocardium, which is believed to reflect their metabolic turnover in the β-oxydation pathway. Apart from visualization of infarct areas, abnormal turnover rates of I^{123}-FFA in ischemic and infarcted regions can then be measured (102,106). In very recent publications, doubt has arisen whether the measured change in radioactivity really represents the metabolic turnover of FFA or merely the kinetics of free I^{123} (107,108).

Glucose as the main fuel for energy production during anaerobic glycolysis is theoretically the more desirable substrate to indicate elevated glycolytic flux. Complete study of glycolysis with labelled glucose, have not been entirely possible so far. Fluoro-2-deoxyglucose labelled with F^{18} is trapped after being converted to F^{18}-2-deoxyglucose-6-P and does not enter the glycolytic pathway. It therefore only indicates the rate of cellular uptake and subsequent phosphorylation. Although the latter is related to the degree of glycolysis it also is dependent on glycogen formation. In view of its long half-life (109.7 min, B+ 97%), the value of its use is dubious, especially in the event of a progressive reduction in regional coronary flow.

Myocardial necrosis is visualized with Tc^{99m}-pyrophosphate or tetracycline complexes, preferably administered 24-72 hours after onset of infarction (109-113). Uptake is determined by

the presence of myocardial necrosis and presumably by calcium
deposits in the infarcted area (114,115), although in later
animalstudies pyrophosphate uptake was shown not to correlate
with calcium uptake (116). The time interval after onset of
infarction and optimal pyrophosphate uptake, is presumably
due to the development of collateral flow into the infarcted
area. With this technique transmural infarcts consisting of
more than 3 grams necrotic tissue can be demonstrated, as well
as acute subendocardial infarcts in the majority of instances
(110,117). Small nontransmural necrotic areas and inferior or
true posterior infarcts can be missed by this imaging technique (112,121). Although in most infarcts a positive Tc^{99m}-
pyrophosphate scan becomes negative after approximately one
week it can persist for months in some patients (118,119).
Also, positive scans may be found in patients with unstable
angina without definite clinical signs of infarction (119,
120). In these cases small multifocal areas with coagulation
necrosis, myocytolysis or, with elder lesions, fibrosis have
been found (121).

A good correlation between estimated infarct size and
Tc^{99m}-pyrophosphate was observed in experimental anterior
infarcts, however, less consistent in subendocardial and
inferior infarcts (122,123). The correct estimation of infarct
size will be rather difficult in clinical practice because of
imaging problems, when not utilizing a tomograph system, and
the dependence of the infarct-avid isotope on (changing)
collateral flow.

Myocardial function
Isotope methods for the assessment of myocardial function
include first pass and dual or multigated equilibrium techniques which allow for the determination of overall ejection
fraction, heart volumes and local ventricular wallmovement
(124-135). In the detection of myocardial ischemia which is
essentially a regional disease the study of local changes in
contractility and relaxation and thus in regional wallmotion
seems most important. The multigated blood-pool scan with

38

Tc^{99m} labelled erythrocytes and sufficient computer facilities provides an excellent opportunity for the non-invasive study of myocardial function, which compares well with angiographic techniques (129,136,137).

A disadvantage here is the superposition of other intra-vascular structures, especially the right ventricle when investigations are performed in the antero-posterior or right anterior-oblique position. This problem is bypassed using the first pass technique, which permits the independent study of left and right ventricle due to temporal separation. The use of Tc^{99m} as radionuclide however, permits only a few studies to be carried out at short intervals (138). Recently, Au^{195m} has been introduced with a very short half-life of 30.5 sec produced from a Hg^{195m}/Au^{195m} generator (139). Multiple investigations using the first pass method are possible with an interval of 1.5 - 3 min with promising results in animal studies as well as in man (140,141).

Potential drawbacks in patient studies are the contamina-tion with its motherproduct Hg^{195m} (half-life 41.6 hours) and its photopeak of 262 KeV, which is not ideal using the 1/4 inch single crystal cameras currently employed in cardiology work (142).

Conclusion

Nuclear cardiology offers the clinical cardiologist a wide spectre of diagnostic possibilities. Its still growing potentials are made possible by the introduction of new radio-pharmaceuticals and the development of instrumentation. It contributes to the diagnosis of the main pathophysiological areas in myocardial ischemia: i.e. coronary blood-flow, myo-cardial perfusion, metabolism and myocardial hemodynamic function. However, various limitations, especially concerning the presently used radiopharmaceuticals, exist influencing their optimal application. Although positron-emitting radio-nuclides offer greater possibilities in the study of myocard-ial perfusion and metabolism, their use remains limited to only a few centers. Further research and development of new gamma-emitting radiopharmaceuticals is therefore necessary. New developments in this field are being discussed in this volume.

40

REFERENCES

1. Rubio R, Berne RM, Release of adenosine by the normal myocardium in dogs and its relationship to the regulation of coronary resistance. Circ. Res. 25:407, 1969.

2. Rubio R, Berne RM, Dobson JG, jr, Sites of adenosine production in cardiac and skeletal muscle. Amer. J. Physiol. 225:938, 1973.

3. Berne RM, Rubio R, Regulation of coronary bloodflow. Advanc. Cardiol. 12:303, 1974.

4. Olsson RA, Davis CJ, Khouri EM, Patterson RE, Evidence for an adenosine receptor on the surface of dog coronary myocytes. Circulat. Res. 39:93, 1976.

5. Olsson RA, Changes in content of purine nucleosides in canine myocardium during coronary occlusion. Circulat. Res. 26:301, 1970.

6. Fox AC, Reed GE, Glassman E, et al, Release of adenosine from human hearts during angina induced by rapid atrial pacing. J. Clin. Invest. 53:1447, 1974.

7. De Jong JW, Verdouw PD, Remme WJ, Myocardial nucleoside and carbohydrate metabolism and hemodynamics during partial occlusion and reperfusion of pig coronary artery. J. Mol. Cell. Cardiol. 9:297, 1977.

8. Remme WJ, De Jong JW, Verdouw PD, Effects of pacing induced myocardial ischemia on hypoxanthine efflux from the human heart. Amer. J. Cardiol. 40:55, 1977.

9. Remme WJ, De Jong JW, Verdouw PD, Changes in purine nucleoside content in human myocardial efflux during pacing-induced ischemia. In: Recent advances in studies on cardiac structure and metabolism. Vol. 12: Cardiac adaptation. Kobrynski T, Ito Y, Rowa G, (eds), University Park Press, Baltimore, p 409, 1978.

10. Kugler G, Myocardial release of lactate, inosine and hypoxanthine during atrial pacing and exercise-induced angina. Circulation 59:43, 1979.

11. Schaper W, Regulation of coronary bloodflow. In: The pathophysiology of myocardial perfusion. Schaper W, (ed), Elsevier/North-Holland Biomedical Press, Amsterdam, p 181, 1979.

12. Bretschneider HJ, Die hemodynamische Determinanten des myokardialen Sauerstoff verbrauchs. In: Die therapeutische Anwendung sympathicolytischer Stoffe. Dengler (ed), Schattauer Verlag, Stuttgart, 1972.

13. Opherk D, Zebe H, Weihe E, Mall G, Dürr C, et al, Reduced coronary dilatory capacity and ultrastructural changes of the myocardium in patients with angina pectoris but normal coronary arteriograms. Circulation 63:817, 1981.

14. Gould KL, Lipscomb K, Hamilton GW, Physiology basis for assessing critical coronary stenosis. Amer. J. Cardiol. 33:87, 1974.

15. Schwartz JS, Carlyle PF, Cohn JN, Decline in bloodflow in stenotic coronary arteries during increased myocardial energetic demand in response to pacing induced tachycardia. Amer. Heart J. 101:435, 1981.

16. Schaper W, Lewi P, Flameng W, et al, Myocardial steal produced by coronary vasodilatation in chronic coronary artery occlusion. Basic

Res. Cardiol. 68:3, 1973.

17. Becker LC, Conditions for vasodilator-induced coronary steal in experimental myocardial ischemia. Circulation 57:1103, 1978.

18. McKeever WP, Gregg DE, Canney PC, Oxygen uptake of the non-working left ventricle. Circulat. Res. 6:612, 1958.

19. Prinzmetal M, Kennamer R, Merliss R, et al, Angina pectoris, I. A variation form of angina pectoris. Amer. J. Med. 27:375, 1959.

20. Maseri A, Chierchia S, Coronary artery spasm: Demonstration, definition, diagnosis and consequences. Progr. cardiovasc. Dis. 25, no.3: 169, 1982

21. Vatner SF, Alpha-adrenergic regulation of the coronary circulation in the conscious dog. Amer. J. Cardiol. 52, no.2:15a, 1983.

22. Hamberg M, Svensson J, Samuelsson B, Thromboxanes: A new group of biologically active compounds derived from prostaglandin enderoperoxides. Proc. nat. Acad. Sci. USA. 72:2994, 1975.

23. Moncada S, Vane JR, Unstable metabolites of arachidonic acid and their role in haemostasis and thrombosis. Brit. Med. Bull. 34:129, 1978.

24. Martin IJ, Smith IL, Noland RD, et al, Prostanoids in platelet-vascular interactions. Amer. J. Cardiol. 52, no.2:22a, 1983.

25. Dalen JE, Ockene MD, Alpert JS, Coronary spasm, coronary thrombosis and myocardial infarction. A hypothesis concerning the pathophysiology of acute myocardial infarction. Amer. Heart J, 104:1119, 1982.

26. Liedtke AJ, Alterations of carbohydrate and lipid metabolism in the acutely ischemic heart. Progr. cardiovasc. Dis. 23, no.5:321, 1981.

27. Spitzer JJ, Effect of lactate infusion on canine free fatty acid metabolism in vivo. Amer. J. Physiol. 226:213, 1974.

28. Stein O, Stein Y, Lipid synthesis, intracellular transport and storage. J. Cell. Biology 36:62, 1968.

29. Vasdev SC, Kako KJ, Incorporation of fatty acids into rat heart lipids. In vivo and in vitro studies. J. Mol. Cell. Cardiol. 9:617, 1977.

30. Kobayaski K, Neely JR, Control of maximum rates of glycolysis in rat cardiac muscle. Circulat. Res. 44:166, 1979.

31. Idell-Wenger JA, Neely JR, Effects of ischemia on myocardial fatty acid oxidation. In: Pathophysiology and therapeutics of myocardial ischemia. Lefer AM, Kelliher GJ, Rovetto MJ (eds), Spectrum Publications, New York, pp 227-238, 1976.

32. Opie LH, Effects of regional ischemia on metabolism of glucose and fatty acids. Circulat. Res. (suppl. 1) 38:52, 1976.

33. Whitmer JT, Idell-Wenger JA, Rovetto MJ, et al, Control of fatty acid metabolism in ischemic and hypoxic heart. J. biol. Chem. 253: 4305, 1978.

34. Shrago E, Shug AL, Sul H, Bittar N, et al, Control of energy production in myocardial ischemia. Circulat. Res. (suppl. 1) 38:75, 1976.

35. Wood JM, Bush B, Pitts BJR, et al, Inhibition of bovine heart Na^+, K^+-ATP-ase by palmitylcarnitine and palmityl-CA. Biochem. biophys. Res. Commun. 74:677, 1977.

36. Cohen D, Wang T, Sumida M, et al, Effect of palmitylcarnitine on cardiac and skeletal sarcoplasmatic reticulum. Fed. Proc. 37:376, 1978.

37. Borst P, Loos JA, Christ EJ, et al, Uncoupling activity of long-chain fatty acids. Biochim. biophys. Acta 62:509, 1962.

38. Pande SV, Mead JF, Inhibition of enzyme activities by free fatty acids. J. biol. Chem. 243:6180, 1968.

39. Cornblath M, Randle PJ, Parmeggiani, et al, Regulation of glycogenolysis in muscle: Effects of glucagon and anoxia on lactate production, glycogen content and phosphorylase activity in the perfused rat heart. J. biol. Chem. 2339:1592, 1963.

40. Braasch W, Cubjarnason S, Puri PS, et al, Early changes in energy metabolism in the myocardium following acute coronary artery occlusion in anesthetized dogs. Circulat. Res. 23:429, 1968.

41. Remme WJ, Krauss XH, Storm CJ, et al, Improved assessment of lactate production during pacing-induced ischemia. J. Mol. Cell. Cardiol. 13:76, 1981.

42. Rovetto MJ, Neely JR, Carbohydrate metabolism during ischemia. In: Pathophysiology and therapeutics of myocardial ischemia. Lefer AM, Kelliher GJ, Rovetto MJ, (eds), Spectrum Publications, New York, 1976.

43. Mochizuki S, Neely JR, Control of glyceraldehyde-3-phosphate dehydrogenase in cardiac muscle. J. Mol. Cell. Cardiol. 11:221, 1979.

44. Katz AM, Mechanism and control of the cardiac contractile process. In: Physiology of the heart. Katz AM (ed), Raven Press, New York, 1977.

45. Dudel J, Rudel R, Voltage and time dependence of excitatory sodium current in cooled sheep fibers. Pflügers Eur. J. Phys. Arch. 315:136, 1970.

46. Beeler GW, jr, Reuter K, Voltage clamp experiments on ventricular myocardial fibers. J. Physiol. 207:165, 1970.

47. Langer GA, Effects of digitalis on myocardial ionic exchange. Circulation 46:180, 1972.

48. Zimmer L, McCall D, D'Addabbo L, et al, Kinetics and characteristics of Thallium exchange in cultured cells. Circulation 59-60 II:138, 1979.

49. Keung ECK, Aronson RS, Physiology of calcium current in cardiac muscle. Progr. cardiovasc. Dis. 25:279, 1983.

50. Katz AM, Calcium fluxes during excitation-contraction coupling. In: Physiology of the heart. Katz AM (ed), Raven Press, New York, 1977.

51. Boucher CA, Zir LM, Beller CA, et al, Increased lung uptake of Thallium-201 during exercise myocardial imaging: Clinical, hemodynamic and angiographic implications in patients with coronary artery disease. Amer. J. Cardiol. 46:189, 1980.

52. Katz AM, Effects of ischemia on the contractile processes of heart muscle. Amer. J. Cardiol. 32:456, 1973.

53. Schwartz A, Wood JM, Allen JC, et al, Biochemical and morphologic correlates of cardiac ischemia. I. Membrane systems. Amer. J. Cardiol. 32:46, 1973.

54. Leaf A, Cell swelling, a factor in ischemic injury. Circulation 48:455, 1973.

55. Braasch W, Gubjarnason S, Puri PS, Ravens KB, Bing RJ, Early changes in energy metabolism in the myocardium following acute coronary artery occlusion in anesthetized dogs. Circulat. Res. 23:429, 1968.

56. Jennings RB, Reimer KA, Biology of experimental, acute myocardial ischemia and infarction. In: Enzymes in cardiology, diagnosis and research. Hearse DJ, De Leiris J, (eds), John Wiley and Sons, Chichester, p 35, 1979.

57. Reimer KA, Lowe JE, Rasmussen MM, et al, The wavefront phenomenon of ischemic cell death. I. Myocardial infarct size vs duration of coronary artery occlusion in dogs. Circulation 56:786, 1977.

58. Jennings RB, Reimer KA, Biology of experimental, acute myocardial ischemia and infarction. In: Enzymes in cardiology, diagnosis and research. Hearse DJ, De Leirus J, (eds), John Wiley and Sons, Chichester, pp 50-51, 1979.

59. Domenech RJ, Hoffman JIE, Noble MIM, et al, Total and regional coronary bloodflow measured by radioactive microspheres in conscious and anesthetized dogs. Circulat. Res. 25:581, 1969.

60. Ashburn WL, Braunwald E, Simon AL, et al, Myocardial perfusion imaging with radioactive labelled particles injected directly into the coronary circulation of patients with coronary artery disease. Circulation 44:851, 1971.

61. Weller DA, Adolph RJ, Wellman HN, et al, Myocardial perfusion scintigraphy after intracoronary injection of Tc-99m-labelled human albumin microspheres. Circulation 46:963, 1972.

62. Jansen C, Judkins MP, Grames GM, et al, Myocardial perfusion color scintigraphy with MMA. Radiology 109:369, 1973.

63. Ritchie JL, Hamilton GW, Gould KL, et al, Myocardial imaging with Indium-113m and Technetium-99m-macroaggregated albumin. Amer. J. Cardiol. 35:380, 1975.

64. Bing RJ, Hammond MM, Jandelsman JC, et al, Measurement of coronary bloodflow, oxygen consumption and efficiency of the left ventricle in man. Amer. Heart J. 38:1, 1949.

65. Rau C, Messung der Koronardurchblutung mit der Argon-Fremdgasmethode. Arch. Kreisl. Forsch. 58:322, 1969.

66. Tauchert M, Kochsiek K, Heiss HW, et al, Measurement of coronary bloodflow in man by the argon method. In: Myocardial bloodflow in man. Maseri A, (ed), Minerva Medica, Turin, p 139, 1972.

67. Pitt A, Friesinger GC, Ross RS, Measurement of bloodflow in the right and left coronary artery beds in humans and dogs using the 133 Xenon technique. Cardiovasc. Res. 3:100, 1969.

68. Cannon PL, Dell RB, Dwyer EM, jr, Measurement of regional myocardial perfusion in man with 133 Xenon and a scintillation camera. J. clin. Invest. 51:964, 1972.

69. Engel HJ, Assessment of regional myocardial bloodflow by the precordial 133 Xenon clearance technique. In: The pathophysiology of myocardial perfusion. Schaper W, (ed), Elsevier/North-Holland Biomedical Press, Amsterdam, p 58, 1979.

70. McIntyre WJ, Cannon PJ, Ashburn WL, Measurement of regional myocardial perfusion. In: Quantitative nuclear cardiology. Pierson RH, jr, Kriss JP, Jones RH, McIntyre WJ, (eds), Wiley and Sons, New York, p 170, 1975.

71. Cannon PJ, Measurements of regional myocardial perfusion by intra-coronary injection of xenon-133. In: Clinical nuclear cardiology. Berman DS, Mason DI, Grune and Stratton, New York, p 119, 1981.

72. Kaplan E, Mayron LW, Friedman AM, Gindler JE, Frazin L, Moran JM, Loeb H, Gunnar RM, Definition of myocardial perfusion by continuous infusion of Krypton-81m. Amer. J. Cardiol. 37:878, 1976.

73. Selwyn AP, Jones T, Turner JH, Pratt T, Clark J, Lavender P, Contiuous assessment of regional myocardial perfusion in dogs using Krypton-81m. Circulat. Res. 42:771, 1978.

74. Selwyn AP, Steiner R, Kivisaari A, Fox KM, Forse G, Krypton-81m in the physiologic assessment of coronary artery stenosis in man. Amer. J. Cardiol. 43:547, 1979.

75. Selwyn AP, Forse G, Fox KM, Jonathan A, Steiner R, Pattern of disturbed myocardial perfusion in patients with coronary artery disease. Circulation 64:83, 1981.

76. Remme WJ, Cox PH, Krauss XH, Continuous myocardial bloodflow distribu-tion imaging in man with Krypton-81m intracoronary (abstract). Amer. J. Cardiol. 49:979, 1982.

77. Remme WJ, Kruyssen HA, Cox PH, Krauss XH, Assessment of functionally significant coronary artery disease during continuous intracoronary administration of Krypton-81m. Eur. Heart J. 4:32, 1983.

78. Remme WJ, Cox PH, Krauss XM, et al, Continuous myocardial bloodflow imaging with Krypton-81m selective intracoronary. In: Radioisotopes in Cardiology. Salvatore M, Porta E, (eds), Plenum Press, New York, p 155, 1983.

79. Remme WJ, Cox PH, Krauss XH, Visualization of myocardial blood-flow changes with intracoronary 81mKr (this volume).

80. Lebowitz E, Greene MW, Bradley-Moore P, et al, Tl-201 for medical use. J. nucl. Med. 14:421, 1973.

81. Pohost GM, Zir LM, Moor RK, et al, Differentiation of transiently ischemic from infarcted myocardium by serial imaging after a single dose of Tl-201. Circulation 55:294, 1977.

82. Beller GA, Pohost GM, Mechanism for Tl-201 redistribution after transient myocardial ischemia. Circulation 56:141, 1977.

83. Ritchie JL, Zaret BL, Strauss HW, et al, Myocardial imaging with Thallium-201: A multicenter study in patients with angina pectoris or acute myocardial infarction. Amer. J. Cardiol. 42:345, 1978.

84. Berman DS, Garcia EV, Maddahi J, Thallium-201 myocardial scintigraphy in the detection and evaluation of coronary artery disease. In: Clinical nuclear cardiology. Berman DS, Mason DT, Grune and Stratton, New York, p 49, 1981.

85. Winkler B, Schaper W, Tracer kinetics of Thallium, a radionuclide used for cardiac imaging. In: The pathophysiology of myocardial perfusion. Schaper W (ed), Elsevier/North-Holland Biomedical Press, Amsterdam, p 102, 1979.

86. Glaser J, Crystal and molecular structure of trisodium hexachloro-thallium (111) and dodekahydrate, $Na_3TlCl_6 12H_2O$. Acta Chem. Scand. a34:141, 1980.

87. Cox PH, The comparative radiopharmacology of Thallium-201 in relation to potassium. In: Progress in Radiopharmacology. Cox PH, (ed), Elsevier/North-Holland Biomedical Press, Amsterdam, p 19, 1981.

88. Maddahi J, Garcia EV, Berman DS et al, Improved noninvasive assessment of coronary artery disease by quantitative analysis of regional stress myocardial distribution and washout of Thallium-201. Circulation 64:924, 1981.

89. Vogel RA, Kirck DL, Lefree MT, et al, Thallium-201 myocardial perfusion scintigraphy: Results of standard and multi-pinhole tomographic techniques. Amer. J. Cardiol. 43:787, 1979.

90. Selwyn AP, Allan RM, l'Abbate A, et al, Relation between regional myocardial uptake of Rubidium-82 and perfusion: Absolute reduction of cation uptake in ischemia. Amer. J. Cardiol. 50:112, 1982.

91. Phelps ME, Hoffman EJ, Coleman RE, et al, Tomographic images of blood-pool and perfusion in brain and heart. J. nucl. Med. 17:603, 1976.

92. Schelbert HR, Phelps ME, Hoffman EJ, et al, Regional myocardial perfusion assessed with N-13 labelled ammonia and positron emission computerized axial tomography. Amer. J. Cardiol. 43:209, 1979.

93. Ter Pogossian MM, The assessment of myocardial integrity by positron emission computerized tomography. In: The pathophysiology of myocardial perfusion. Schaper W, (ed), Elsevier/North-Holland Biomedical Press, Amsterdam, p 113, 1979.

94. Davidson S, Sonnenblick EH, Glutamine production by the isolated perfused rat heart during ammonium chloride perfusion. Cardiovasc. Res. 9:295, 1975.

95. Chazov E, Smirnov VN, Mazaev AV, et al, Myocardial ammonia metabolism in patients with heart disease as revealed by coronary sinus catheterization study. Circulation 47:1327, 1973.

96. Bergmann SR, Hack S, Tewson T, et al, The dependence of accumulation of $^{13}NH_3$ by myocardium on metabolic factors and its implications for quantitative assessment of perfusion. Circulation 61:34, 1980.

97. Weiss ES, Hoffman EJ, Phelps ME, et al, External detection and visualization of myocardial ischemia with C-substrates in vitro and vivo. Circulat. Res. 39:24, 1976.

98. Schelbert HR, Henze E, Phelps ME, et al, Assessment of regional myocardial ischemia by positron-emission computed tomography. Amer. Heart J. 103:588, 1982.

99. Schön HR, Schelbert HR, Najafi A, et al, C-11 labelled palmitic acid for the noninvasive evaluation of regional myocardial fatty acid metabolism with positron-computed tomography. II. Kinetics of C-11 palmitic acid in acutely ischemic myocardium. Amer. Heart J. 103:548, 1982.

100. Machulla HJ, Stöcklin G, Kupfernagel C, et al, Comparative evaluation of fatty acids labelled with C-11, CL-34m, Br-77 and J-123 for metabolic studies of the myocardium: concise communication. J. nucl. Med. 19:298, 1978.

46

101. Westera G, Labelled fatty acids. Synthesis and biological behaviour.
A review. In: Progress in radiopharmacology. Cox PH, (ed), Elsevier/
North-Holland, Biomedical Press, p 29, 1981.

102. Freundlieb C, Höck A, Vyska K, et al, Ânwendung von I-123 markierten
langkettigen Fettsaüren zum Studium des Herzmuskelstoffwechels. In:
Radioaktive Isotope in Klinik und Forschung. R. Höfe (ed), Wien,
p 265, 1978.

103. Van der Wall EE, Heidendal GAK, Den Hollander W, et al, ^{123}I labelled
hexadecanoic acid in comparison with ^{201}Tl for myocardial imaging
in coronary heart disease. Eur. J. Nucl. Med. 5:401, 1980.

104. Feinendegen LE, Vyska K, Freundlieb C, et al, Non-invasive analysis
of metabolic reactions in body tissues. The case of myocardial fattt
acids. Eur. J. Nucl. Med. 61:191, 1981.

105. Dudczak R, Schmoliner R, Angelberger P, et al, Myocardial scintigraphy using 123-I-phenylpentadecanoic acid. In: Radioisotopes in
Cardiology. Salvatore M, Porta E, (eds), Plenum Press, New York,
p 147, 1983.

106. Reske SN, Koischwitz D, Machulla KJ, et al, Myocardial extraction
fraction and metabolism of W-P-I123-phenylpenta decanoic acid (IPPA)
in patients with coronary artery and valvular heart disease. In:
Radioisotopes in cardiology. Salvatore M, Porta E, (eds), Plenum
Press, New York, p 255, 1983.

107. Okada RD, Elmalek D, Werre GS, et a,, Myocardial kinetics of [123]I
labelled 16-hexadecanoic acid. Eur. J. Nucl. Med. 8:211, 1983.

108. Visser FC, Westera G, Van der Wall EE, et al, Does the turnover rate
of 123I-FFA reflect cardiac FFA metabolism? Eur. Heart J. 4:92
(suppl E), 1983.

109. Parkey RW, Bonte FJ, Meyer SL, et al, A new method for radionuclide
imaging of acute myocardial infarction in humans. Circulation 50:
540, 1974.

110. Willerson JT, Parkey RW, Bonte FJ, et al, Acute subendocardial myocardial infarction in patients: Its detection by Technetium-99m
stannous pyrophosphate myocardial scintigrams. Circulation 51:436,
1975.

111. Holman BL, Tanaka TT, Lesch M, Evaluation of radiopharmaceuticals
for the detection of acute myocardial infarction in man. Radiology
121:427, 1976.

112. Willerson JT, Parkey RW, Bonte FJ, et al, The use of Technetium-99m
stannous pyrophosphate myocardial scintigraphy to establish the
presence of acute myocardial necrosis. In: Clinical nuclear cardiology.
Berman DS, Mason DT, (eds), Grune and Stratton, New York, p 155, 1981.

113. Holman BL, Lesch M, Zweiman FG, et al, Detection and sizing of acute
myocardial infarcts with Tc-99m-(Sn) tetracycline. New Engl. J. Med.
291:159, 1974.

114. Buja LM, Parkey RW, Stokeley EM, et al, Pathophysiology of Techne-
tium-99m stannous pyrophosphate and Thallium-201 scintigraphy of
acute anterior myocardial infarcts in dogs. J. Clin. Invest. 57:1508,
1976.

115. Buja LM, Tofe AJ, Mukkerjee A, et al, A role of elevated tissue calcium in myocardial infarct scintigraphy with Technetium phosphorus radiopharmaceuticals. Circulation 54:219 (suppl2), 1976.

116. Schelbert H, Ingwall J, Sybers H, et al, Uptake of Tc-99m pyrophosphate and calcium in irreversibly damaged myocardium. J. nucl. Med. 17:534, 1976.

117. Poliner LR, Buja LM, Parkey RW, et al, Comparison of methods of infarcts sizing during myocardial infarction. J. nucl. Med. 18:517, 1977.

118. Poliner LR, Hutcheson D, Buja LM, et al, Persistently positive Technetium-99m stannous pyrophosphate myocardial scintigram after acute myocardial infarction. Clin. Res. 25:7a, 1977.

119. Willerson JT, Parkey RW, Bonte FJ, et al, Technetium stannous pyrophosphate myocardial scintigrams in patients with chest pain of varying etiology. Circulation 51:1046, 1975.

120. Abdulla AM, Canedo MJ, Cortez BC, et al, Detection of unstable angina by 99m-Technetium pyrophosphate myocardial scintigraphy. Chest 69: 168, 1976.

121. Poliner LR, Buja ML, Parkey RW, et al, Clinicopathologic findings in 52 patients studied by Technetium-99m stannous pyrophosphate myocardial scintigraphy. Circulation 59:257, 1979.

122. Stokely EM, Buja LM, Lewis SE, et al, Measurement of acute myocardial infarcts in dogs with Tc-99m-stannous pyrophosphate scintigrams. J. nucl. Med. 17:1, 1976.

123. Willerson JT, Parkey RW, Harris RA, et al, Sizing acute myocardial infarction utilizing Technetium stannous pyrophosphate myocardial scintigrams in dogs and man (abstr) Clin. Res. 23:214a, 1975.

124. Strauss HW, Zaret BL, Hurley PJ, et al, A scintigraphic method for measuring left ventricular ejection fraction in man without cardiac catheterization. Amer. J. Cardiol. 28:575, 1971.

125. Van Dijke D, Anger HO, Sullivan RW, et al, Cardiac evaluation from radioisotope dynamics. J. nucl. Med. 13:585, 1972.

126. Schelbert HR, Verba JW, Johnson AD, et al, Non-traumatic determination of left ventricular ejection fraction by radionuclide angio-cardiography. Circulation 51:902, 1975.

127. Berman DS, Salel AF, De Nardo GL, et al, Clinical assessment of left ventricular regional contraction patterns and ejection fraction by high resolution gated scintigraphy. J. nucl. Med. 16:865, 1975.

128. Green MV, Ostrow HG, Douglas MA, et al, High temporal resolution ECG-gated scintigraphic angiocardiography. J. nucl. Med. 16:95, 1975.

129. Burow RD, Strauss HW, Singleton R, et al, Analysis of left ventricular function from multiple gated acquisition cardiac bloodpool imaging: Comparison to contrast angiography. Circulation 56:1024, 1977.

130. Bodenheimer MM, Banka VS, Fooshee CM, et al, Quantitative radionuclide angiography in the right anterior oblique view: Comparison with contrast ventriculography. Amer. J. Cardiol. 41:718, 1978.

131. Tobernick E, Schelbert H, Henning H, et al, Right ventricular ejection fraction in patients with acute anterior and inferior myocardial infarction assessed by radionuclide angiocardiography. Circulation 57:1078, 1978.

132. Hecht HS, Mirell SG, Rolett EL, et al, Left ventricular ejection fraction and segmental wall motion by peripheral first-pass radionuclide angiography. J. nucl. Med. 19:17, 1978.

133. Jengo JA, Oren V, Conant R, et al, Effects of maximal exercise stress on left ventricular function in patients with coronary artery disease using first pass radionuclide angiocardiography: A rapid, non-invasive technique for determining ejection fraction and segmental wall motion. Circulation 59:60, 1979.

134. Slutsky R, Karliner J, Ricci D, et al, Response of left ventricular volume to exercise in man assessed by radionuclide equilibrium angiography. Circulation 60:565, 1979.

135. Pantaleo N, Freeman M, Van Train K, et al, A simple, objective method for measurement of absolute left ventricular end-diastolic volume with multiple gated equilibrium scintigraphy. Clin. Nucl. Med. 5:329, 1980.

136. Folland ED, Hamilton GW, Larson SM, et al, The radionuclide ejection fraction: A comparison of three radionuclide techniques with contrast angiography. J. nucl. Med. 18:1159, 1977.

137. Maddahi J, Berman DS, Silverberg R, et al, Validation of a two minute technique for multiple gated scintigraphic assessment of left ventricular ejection fraction and regional wall motion. J. nucl. Med. 19:669, 1978.

138. Gordon GD, Ashburn WL, Slutsky AR, Assessment of ventricular function by first-pass radionuclide angiography. In: Clinical nuclear cardiology. Berman DS, Mason DT, (eds), Grune and Stratton, New York, p 204, 1981.

139. Wackers FJ, Giles RW, Hoffer PB, et al, Gold-19501, a new generator-produced short-lived radionuclide for sequential assessment of ventricular reformance by first pass radionuclide angiocardiography. Amer. J. Cardiol. 50:89, 1982.

140. Wackers FJT, Berger HJ, Hoffer PB, Lange RC, Zaret BL, [195m]Gold for assessment of cardiac function (this volume).

141. Dymond C, Caplin J, Flatman W, et al, The cold pressor test: Serial evolutionary changes in left ventricular function assessed with Gold-195m (T½ 30.5 sec). Eur. Heart J. 4:65 (suppl E), 1983.

142. Shapiro B, Pillay M, Cox PH, et al, First-pass left ventricular ejection fraction with Au-198m on a 1/4" crystal gamma camera. Eur. J. Nucl. Med. (to be published) 1984.

DATA PROCESSING IN NUCLEAR CARDIOLOGY

R. KNOPP, C. WINKLER

INTRODUCTION

The introduction of digital data processing into nuclear
medicine dates back to 1963/64 when first reports on the
development of computer scintigraphic systems were published
(1-4). With regard to dynamic cardiac studies, connecting the
gamma camera to a dedicated computer was a major breakthrough
in the late 60's (5-7). The linkage allowed data to be acquired
in a digital format and subsequently analyzed to give quantitative information on parameters of ventricular function.
The latest generation of mini- and microcomputers have provided
us with high speed data transfer rates and tremendous data
storage capacity (8). These technological achievements have
led to rapid advances in nuclear cardiology, which is more
dependant on the computer than are any other areas of nuclear
imaging.

The purpose of the present survey is to outline some of
the most important facts regarding currently available data
processing techniques for scintigraphic evaluation of myocardial performance.

Data collection

By means of a gamma camera computer system the cardiac
cycle can be scintigraphically framed into nummerous segments,
each of which represents a different ventricle position in the
course of the heart beat. For this purpose ECG-triggered
imaging may be performed either during the first pass of a
radiotracer through the heart chambers following its intravenous injection as a bolus, or later, after the tracer has

equilibrated within the vascular system. The most commonly
used types of data acquisition are the multi-gated frame mode
(MUGA) and the list mode techniques. Although for some practical reasons the MUGA technique is in widespread use, there is
no doubt that list mode acquisition is much more flexible and
thus superior to MUGA in crucial respects.

Multi-gated frame mode acquisition

Since, after tracer equilibration in the entire blood-pool
the activity content in the ventricles is too low to give
adequate count rates for segmental frame formation during one
cardiac cycle alone, the scintigraphic data of several hundred
cycles have to be accumulated. In this way, composite images
of the ventricular blood-pool can be made in the different
stages of the heart's contraction or relaxation. The R-waves
of the ECG serve as triggers to define the cardiac cycle
length which is divided into a number of time increments
(16-64).

Each time when trigger pulses occur a pointer is set to
the storage location of the first frame in the memory. All
gamma camera data is then stored into this array during the
defined time interval. Subsequently the pointer is advanced to
start the next frame in the memory and the incremental data
sorting process continues until the next trigger pulse occurs.
Now the pointer is reset to repeat the acquisition process in
the same fashion. The sequence is stopped after reaching a
predefined number of cardiac cycles (300-500) and the data
set can be directly used for analyzing ventricular function.
Advantages of the MUGA technique are:
1) only relatively little storage capacity is required,
2) frames are generated in real time and are ready for
   analysis immediately after terminating the study,
3) since the method is fully automated, no operator interactions are necessary.
There are, however, considerable limitations of the MUGA
technique so that accurate results can be achieved only under
special conditions. When there are arhythmias, for example,

the calculated ventricular function parameters may be mis-
leadingly low. But even with normal sinus rhythm, statistical
variations in R-R-intervals can lead to inaccurate assessment
of the diastolic portion of the cardiac cycle and its functional parameters.

In order to overcome the latter disadvantages of MUGA, two
modifications of the technique have been introduced:

1) Data acquisition is buffered so that the computer is
   enabled to collect heart cycles of preselected R-R-intervals in order to minimize statistical variations. For this
   means, however, twice as much memory capacity is needed
   in comparison to the simple MUGA technique.

2) The program for data acquisition is modified to allow
   image collection with constant frame rate per second
   instead of a constant number of frames per heart cycle.
   A time correction for acquiring the diastolic data according to the statistical distribution of the R-R-intervals
   is hereby rendered possible. Although the procedure leads
   to satisfactory results in cases of normal sinus rhythm
   it does not allow falsified parameters to be avoided
   completely (9).

List mode acquisition

In list mode acquisition technique the individual scintillation co-ordinates are fed sequentially into the memory of the
computer, usually in a 7 bit format for x and y. In addition,
time markers and R-wave markers have to be stored so that the
co-ordinates of the scintillations can be subsequently attached
to different time increments or heart cycles. Time markers may
be stored by an internal clock in either 1ms or 10ms intervals
providing temporal resolution equal to 1000 or 100 frames/s,
respectively. Since the 7-bit x-, y-co-ordinate pair is stored
on the disc as a 16-bit-word, there are two bits available
serving as time marker and R-wave marker (10).

List mode data acquisition necessitates data formatting
and sorting into image sequences after the acquisition is
complete. The ability to sort the data and generate composite

image sequences once the R-R-interval is known provides great flexibility in rejecting data from disparate cardiac cycles and in selecting data from defined representative cycles. However, because each scintillation event requires a separate memory location, list mode acquisition of gamma camera data calls for a large storage space in computer memory, depending on the clinical applications (see below).

First pass list mode acquisition

ECG gated list mode acquisition is excellently suited for use, both, with first pass technique and with tracer equilibrated in the blood-pool. In ECG gated first pass acquisition, the data are collected following the intravenous injection of a compact bolus of radiotracer. Data acquisition starts as the tracer enters the right atrium and stops when it leaves the left ventricle. Generally up to 40000 to 60000 counts/sec are registered from a single crystal gamma camera during the measure time of about 20 seconds. The resultant volume of data from 500000 to 900000 counts requires up to 2 Mbytes of data storage. Thus, first pass studies can be performed by means of data systems with relatively small disc capacity of say 5 Mbytes without storage problems.

In contrast to the gated frame mode technique, all list mode studies must be reformatted before calculation of the cardiac function parameters and evaluation of ventricular wall motion. Reformatting of such a study requires considerable operator interaction and takes about 20 min. First a rough frame sequence, each frame representing one sec time intervals, must be reformatted and displayed so that the tracer transit through the heart chambers and the lungs can be recognized. The next step is the construction of a heart cycle length histogram from the registered R-wave intervals. The vertical axis of the histogram represents the number of cycles with similar R-R-intervals and the horizontal axis the cycle length. By means of the histogram cycle length limits are chosen for use in further processing. Thus, any ectopic beats that have occurred during acquisition may be excluded.

Finally choice of different clock times is necessary for repeated reformatting. For example, if left ventricular function
is to be evaluated, time limits are chosen within which the
tracer activity was noted in the left ventricle. If the determination of right ventricular function is required, time
limits corresponding to maximum activity in the right ventricle
are set.

On the basis of these parameters the computer program
creates a final frame sequence by reformatting the primary
list mode data in a manner identical to the real time formatting of a conventional frame mode study. Only the preselected
cardiac cycles are processed. The resultant frame sequence
usually consists of the sum of 6 to 8 individual beats of
equal beat lengths. It is then ready to be evaluated as in an
equilibrium gated study.

The advantage of the method is that heart imaging can be
performed in any projection desired because right and left
ventricular activity is temporally separated. The low count
rate statistics of such a study is compensated by its high
signal-to-noise ratio.

Equilibrium gated list mode acquisition

In addition to the first pass list mode acquisition technique, methods have also been developed for recording left
ventricular performance after tracer equilibration in the
blood-pool (11-13). Data are again hereby acquired as a series
of X, Y co-ordinates, time-markers and R-wave markers, in the
same way as in the described first pass technique. Accordingly
they have to be reformatted prior to quantitative analysis.
However, reformatting does not require operator interaction to
identify the left and right ventricular phases. Thus, the
reformatting procedure can usually be performed automatically.
Prior to frame generation for producing a composite dynamic
scintigram of a cardiac cycle the variable cardiac beat-length
have to be analysed from the stored R-wave intervals. The
statistical distribution of the different beat lengths is
determined from which a so-called representative cardiac

cycle - usually the most frequently occuring - is selected
(automatically or by operator). Then the cumulative frame
sequence is generated exclusively from cycles which are within
the selected range. Distortion of results, e.g. by extrasystolic
beats, is thus avoided. A high time resolution (frame rate) is
obtainable since a great number of cardiac cycles can be
cumulated with sufficient statistical accuracy. Usually a
frame rate of 50 to 100 frames per sec is selected (frame size
of 64 x 64) and up to 300 cycles are cumulated.

Special frame generation by Fourier transform
By means of discrete Fourier transform a time series can
be substituted exactly or approximately by a trigometric
progression according to

$$F(t) \cong \frac{a_o}{2} + \sum_{n=1}^{n} (a_n \cdot COS(n. \frac{2\Pi}{T} .t) + b_n \sin(n. \frac{2\Pi}{T} .t))$$

The time series substitution can be calculated for each pixel
of a scintigram, whereby the Fourier coefficients a_o, a_n and
b_n may be, for instance, matrices of the size 64 x 64.
T indicates the number of harmonic waves, base frequency being
$2\Pi/T$. Since in radionuclide ventriculography 3 or 4 harmonic
waves are sufficient to describe the ventricular volume curves
and wall motion changes, the scintigram sequence is represented
fully by only a few Fourier coefficient matrices. These matrices
are calculated according to the equations

$$a_n = \frac{2}{T} . \sum_{k=1}^{T} I(k) \cdot COS(n. (k-1)\frac{2\Pi}{T}); \quad b_n = \frac{2}{T} . \sum_{k=1}^{T} I(k) . \sin(n(k-1)\frac{2\Pi}{T})$$

I(k) indicates the counts in one pixel during the time in-
crement (k). It is obvious that the use of these equations
does not necessitate previous frame formatting. In contrast
the a_n and b_n matrices can also be calculated from the unformatted list mode data. We have developed a respective

program for frame generation and regional Fourier transform
from list mode data (14,15).

In a first step this program calculates the base frequency
during selected "representative" heart cycle. The second step
is the pixel by pixel calculation of the matrices of Fourier
coefficients according to Fourier's formula. This is performed
by only a single run through the list mode data file. Finally
a series of frames - time increments being 20 ms - is generated
by means of Fourier resynthesis.

This method of Fourier image generation results in a
considerable improvement of image quality or in a substantial
reduction of acquisition time. Needless to say, it is frequently of utmost interest to shorten the time of investigation,
especially in the case of severely ill patients, who can only
be exposed to relatively short ergometer exercise.

Conclusions

Once formatted into a single cardiac cycle, the list mode
study provides the same options made available for analysis by
multi-gated ventriculography, including global volume curve
analysis, parametric imaging of ejection fraction, stroke
volume, and Fourier coefficients. When special analysis of
diastolic function is required, so-called backward gating can
be useful (9).

List mode acquisition at equilibrium requires an enormous
amount of computer storage capacity. For example, if data are
acquired at a rate of 30000 counts per sec for two min the
storage requirement exceeds that provided by the standard 2,5
Mbyte disk which is part of many computer systems. Even a 80
Mbyte disk allows acquisition of only about 25 min. Furthermore, reformatting in most of the usual data systems takes as
long as the acquisition time or even more. However, gated list
mode technique increases flexibility in the examination of
individual patients by tailoring the acquisition method to the
respective problem. If a patient has no arhythmias, any method
can be chosen. If a patient does have arhythmias, however,
gated list mode technique provides the assessment of all

distinct types of cardiac cycles (e.g. interrupted sinus beats, post extrasystolic or ventricular primature beats etc). Heart cycles not belonging to the selected group can be excluded effectively.

Evaluation of cardiac studies

Global function parameters. Global parameters of ventricular performance are derived from the ventricular volume curve as attained from a composite frame sequence. The precise correction of extraventricular back-ground activity is absolutely necessary although problematic. Several groups have developed adequate procedures for back-ground correction combined with automatic or semi-automatic selection of respective ROI's using edge detecting algorithms or phase analysis (11,16,17).

The back-ground activity represents about 50% of the maximum activity within the left ventricle region in standard LAO-view. A region surrounding the inferior and lateral walls is often used to estimate the back-ground. One method of ascertaining that this region does not include from the ventricle is to note that the time-activity curve from the back-ground ROI does not change during the cardiac cycle. Because of background inhomogeneity it is important to apply strict criteria for selecting the back-ground ROI. For this reason it seems advisable to use computer controlled back-ground ROI's.

A firmly established method of selecting the back-ground is based on the fact that the activity at the endsystole in the area between the endsystolic and enddiastolic contour must originate from back-ground exclusively and can be subtracted as a constant rate from the incorrected time-activity curve. This so-called systolic-diastolic area difference can easily be ascertained by masking the enddiastolic ventricle ROI by means of the endsystolic frame whereby all pixels within the endsystolic contour are excluded (18).

Two methods can be used to define the left ventricular ROI: either a constant ROI of the enddiastolic area is used throughout the entire cardiac cycle or the ROI varies according to the ventricular contraction. If the back-ground can be adequately computed and if all of the ROI's include the entire left ventricle with no activity from other large blood-pools, then both of the methods should yield the same results (19). In fact, the two methods have been applied quite satisfactorily in clinical practice. One approved method for selecting the left ventricle ROI uses parametric amplitude and phase images (11). In the amplitude image moving structures - such as the ventricle and atria - show amplitudes which differ significantly from zero. Non-moving structures have amplitudes of less than two standard deviations and can therefore be easily removed. The phase image makes it possible to differentiate between ventricles and atria as well as large vessels, due to their different activity changes. The septum and also akinetic regions may be detected by comparing the parametric images with the enddiastolic picture.

Because of the statistical noise, the back-ground corrected volume curves necessitate smoothing procedures, especially when determining the differentials $\frac{dV}{dt}$ max and $\frac{dV}{dt}$ min (filling and ejection rate). Smoothing by means of the simple sliding average method causes a systematic distortion of the systolic minimum. The curves smoothed in this way do not converge towards the original curve. Resynthesis after Fourier transform appears to be an ideal method of smoothing because of its convergence in the minimum quadratic error for the type of function concerned (20-22). Corresponding investigations have proven that resynthesis including four harmonic waves is sufficient, since higher frequencies represent only noise and do not contribute to the signal (23).

Regional function parameters

The simplest method for visualizing ventricular wall motion is the so-called cinematic display. For this purpose an endless loop of a series of images is used. Because of the large volume of data, the cinematic display causes special problems for the data system. If the display memory is large enough and if the study is sufficiently small then the entire cinematic data can be stored in the display memory. Otherwise the frame sequence must be shortened by combining consecutive frames so that the new sequence - spanning one heart cycle - can be stored. In most cases it is advisable to display the currently varying ventricle contour combined with the fixed enddiastolic contour instead of displaying the unprocessed frames representing the current activity distribution.

Functional imaging

Further possibilities for the assessment of regional cardiac function parameters can be achieved by frame-arithmetic procedures. After certain arithmetic operations on a pixel-by-pixel basis have been performed the resultant image (or images) do not exhibit anatomical structures but are representative of certain physiological functions. For example, a regional ejection fraction image is formed by dividing the image data of stroke volume (enddiastolic minus endsystolic image) by data of a back-ground -corrected image of the enddiastolic. In such an image the pixel intensities correspond to a function, which is - in this case - the regional ejection fraction and not, however, the original activity distribution. These calculated images relating to physiological functions or mathematical parameters are usually called functional or parametric images (19).

Among the procedures of functional imaging Fourier analysis has proved to be of great significance for data compression resulting in phase and amplitude images. This technique was developed in the early 1970's and has become firmly established as a useful instrument in nuclear cardiology during the last five years (11,24,25).

Since the cardiac cycle represented by a gated radionuclide ventriculogram is periodic the mathematical analysis known as Fourier transform is ideally suited to describe such a function by means of a set of cosine and sine waves. Using the Fourier transform the time-activity changes of each pixel of the image are approximated by the Fourier's formula (see above). As mentioned, the calculation of the Fourier coefficients a_n and b_n can be performed directly from the unformatted list mode data or from a reformatted or acquired frame sequence, respectively. Two significant parameters can be extracted from the first harmonic coefficients:

$$\text{Phase angle} = \text{arctg} \left(\frac{b_n}{a_n}\right) \quad \text{and} \quad \text{Amplitude} = \sqrt{a_n^2 + b_n^2}$$

The phase angle is arbitrarily chosen as the time distance between the peak of the approximately wave and the R-wave. The amplitude corresponds approximately to one-half the stroke volume. As the back-ground pixels have random phase angles and small amplitudes, compared to the pixels in the heart and great vessels, they can be excluded by masking all pixels with amplitudes of less than a predetermined value, e.g. twice the standard deviation of the amplitudes within the heart.

The resultant phase image is a temporal map of the sequence of cardiovascular chamber emptying. Another display mode which has been realized in some nuclear medicine data systems present the phase angle information in the form of a propagating colour wave-front, that sweeps through the image linking pixels with similar phase angles moving from the earliest to the latest phase angles. Both the colour-codes "static" and the "dynamic" wave front displays allow for an effective visual presentation of the relative sequence of chamber emptying in the cardiovascular system during the cardiac cycle.

The amplitude image is a picture of the "stroke volumes" of individual pixels. This image indicates the amplitudes independent from their time of peak.

Since parametric images are derived from numerical values the quantification of regional wall motion is possible in order to assess the extent, grade and statistical significance of wall motion abnormalities. Quantification can be performed in two different ways (11,26):

1) Distribution curves of the calculated parameters within the left ventricular area assessed and compared with the respective curves of a group of normal subjects.

2) The enddiastolic left ventricular area is divided into segments or sectors, respectively. The values of the

parameters are averaged within the segments or sectors
and compared with those of a group of normal subjects.
However, for inter- and intra-individual comparisons normalization of the parametric images is necessary.

To summarize, parametric images show the regional distribut-
tion of one parameter in the heart. Of special interest are
amplitude and phase of the base frequency of the Fourier transform. The amplitude image allows diagnosis, localization and
extent of regional wall motion abnormalities with high accuracy.
The phase image makes the delineation of a dyskinetic area as
well as unco-ordinated myocardial contraction possible. Thus,
parametric cardiac imaging enables the exact definition of wall
motion abnormalities with respect to localization, extent, form
and type.

REFERENCES

1. Brown DW, Digital computer analysis and display of the radioisotope scan. J. nucl. Med. 5:802, 1964.

2. Winkler C, Neue Methoden in der Szintigraphie. In: Atomstrahlung in der Medizin und Technik. München p 137, 1963.

3. Schepers H, Winkler C, An automatic scanning system using a tape perforator and computer techniques. In: Medical Radioisotope Scanning. IAEA Wien p 321, 1964.

4. Winkler C, Szintigraphischer Nachweis minimaler Aktivitätsdifferenzen infolge von Parenchymdefekten in Schilddrüse, Leber, Nieren und Pankreas. Sd. Bd. Dtsch. Röntgenkongr. Fortschr. Röntgenstr. p 59, 1964.

5. Pizer SM, Vetter HG, Processing radioisotope scans. J. nucl. Med. 10:150, 1969.

6. Winkler C, Digitalregistrierung,- speicherung und Computerauswertung von Meszergebnissen einer Szintillationskamera. Atompraxis, Direct Information p 3, 1966.

7. Winkler C, Radionuklid-Diagnostik mit Szintillationskamera und Computermethoden. Kerntechnik 11:328, 1969.

8. Bacharach SL, Nuclear cardiology instrumentation. In: Radioisotopes in cardiology. Salvatore M, E. Porta (eds), Plenum Press, New York, p 11, 1983.

9. Knopp R, Bähre M, Breuel HP, Winkler C, Die Methoden der Datenakquisition bei der Herzfunktionsszintigraphie - Vor- und Nachteile, diagnostische Wertigkeit. Nuklearmedizin 19:155, 1980.

10. Knopp R, Quantitative heart scintigraphy - Technical basis and clinical results. In: Medinfo 80. Proc. III World Conf. Med. Inform. Tokyo 1980. Lindberg DAB, Kaihara S (eds), North-Holland Publ. Comp. Amsterdam, p 200, 1980.

11. Bitter F, Adam WE et al, Nuclear Medicine: Synchronized steady state heart investigations. Int. Symp. on Fundamentals in Technical Progress. Cmt. rend. Vol. III, Presses Univ. Liege, 1979.

12. Knopp R, Breuel HP, Schmidt H, Winkler C, Funktionsszintigraphie des Herzens, I. Datentechnische Grundlagen und Methodik. Fortschr. Röntgenstr. 128:44, 1978.

13. Breuel HP, Simon H, Bähre M, Otten M et al, Die Funktionsszintigraphie der Herzens nach Indikatorgleichverteilung zur nicht invasiven Beurteilung der linksventrikulären Funktion. Klin. Wochenschr. 57:839, 1979.

14. Knopp R, Schmidt H, Reichmann K, Biersack HJ, Winkler C, Herzfunktionsszintigraphie durch Fourier Analyse nicht formatierter list mode Daten. NucCompact 12:275, 1981.

15. Knopp R, Schmidt H, Reske SN, Biersack HJ, Winkler C, A new method for frame generation in sequential scintigraphy of the heart. In: Nuclear medicine and biology. III World Congr. Nucl. Med. and Biol. Raynaud C (ed), Pergamon Press, p 2347, 1982.

16. Bourgignon MH, Douglas KH, Links JM, Wagner HN, Fully automated data acquisition, processing and display in equilibrium radioventriculo-

graphy. Eur. J. Nucl. Med. 6:343, 1981.

17. Chang W, Henkin RE, Hale DJ, Hall D, Methods for detection of left ventricular edges. Sem. Nucl. Med. Vol. X, Noi, p 39, 1980.

18. Breuel HP, Knopp R, Winkler C, Backgroundkorrektur bei der Funktions-szintigraphie des linken Ventrikels. NucCompact 8:77, 1977.

19. Holman BL, Parker JA, Computer-assisted cardiac nuclear medicine. Little, Brown and Comp, Boston, 1981.

20. Fischer M, Knopp R, Breuel HP, Zur Anwendung der harmonischen Analyse bei der Funktionsszintigraphie des Herzens. Nuklearmedizin 18:167, 1979.

21. Rahmann H, Untersuchungen zur Fourierglättung von nuklearmedizinisch gewonnenen Volumenkurven des linken Ventrikels. Diss. Bonn, 1982.

22. Zillikens B, Nuklearmedizinisch bestimmte Volumenkurven des linken Ventrikels - Untersuchungen zur zeitlichen Auflösung. Diss. Bonn, 1983.

23. Spiller P, Quantitative Lävokardiographie. Urban und Schwarzenberg, München, 1978.

24. Links JM, Douglas KH, Wagner HN, Patterns of ventricular emptying by Fourier analysis of gated blood pool studies.

25. Clare J, Chan W, Kalff V et al, Use of phase images in the display of condaction and contraction abnormalities. J. nucl. Med. Technol. 9:111, 1981.

26. Hör G, Myokard- und Ventrikelszintigraphie. Radionuklid-Ventrikulo-graphie bei koronarer Herzkrankheit. Therapiewoche 32:6256, 1982.

RADIOPHARMACEUTICALS

P.H. COX

INTRODUCTION

A diversity of radiopharmaceuticals have been developed
to cover the wide spectrum of in vivo nuclear medical procedures which have been applied to the study of cardiac disease.
In order to examine their pharmaceutical and pharmalogical
properties it is convenient to classify them into a number of
functional groups:

a. Reagents for imaging the cardiac blood-pool.

b. Reagents for imaging the myocardial blood-pool.

c. Myocardial metabolites.

d. Non metabolites with an affinity for the myocardium.

e. Reagents with an affinity for infarcted tissue.

The first three groups are primarily utilized to evaluate
the physiological status of the heart, primarily of the left
ventricle, by providing information about the efficiency of
the heart as a pump during stress and at rest, by showing up
anomalies in wall motion, changes in regional myocardial
blood-pool distribution or finally by delineating regional
changes in cell metabolism. Reagents in group d show an
affinity for normal myocardial cells. Their distribution is
influenced by both changes in blood-pool distribution and cell
metabolism whilst not being a true measure of either. Nevertheless a number of substances, exemplified by Thallium, have
been used with some success to distinguish between grades of
ischemia and infarcted tissue even to the extent of predicting
tissue viability prior to undertaking operative treatment.
This important group of substances will be dealt with separately.

The last group of reagents show an avidity for infarcted

tissue and can be of value to identify infarcts at an early
stage but which are less effective with older infarcts for
reasons which will be examined in due course. Let us now turn
our attention to each group in turn.

Reagents for imaging the cardiac blood-pool

The heart is a dual pump system, the right side receiving
systemic blood and pumping it via the right ventricle to the
lungs for oxygenation. The left side receives blood from the
lungs and pumps it via the left ventricle to the systemic
circulation. It is self evident that the capacity and work
load of the left ventricle exceeds that of the right and indeed
the most functional studies are carried out to evaluate the
left ventricle.

In studies involving the visualization of the cardiac
blood-pool the activity in the left ventricle dominates and
makes it difficult to see the other chambers. However as we
shall see by a suitable choice of reagent and route of administration it is possible to evaluate right ventricular function
successfully.

Studies involving the cardiac blood-pool can be divided
into two categories the so-called first pass study which
requires a high level of activity for a short period of time,
in the form of a bolus, or the gated equilibrium study which
requires an even distribution of activity throughout the blood
maintained at a constant level for a considerable period of
time but with a low radiation dose. With the use of Technetium
labelled compounds it is possible to achieve both aims although
the first pass study can then only be carried out effectively
once.

Bolus injections for first pass studies. The cheapest
reagent available for bolus injection is Sodium Tc^{99m} pertechnetate which can be obtained in high specific activities in very
small volumes from all modern generators but for a limited
number of patients at certain hours of the day, nevertheless,
every day of the week. The drawback associated with pertechnetate is that it has a relatively slow blood-clearance and the

thyroid has to be blocked. A slow blood-clearance has the inherent disadvantage that at the most one repeat bolus injection can be given during a period of hours and this would be rendered less effective by the back-ground activity.

A possible way around this, which has not been implemented in practice, would be to use a Technetium complex which is rapidly cleared from the blood to another target organ (1). Technetium diethyl ida or tin colloid are examples of such reagents which show a rapid clearance to the liver (T max in the liver of ± 12 min in both cases). The only drawback to this proposal is the high radiation dose to the target organ from multiple first pass studies.

Combined single first pass studies followed by gated equilibrium blood-pool studies can be conveniently carried out using Tc^{99m} albumin the characteristics of which will be discussed later.

Despite these possibilities however there has been an expressed desire for a short lived radiopharmaceutical suitable for bolus injections to carry out first pass studies and this has led to the recent introduction of short lived generator products.

The mercury-gold generator. Mercury^{195m} produces ultra short lived Gold^{195m} by the decay reaction:

$$^{195m}Hg \xrightarrow[40.5 \text{ hr}]{EC} \; ^{195m}Au \xrightarrow[30.5 \text{ sec}]{IT} \; ^{195}Au$$

The long half life of mercury and the short life of the daughter make this an excellent system for generator production (2). At the energies used in the cyclotron no other significant mercury isotopes are produced.

Recently two such generators have become available for clinical study both of which have a three day effective shelf life. In the generator described by Bett et al (3) the mercury is absorbed as sulphide on to a column of vicinal dithiol cellulose a material which has been previously used to sequestrate mercurial ions from aqueous solutions (4). Gold^{195m} is eluted from the column using a highly diluted sodium cyanide solution to give up to 15 mCi in an eluate volume of 0.5 ml with a gold/mercury ratio of $1:10^{-5}$. A good correlation between ejection fractions calculated from first pass studies was obtained in comparison with Technetium studies in the same patients (5).

An alternative generator system has been described by De Jong et al (6) which is now available for clinical evaluation. In this system the mercury^{195m} and its daughter product mercury^{195} is deposited as mercuric sulphide on a silica gel column. The Gold^{195m} is eluted by means of 2 ml eluates of Sodium thiosulphate solution.

Radiation dose. There are a number of technical aspects related to the mercury/gold generator which warrant further discussion as they are also relevant to other potential generator systems likely to be used in cardiology. One of these is the radiation dose to the personel. In the clinical environment it is recommended to place the generator in a lead castle 6-8 cm thick which gives a total shielding of 9-11 cm. Under these conditions De Jong et al (6) have estimated the total absorbed radiation dose, for three days of clinical use, to be:

for hotroom analyst:

        (assembly and testing) : 8.9 mrem/week

for clinical personel:

    a) radiographer   : 16   mrem/week

    b) supervising
       specialist   : 22   mrem/week

With respect to the patient Ackers and De Jong (7) have reported the radiation dose resulting from six consecutive eluate administrations as being:

kidneys	1.5 rad (15 mGy)
gonads	0.1 rad (1 mGy)
total body	0.07 rad (0.7 mGy)

Pharmaceutical considerations. The mercury/gold generator presents some interesting pharmaceutical problems. At the time of use the column contains a mixture of ^{195}Hg, ^{195m}Hg, ^{195m}Au and ^{195}Au. The eluated bolus is injected immediately and therefore there is no time to control the degree of mercury breakthrough. Hence the design characteristics and reliability of performance of the generator is all important. It is inevitable that some mercury breakthrough will occur because the elution media have a solubilising action on mercury salts, even insoluble mercuric sulphide. This is minimized by flushing the column prior to use and after long periods of non usage. Depending upon the system flushing may take up to 30 min to complete and during the periode of usage of the generator 70-100 ml of washings may be accumulated which contain ^{195}Hg, ^{195m}Hg and ^{195}Au. These pre-washings can be controlled for untoward mercury concentrations, by means of a germanium-lithium detector, prior to commencing clinical studies.

A direct test for pyrogenicity can be carried out daily by means of the one step limulus test. Sterility however can only be controlled in retrospect. Radioactive materials are normally tested for sterility when they have become cold. This is a potential difficulty because the eluate contains mercury^{195m} with a half life of 41.6 hours. However the problem can be surmounted by passing the eluate sample over a sterile 200 nm membrane filter, which traps the bacteria, and incubating the filter with fluid culture medium. In this way the time lapse between sampling and test result can be reduced to normal proportions.

Gold^{195m} does not adhere to catheter or blood-vessel walls and the bolus is adequate for first pass studies. The gamma energy is excellent for multicrystal cameras but is not optimal for the standard cameras in use in most cardiology units. It is too soon to express a definitive opinion as to the value of this reagent as a clinical tool.

The osmium iridium generator. The osmium[191] - iridium[191m] generator developed for cardiology studies by Cheng et al (8) has a number of potential advantages over the mercury/gold system. Osium[191] can be produced rapidly and economically in a reactor. It has a half life of 15.4 days which allows ample time for the manufacture, control and delivery of the generator to centres at a distance from the manufacturer and yet still provide a useful clinical shelf life of two weeks.

Iridium[191m] has a half life of 4.9 sec, decays to stable Iridium[191] with the emission of 129 KeV γ photons and 65 KeV X rays. These energies provide a high photon flux and are highly suited for use with standard gamma cameras particularly the thin crystal portable cameras in common use for cardiological work.

The osmium[191] is loaded on to a column containing Biorad AGMP 1 anion exchange resin. The eluate is passed over a second column containing Dowex 2 x 10/pyrocatechol to prevent osmium breakthrough. The eluant volume is 0.6 - 1 ml and contains high specific activity [191m]Ir. This generator has been used successfully, in both adult and paediatric patients, for first pass studies at dose levels of 25 - 80 mCi [191m]Ir (9). The total osmium breakthrough is claimed to be less than 1 µg/ml and the radiation dose to the patient is small since the osmium is the main contributing factor. A 25 mCi [191m]Ir dose administered to a one year old patient has been calculated to give a whole body adsorbed radiation dose of 35.4 mrad of which 0.4 mrad is attributed to [191m]Ir and 35 mrad to the osmium[191]. The critical organ is the vein receiving the injection which receives ± 500 mrad. For comparison a 3 mCi dose of Technetium pertechnetate in a similar patient gives a whole body dose of 195 mrad. Treves et al (9,10) have shown this generator to be suitable for visualizing both the right and left heart and for the evaluation of shunting. The long shelf life and favourable radiation characteristics of the generator make it an extremely interesting and economically viable radiopharmaceutical system.

The fluid krypton[81m] system. Krypton[81m] is an inert freely diffusable gas with a half life of 13 sec and an emission of 190 KeV γ radiation which is well suited for gamma camera studies. It can be obtained in solubilised form from a generator system in which the parent nuclide rubidium[81] is absorbed on an ion exchange column. The krypton[81m] is eluted by means of 5% glucose solution and provided no ionic substances are present the rubidium breakthrough is negligible. This system is more suited to continuous perfusion than bolus injection but its use for intermittent studies has also been reported. Krypton[81m] has been used to study pulmonary and cerebral blood-flow and, of course as gas, pulmonary ventilation.

It has been used to study right ventricular function (11) by continuous perfusion directly from the generator via the antecubital vein. In the equilibrium situation insufficient activity reaches the left ventricle to interfere with the study and good results have been reported. The most important use for fluid krypton in cardiology has been its application to the study of regional myocardial perfusion and this will be discussed shortly. Let us now however turn our attention away from bolus injections to blood-pool imaging in the equilibrium state.

Reagents for equilibrium blood-pool studies. For MUGA studies the optimal radiopharmaceutical will be homogenously distributed through the blood-pool and will remain in equilibrium during the period in which data is acquired.

One of the most elegant methods to label the blood-pool is to allow the patient to inhale ^{11}C carbon monoxide which then becomes fixed in the erythrocytes as carboxyhaemoglobin. This method has the obvious disadvantage of being restricted to centres with a cyclotron and positron scanner (12).

Technetium labelled human serum albumin. The most commonly used reagent until recently has been Tc[99m] labelled human serum albumin. This reagent is readily available in the form of stannous labelling kits but the in vivo stability leaves much to be desired (13,14). Dependent upon the formulation used up to 40% of the injected activity may be lost from the blood-stream in the first hour post injection (15). In general commercially available labelling kits will produce in excess of 90% labelling the remainder being present as free pertech-netate or reduced Technetium in hydrolysed form. The amounts present can be determined by thin layer chromatography using a double solvent development. A primary development of the chromatogram using physiological saline separates hydrolysed Technetium which remains on the start line whilst a secondary development with 85% methanol separates the albumen complex, which remains on the sodium chloride front, from the pertech-netate which runs with the methanol front.

This data, however, whilst relevant to the biodistribution, does not fully relate to the rate of blood-clearance. Miller et al (16) examined the radiochemical purity of four commercial-ly available stannous HSA kits and found between 73 - 93% labelling in vitro. The blood-pool retention after intravenous injection varied between 59.4% and 76.2% of the injected dose at 30 min post injection the lowest figure related to a product with 84% labelling whilst the product with the 73% labelling had a retention of 70.7%. There appears to be no relationship between vitro and vivo data which suggests that the albumin may be denatured to varying degrees by the various kits.

Evidence to support this is offered by Miller in the same study by the fact that electrolytic labelling of Technetium albumin in two different kits, both using zirconium electrodes, produced a significantly more stable product with respect to biodistribution with 30 min blood-retention of 94.7 and 93.3% injected dose respectively. The electrolytic labelling tech-nique is chemically less aggressive than stannous labelling and the final product is buffered to a neutral pH which may also be significant. In view of this data it is regrettable that electrolytic labelling kits are no longer available.

Technetium labelled erythrocytes. Technetium labelled albumin has now been largely replaced for blood-pool imaging by the use of Technetium labelled erythrocytes (13) which may be labelled in vivo (17) or in vitro (14). Technetium labelled erythrocytes have an effective half life in the blood of six hours, equivalent to the physical half life of the label, and are ideal for gated equilibrium studies. A number of reagents have been used as labelling aid such as stannous citrate, DTPA and iminodiphosphonate but the most widely used is stannous pyrophosphate.

In both the in vivo and in vitro labelling procedure the stannous ions are added to the erythrocytes prior to adding the pertechnetate. The in vivo procedure is the one of choice because it is simpler and does not involve taking and re-injecting a blood-sample. Further the pertechnetate can be injected as a bolus if desired so that a first pass study can be carried out prior to the MUGA study. The mechanism of stannous labelling has not as yet been resolved both in vitro and in vivo labelling results in a binding to the erythrocytes in excess of 80%. Binding to the choroid plexus also occurs with in vivo labelling (17-19).

The amount of stannous ion injected is important for in vivo labelling the degree of labelling being related exponentially to the tin concentration up to concentrations of 10 - 15 µg/kg body weight above which saturation occurs (19). The injected stannous ion has a biological half life of several days in the blood-stream (15) hence reinjection of pertechnetate will result in relabelling.

Miscellaneous agents for blood-pool studies. The possibility of using ^{11}C carbon monoxide for cardiac blood-pool imaging has already been mentioned, carbon dioxide has also been prepared labelled with ^{11}C of ^{15}O and used for cardiac studies by Jones et al (20). When administered by inhalation it passes directly from the lungs to the left heart no activity reaches the right heart thus making it an optimal reagent to study the left ventricle. Such studies remain, however, limited to a few specialized centres.

An alternative to Technetium is generator produced Indium ^{113m} which is readily available from a ^{113}Sn - ^{113m}In generator. Indium eluates can be obtained with a high specific activity which can be directly injected. The Indium binds to serum transferrin firmly which makes it an excellent reagent for gated blood-pool studies. Hosain et al (21), particularly in view of its 100 min physical half life. Indium ^{113m} DTPA has also been used because of its rapid blood-clearance which facilitates repeat studies (22).

Reagents for the study of myocardial blood-pool

The study of the blood-pool kinetics of the cardiac chambers and associated phenomena such as wall motion, particularly of the left ventricle, provides valuable information concerning the efficiency of the heart as a pump. In order to obtain data of prognostic value to estimate the response of diseased myocardium to treatment more detailed information is required amongst other things about myocardial perfusion.

The techniques used in the study of myocardial perfusion may be classified as invasive and non-invasive.

Invasive techniques. Gaseous washout. The intracoronary injection of radiopharmaceuticals to evaluate myocardial perfusion in patients undergoing catheterization has provided useful information concerning both perfusion patterns and blood-flow. Tc^{99m} pertechnetate and HSA have been used for this purpose (15). Solubilized inert gases such as Xenon^{133}, Xenon^{127} and Krypton^{85} diffuse rapidly across capillary walls and into the cells. The degree of distribution is related to blood-flow, capillary permeability and cell membrane permeability. Ross et al (23) reported the myocardial to blood partition co-efficients for Krypton and Xenon to be 1.0 and 0.72. The rate of build up in the tissue is thus related to the blood-flow but is also affected by the other factors. The rate of washout on the other hand is proportional to the relative blood-flow in different myocardial regions hence quantitative studies can be used as a measure of regional blood-flow. In such cases the gas is introduced into the myocardium by intra coronary catheter or direct intra myocardial injection (23,24).

Krypton^{85} is a β emitter and only suitable for sampling methods whilst ^{133}Xe has a long half life (5.3 days) which entails the use of trapping systems to recover exhaled gas. It is also poorly soluble which gives rise to storage problems and its γ energy (79 KeV X-ray) whilst adequate for scintilla-

tion counting is not optimal for gamma camera imaging. ^{127}Xe
is better in this respect but has a long half life of 36 days
which gives problems with storage and waste disposal (15).

Microspheres. Technetium labelled microspheres or macroaggregates injected by intracoronary injection become fixed
in the capillaries in concentrations directly related to
blood-flow patterns and have been successfully used in human
subjects (26-28). Anomalous results may be observed however if
the main branch of the coronary artery is short and prevents
homogenous mixing (29). Both microspheres and macroaggregates
are obtainable from commercial sources with carefully standard-
ized particle size ranges and it is possible to label with a
number of nuclides to facilitate repeat studies at short intervals of time or to carry out concurrent studies of the distribution in different branches of the coronary system. Indium^{113m},
and by implication Indium^{111}, and Lead^{203} have been successfully used as well as Technetium (28).

Human serum albumin microspheres have the disadvantage that
they are not cleared from the capillaries although the Technetium label washes off. Macroaggregates on the other hand
undergo physical disintegration and eventually pass through
the capillaries to be taken up in the RES.

When considering organs with end-arteries, such as the
heart, the question as to what is a safe dose level before
alterations in perfusion are induced by the reagent is one
which constantly arises. Chervu (15) reviewed the relevant
literature and came to the conclusion that the injection of
up to 200,000 particles was safe provided that the particle
size range lay between 10 - 60μ (≃ 0.4 mg HSA) and they were
administered by slow intracoronary injection in a small volume
of injection medium (up to 0.5 ml). At such dose levels no
significant side effects have been observed but nevertheless
the potential risk of an allergic response and the theoretical
danger of embolus induction has inhibited the use of these
reagents in clinical diagnosis.

Gaseous perfusion. Continuous perfusion with solubilized
Krypton^{31m} via selective catheterization has proved to be a
useful technique which has yet to be implemented on a large

scale. Two methods of approach have been reported in the literature. Selwyn (30,31) introduced Krypton[81m] by continuous perfusion into the aortic sinuses. At equilibrium a constant quantity of Krypton will enter the coronary vessels in relation to blood-flow and it is possible to make quantitative studies. This approach however suffers from the technical disadvantages that small alterations in the catheter position may cause streaming and alterations in the mixing pattern with subsequent artefacts in myocardial distribution. Further, more than 90% of the infused activity passes directly into the circulation a less than optimum useage of the radiopharmaceutical. The alternative approach, which has been used to some advantages, is continuous perfusion with Krypton[81m] combined with selective coronary-catheterization (32-35). With this method all of the eluted activity enters the coronary circulation irrespective of the blood-flow. Depending on the degree of selective with which the catheter has been placed all or part of the coronary bed will be perfused. The distribution of Krypton within the perfused region reflects the physiological status of the vessels but is not a true measure of blood-flow.

Nevertheless regional changes in perfusion are easily identified as redistribution of activity to or from perfused regions. With a 14-20 mCi generator and an elution rate of 600 ml/hr satisfactory perfusion of the coronary vessels is obtained with negligible background activity.

Potassium analogues and myocardial metabolites. It has often been claimed that potassium analogues and labelled myocardial metabolites reflect myocardial blood-pool kinetics in their distribution patterns. In essence this is correct but it is also a fact that the myocardial accumulation of these substances is affected by other factors such as cell membrane permeability, capillary permeability, diffusion patterns, the degree of intactness of the sodium/potassium pump and the availability of intra cellular binding sites. At the time a given study is made these factors may be affected for reasons unrelated to regional blood-flow and therefore some caution should be exercised in interpreting results.

N[13] labelled ammonia, a positron emitter, has been claimed to be a useful reagent in this respect (36,37) since ammonia is rapidly cleared in the myocardium and enters the glutamine amino-acid protein pool where-upon no redistribution occurs.

Knoebel et al (38) found a good correlation between rubidium[84] distribution and microspheres at different myocardial flow rates and concluded that the inequalities of extraction ratios which were observed did not invalidate the findings of the rubidium studies. Similar findings have also been reported for Thallium (39).

These reagents will be considered further in another context.

The internal generator. An interesting concept for evaluating myocardial blood-flow is the use of a so called internal generator. In this concept a mother element is required which decays to an radioactive inert daughter element which is then partially eluted from the myocardium in proportion to the degree of perfusion. Anomalies due to inhomogenous distribution of the mother element can be corrected for by measuring regional Rb/Kr ratio. This ratio can then be used to examine both inter-regional differences and also intra-regional changes in blood-flow with time.

Rubidium[81] a positron emitter with a half life of 4.6 hr and a γ emission at 253 KeV produces a daughter element krypton[81m], with a half life of 13 seconds and a γ emission at 190 KeV, which is biologically inert and therefore potentially ideal for this purpose (40). It has however not until now been implemented in clinical practice.

Myocardial metabolites

The accumulation of ionic substances, such as potassium in the myocardium is related to a number of biochemical parameters and as such it is an indirect measure of myocardial metabolism. It is self evident that the evaluation of the turnover of a true metabolite is the most likely objective measure of cell damage and of the recovery potential of ischaemic cells.

Fatty acids are rapidly assimilated by the myocardium

where they are converted into triglycerides by β oxidation thus providing a readily available source of energy. In ischaemic myocardium the prevailing anoxia inhibits this process and the myocardial cells switch to glucose metabolism as their primary energy source. It is therefore not surprising that a great deal of attention has been paid to the possibility of using labelled fatty acids and glucose derivatives to visualize the myocardium and detect metabolic defects.

Fatty acids. A variety of radionuclides have been utilized to label fatty acids including: Se^{75}, Br^{75}, I^{131}, I^{123}, Tc^{99m}, Tc^{123m}, Cl^{34m}, N^{13} and C^{11}. Acids with a chain length of up to C21 exhibit an enhanced uptake in the myocardium suitable for imaging studies, those with chain length greater than this are less effective. There has been some recent evidence (41) that much of the iodine turnover from fatty acids results from enzymatic removal of the iodine and not from true fatty acid metabolism although the results obtained mirror the clinical condition. The use of ω-phenyl fatty acid to surmount this problem has been proposed by Machulla (42).

Fatty acids are rapidly accumulated in the myocardium where they are primarily converted into triglycerides. Energy is released by β oxidation under normal conditions but in anoxia this is not possible and therefore the turnover rate of fatty acids is greatly reduced in ischaemic myocardium (43). Fatty acid studies therefore show ischaemic areas as regions with reduced uptake which show a slower turnover when time activity curves are generated.

F^{18} De-oxy glucose. Under anoxic conditions the cell metabolism switches from fatty acid oxidation to glucose metabolism. It is therefore of some interest to evaluate this parameter in relation to ischaemic cells and this is possible by use of $Fluorine^{18}$ labelled de-oxy glucose which partly follows glucose metabolism (44). It is possible that dual isotope studies using fatty acids and this compound may provide the optimum method for evaluation of the viability of ischaemic myocardium. In this context it should also not be forgotten that ^{15}O is also available for positron studies.

Myocardial infarction

When myocardial infarction is suspected scintigraphic techniques can give useful information concerning the location and size of the lesion. Two techniques are available, negative imaging in which the radiopharmaceutical is localized in normal tissue the infarct showing as a cold area and positive imaging when the reagent localizes in the infarcted area and not in normal tissue.

Positive imaging

Some fifteen Technetium labelled complexes have been reported in the literature as localizing in infarcted areas (45). The most widely used have been phosphate complexes and in particular pyrophosphate (46). With these compounds infarct to normal myocardium uptake ratios of around 25.1 have been obtained but imaging is hindered by skeletal uptake (47). It is thought that infarct accumulation is probably associated with increased calcium concentrations in ischaemic cells and a general tendency to localize in necrotic tissue.

Attempts have recently been made to reduce skeletal uptake, to enhance cardiac imaging by administering vitamin D (48,49).

Other Technetium compounds which only localize in necrotic tissue have not proved to be as effective in humans as in experimental animals (45) but many experimental studies are being made and it would appear that the uptake of some compounds such as Tc gluconate is proportional to the severity of the condition (50). Technetium heparin has given good results in dogs (51) but in our hands showed no infarct localization in humans.

A potential drawback with all of these compounds is that they are only effective during the first few days of infarction, after four days no uptake can be observed.

Negative imaging

Thallous[201] chloride localizes in normal myocardium where some degree of intracellular binding occurs (52), ischaemia and infarction show reduced uptake. If the Thallium is injected

under exercise stress a redistribution occurs during recovery
whereby ischaemic areas take up activity but infarcts remain
negative. It has been shown that cells may become saturated
(53) with Thallium so that the redistribution factor may
become affected. Thallium may also be present as a negatively
charged complex (53) which means that it does not always act
as a potassium analogue a factor which may render distribution
studies of dubious value.

Recently Technetium arsine derivatives have been developed
(54) which localize in normal myocardium in animals, these
may well compete with Thallium in the future although the first
results in humans have been disappointing.

Cardiac thrombi

The identification of cardiac thrombi has recently become
possible by using Indium [111] labelled thromcocytes both in the
heart chambers (55) and in extracardiac conduits (56) and
appears to be a useful new technique. Tc labelled plasmin may
also be useful in this respect although the slow blood clearance may yield too high a background activity for cardiac use.

REFERENCES

1. De Schrijver M, (Private Communication), 1980.

2. Yano Y, Radionuclide generators. Current and future applications in Nuclear Medicine. Radiopharmaceuticals. Subramanian G,et al (ed), Soc. of Nucl. Med., New York, pp 236-245, 1975.

3. Bett R, et al, Preparation of a ^{195m}Hg ^{195m}Au isotope generator for medical use. Nucl. Med. Comm. 2:75, 1981.

4. Marchant W, Modified cellulose adsorbent for removal of Hg from aqueous solution. Environ. Sci. and Techn. 8:993, 1971.

5. Dymond DS, et al, First pass radionuclide angiography in man using Au^{195m}. Eur. Soc. of Card. Symp., Vienna, p 23, 1982, (abstr).

6. De Jong RBJ, et al, What to expect from an Au^{195m} generator. Eur. Soc. of Card. Symp., Vienna, p. 22, 1982, (abstr).

7. Ackers JG, De Jong RB, Dosimetry consequences of eluates from Hg^{195m} Am^{195m} generators. Soc. Nucl. Med. Annual Meeting, Miami Beach, 1982, (abstr).

8. Cheng C, et al, A new Osmium^{191} - Iridium^{191m} generator. J. nucl. Med. 21:1169, 1980.

9. Treves S, et al, Iridium^{191} angiocardiography for the detection and quantitation of left to right shunting. J. nucl. Med. 21:1151, 1980.

10. Treves S, et al, Angiocardiography with Iridium^{191m}. Circulation 54:275, 1976.

11. Knapp WH, et al, Kr^{81m} for determination of right ventricular ejection fraction. Eur. J. Nucl. Med. 5:487, 1980.

12. Adam WE, Bitter F, Pathophysiology of the Myocardium. In: Progress in Radiopharmacology, Vol. 2, Cox PH, (ed), Elsevier/North-Holland Biomedical Press, Amsterdam, pp 5-18, 1981.

13. Thrall JH, et al, Clinical comparison of cardiac blood pool visualisation with Tc^{99m} red blood cells labelled in vivo and Tc^{99m} human albumin. J. nucl. Med. 19:796, 1978.

14. Füger GF, Popescu HI, Technetium reagents for cardiac function studies. In: Progress in Radiopharmacology, Vol. 2, Cox PH, (ed), Elsevier/North-Holland Biomedical Press, Amsterdam, pp 85-89, 1981.

15. Chervu LR, Radiopharmaceuticals in cardiovascular nuclear medicine. Sem. Nucl. Med. 1X-241, 1979.

16. Millar AM, et al, An evaluation of six kits of Technetium^{99m} human serum albumin injection for cardiac blood pool imaging. Eur. J. Nucl. Med. 4:91, 1979.

17. Pavel DG, et al, In vivo labelling of red blood cells with ^{99m}Tc. J. Nucl. Med. 18:305, 1977.

18. Ryo U, et al, Evaluation of labelling procedures and in vivo stability of ^{99m}Tc red cells. J. nucl. Med. 17:133, 1976.

19. Hamilton RG, Alderson PO, A comparative evaluation of techniques for rapid and efficient in vivo labelling of red cells with Technetium^{99m}. J. nucl. Med. 18:1010, 1977.

20. Jones T, et al, The use of O^{15} labelled CO_2 for inhalation radio-cardiograms and measurements of myocardial perfusion. In: Dynamic studies with radioisotopes in medicine, IAEA, Vienna, 1971.

21. Hosain P, et al, Measurement of cardiac output with $Indium^{113m}$ labelled transfusion. Brit. J. Radiol. 42:931, 1969.

22. Schicha H, et al, Minimum cardiac transit times as parameters of cardiac function measurements with $Indium^{113m}$. In: Dynamic studies with radioisotopes in medicine, IAEA, Vienna, 1971.

23. Ross RS, et al, Measurements of myocardial blood flow in animals and man by selective injection of radioactive inert gas into the coronary arteries. Circulat. Res. 15:28, 1964.

24. Linder E, Measurements of normal and collateral coronary blood flow by close arterial and intra myocardial injection of Kr^{85} and Xe^{133}. Acta Physiol. scand. 272:5, 1966.

25. Ashburn WL, et al, Myocardial perfusion imaging with radioactive labelled particles injected directly into the coronary circulation of patients with coronary artery disease. Circulation 44:851, 1971.

26. Weller DA, et al, Myocardial perfusion scintigraphy after intra-coronary injection of Tc^{99m} labelled albumin microspheres. Circulation 46:963, 1972.

27. Kirk GA, et al, Particulate myocardial perfusion scintigraphy. Its clinical usefulness in the evaluation of coronary artery disease. Sem. Nucl. Med. 7-67, 1977.

28. Hamilton GW, et al, Myocardial perfusion imaging with Tc^{99m} or In^{133m} macroaggregated albumin, correlation of the perfusion image with clinical angiographic surgical and histological findings. Amer. Heart J. 89:708, 1975.

29. Kolibash AJ, et al, Intra coronary radiolabelled particulate imaging. Sem. Nucl. Med. X, 178:186, 1980.

30. Selwyn AP, et al, Continuous assessment of regional myocardial perfusion in dogs using $Krypton^{81m}$. Circulat. Res. 42:771, 1978.

31. Selwyn AP, et al, Patters of disturbed myocardial perfusion in patients with coronary artery disease. Circulation 64:83, 1981.

32. Remme WJ, et al, Continuous myocardial blood flow imaging with $Krypton^{81m}$ selective intra-coronary. Proc. Intern. Nucl. Card. Symp., Napels, Sept. 1981. Salvatore E, (ed), Plenum Press, New York, 1981a.

33. Remme WJ, et al, $Krypton^{81m}$ imaging of myocardial blood flow in regional ischaemia. Proc. Intern. Symp. on the pathophysiology of angina pectoris and coronary artery spasm. Sevilla, Sept. 1981, 1981b.

34. Cox PH, et al, The correlation between myocardial lactate metabolism and myocardial blood pool during induced ischaemia measured by continuous coronary perfusion with $Krypton^{81m}$. Eur. Soc. of Card. Symp. on Nucl. Card., Vienna, 1982.

35. Cox PH, et al, Continuous coronary perfusion with Kr^{81m} in the evaluation of coronary artery disease. Proc. 6th Ann. Meeting Yugoslavian Soc. of Nucl. Med., Skopje, June 1982.

36. Gould KL, et al, Noninvasive detection of 47% diameter coronary stenosis by myocardial emission computed tomography of N^{13} ammonia

during pharmacology coronary vasodilation in intact dogs. In: Frontiers in Nuclear Medicine, Horst W, Wagner HN, Buchanan JW, (eds), Springer Verlag, Berlin, pp 4-18, 1980.

37. Schelbert HR, et al, Regional myocardial perfusion assessed by N^{13} ammonia. In: Frontiers in Nuclear Medicine, Horst W, Wagner HN, Buchanan JW, (eds), Springer Verlag, Berlin, pp 20-34, 1980.

38. Knoebel SB, et al, Myocardial blood flow as measured by fractional uptake of Rb^{84} and microspheres. J. nucl. Med. 19:1020, 1978.

39. Buja LM, et al, Pathophysiology of Technetium stannous pyrophosphate and Thallium 201 scintigraphy of acute anterior myocardial infarcts in dogs. J. Clin. Invest. 57:1508, 1976.

40. Kaplan E, et al, Continuous radionuclide generation 11 scintigraphic definition of capillary exchange by rapid decay of Kr^{81m} and its applications. J. nucl. Med. 15:874, 1974.

41. Goodman MM, et al, Synthesis and biological evaluation of 17(^{131}I) iodo-9-tellura heptadecanoic acid. A potential myocardial imaging agent. J. Med. Chem. 25:613, 1982.

42. Machulla HJ, Marsmann H, Dutschka K, Biochemical concept and synthesis of radioiodinated phenyl fatty acid for in vivo metabolic studies of the myocardium. Eur. J. Nucl. Med. 5:171, 1980.

43. Feinendegen LE, et al, Noninvasive analysis of metabolic reactions in body tissues, the case of fatty acids. Eur. J. Nucl. Med. 6:191, 1981.

44. Goodman M, et al, F^{18} labelled 3 deoxy 3 fluoro-D-glucose for the study of regional metabolism in the brain and heart. J. nucl. Med. 22:138, 1981.

45. Holman LB, et al, Myocardial imaging with technetium labelled complexes. Sem. Nucl. Med. VII,. 29-36, 1977.

46. Ell PJ, Kahn O, The role of technetium phosphates in the context of acute myocardial infarction. In: Progress in Radiopharmacology, Vol. 2, Cox PH, (ed), Elsevier/North-Holland Biomedical Press, Amsterdam, pp 75-84, 1981.

47. Parkey RW, et al, Myocardial imaging with technetium^{99m} phosphates. Sem. Nucl. Med. VII, 15-28, 1977.

48. Carr EA, et al, Effect of Vit. D_3, other drugs altering serum calcium or phosphorus concentrations, and desoxycorticosterone on the distribution of Tc^{99m} pyrophosphate. J. nucl. Med. 22:526, 1981.

49. Carr EA, et al, The use of adjunctive drugs to alter the uptake of ^{99m}Tc pyrophosphate by myocardial lesions and bone. Life Sci. 22:1261, 1978.

50. Lundqvist H, et al, Scintigraphy induced myocardial infarcts with Tc^{99m} gluconate. Acta Radiol. Diag. 20:569, 1978.

51. Kulkani PV, et al, Technetium labelled heparin: Preliminary report of a new radiopharmaceutical with potential for imaging damaged coronary arteries and myocardium. J. nucl. Med. 19:810, 1978.

52. Schelbert HR, et al, Time course of distribution of Tc^{201} administered during transient ischaemia. Eur. J. Nucl. Med. 7:351, 1979.

53. Cox PH, The comparative radiopharmacology of Tl^{201} in relation to

potassium. In: Progress in Radiopharmacology, Vol. 2, Cox PH, (ed), Elsevier/North-Holland Biomedical Press, Amsterdam, pp 19-28, 1981.

54. Deutsch E, et al, Heart imaging with cationic complexes of technetium. Science 215:85, 1981.

55. Ezekowitz MD, et al, Comparison of Indium 111 platelet scintigraphy and two dimensional echocardiography in the diagnosis of left ventricular thrombi. New Engl. J. Med. 306:1509, 1982.

56. Agarwal KG, et al,Noninvasive radioisotopic technique of quantification of platelet deposition in extracardiac conduits in humans. J. nucl. Med. 22:P30, 1981, (abstr).

THE METABOLISM OF RADIOIODINATED FREE FATTY ACIDS IN
THE HEART. PHYSIOLOGICAL BASIS AND CARDIAC BIOKINETICS

S.N. RESKE

Free fatty acids are of paramount importance for structure
and function of the heart muscle (1-3). They are (a) major
constituents of complex lipids organized in the sarcolemma
and subcellular membrane systems (2); (b) they modulate the
activity of some important enzymes (1,2); and (c) are a major
source of energy for myocardial metabolism. Under physiological conditions, they are the main fuel for biological oxidation, i.e. energy production of the heart (1). Up to 80% of
myocardial oxygen consumption is used for the oxidation of
FFA under fasting conditions (1,2). The quantity of cardiac
FFA-oxidized is primarily dependant of the mechanical-
energetic demand of the heart muscle, the availability of
competitive substrates and oxygen supply (1,2).

In fig 1 the main steps of cardiac energy production are
displayed schematically. The main alternate substrates for
cardiac energy production are glucose and lactate (2). Amino
acids are of minor importance for cardiac energy metabolism
under physiological conditions (1).

During the last 15 years the role of FFA as a source of
energy in cardiac metabolism has stimulated several groups to
work on the development of methods for the non-invasive
evaluation of myocardial lipid metabolism by means of radiolabelled FFA (4-9). FFA can be tagged with isotopes of various
radiohalogen (4-9),for example radioiodine, tellurium (10) or
with positron emitting nuclides (^{11}C, ^{18}F) (11,12). Iodination
of FFA results in 'FFA-analogs' with primarily unknown biological properties, whereas ^{11}C-substitution of a carbon
molecule of FFA does not alter the biological behaviour of
the labelled compounds (11). Evaluation of myocardial metabolism

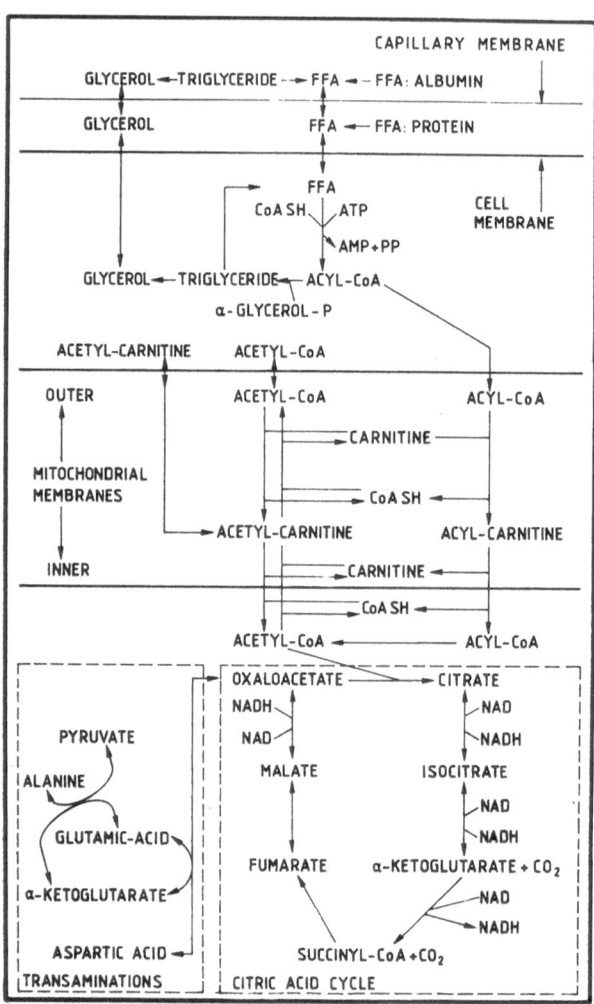

Fig. 1. General metabolic pathway of FFA in the heart muscle (from ref. 1).

with positron-emitting labelled substrates (i.e. ^{11}C-palmatic acid, ^{18}F-fluor-desoxyglucose, ^{13}N-ammonia or ^{11}C/^{18}F-labelled amino acids) is beyond the scope of this chapter but has been the subject of recent excellent reviews (11,13,14).

As early as 1965 Evans and co-workers were able to demonstrate myocardial uptake of ^{131}I-labelled oleic acid in vivo by precordial scanning (4). They demonstrated reduced tracer accumulation in acutely infarcted myocardium (15). The low specific radioactivity of the tracer and the unsatisfactory imaging properties of ^{131}I limited the broad clinical application of this radiolabelled fatty acid analog. However, in 1976 Poe et al (16) were the first to tag FFA with [123]I. With the introduction of this new isotope, considerable progress in the in vivo use of radioiodinated FFA was achieved due to the reduced radiation burden and the superior imaging properties of the labelled FFA (16) and new prospects for the in vivo use of radioiodinated FFA in cardiology were opened.

I-FFA proved to be excellent myocardial imaging agents (4-9, 15-20). Their uptake in heart muscle being closely related to regional tissue perfusion as assessed by K-43 tissue uptake (16) or microspheres (21).

In extensive animal experiments Machulla et al were able to show that terminal radioiodinated 17-I-Iodoheptadecanoic acid (IHA) is accumulated in the heart muscle in similar concentrations to ^{11}C-palmitic acid (6). After rapid cardiac tracer uptake, the concentration of radioactivity of both IHA and ^{11}C-palmitic acid were comparable (6). Preliminary results indicated similar findings in patients (22). It was concluded from these observations that the cardiac metabolism of both compounds was comparable. [123]I was found in increasing amounts in peripheral blood after i.v. IHA-injection (6), indicating deiodination at one - still unknown - step of the metabolic handling of this tracer.

Feinendegen, Vyska, Freundlieb, Höck, Van der Wall, Dudczak and others in extensive clinical studies described a good delineation of left ventricular myocardium after the i.v. injection of IHA and other terminal iodinated aliphatic FFA

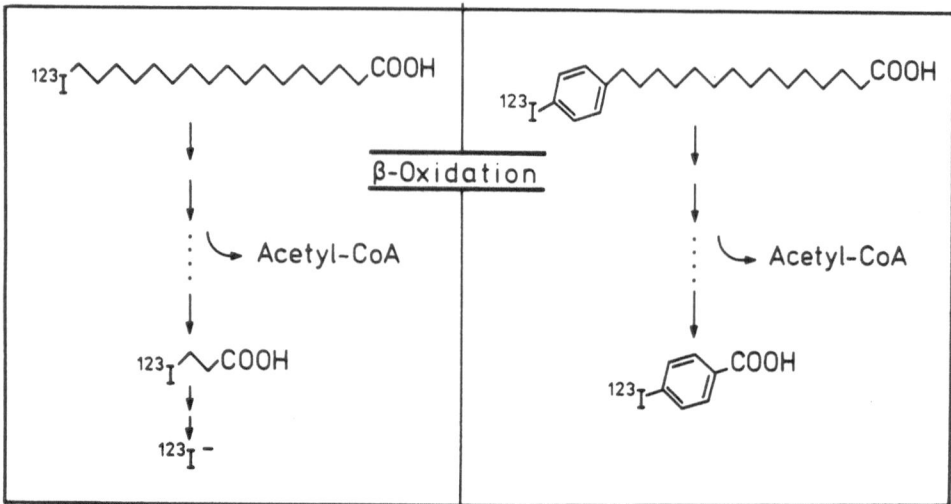

Fig. 2. Schematic catabolism of ω-^{123}I-Heptadecanoic acid and
ω-(p-^{123}I-Phenyl)-Pentadecanoic acid.

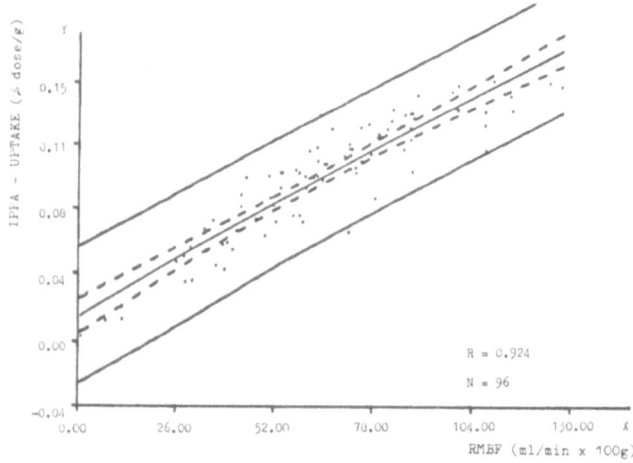

Fig. 3. Relation of maximal cardiac uptake of I-PPA to regional
myocardial blood-flow (RMBF).

(7-9, 17-20). Fast iodide clearance from the heart and probably also from the liver and other tissues (23) produced increasing "back-ground" radioactivity in blood and ECF, thus degrading image quality of myocardial scintigrams (16,17).

Therefore several "back-ground correction" procedures for the correction of extra-cardiac radioactivity, registered in precordial scintigrams, were applied (18,29). High quality cardiac scans with homogenous cardiac tracer uptake were obtained after application of these back-ground correction algorithms (17,18). Acute and chronic myocardial infarcts were characterized by clearly delineated areas of focal reduced tracer uptake. Left ventricular segments supplied by highly stenosed coronary arteries had often reduced tracer uptake. Frequently a mottled tracer uptake pattern has been found in advanced congestive cardiomyopathy (19).

Cardiac radioactivity clearance, determined from properly back-ground corrected I-FFA-scans, has been claimed to reflect a parameter of β-oxidative degradation of these tracers (17). Elimination half times of 20 to 35 min were recorded in healthy volunteers (8,17). Patients with coronary artery disease (CAD) frequently showed prolongations of cardiac tracer elimination in myocardial segments supplied by significantly stenosed coronary arteries (8,17). Prolonged tracer eliminations were found at investigations, performed at rest or immediately after maximal bicycle exercise, from cardiac regions supplied by highly stenosed vessels (8,17). In contrast increased tracer clearance from acutely ischemic myocardium has been reported (20).

Interpretation of these results is hampered by the rapid release of the iodine label from heart muscle tissue (6,24,25). Machulla therefore developed terminal phenyl-substituted fatty acids, labelled in the para-position of the benzene ring (fig 2) (26). This compound is not deiodinated in vivo due to the strong iodine-binding to the terminal benzene ring (26). Indeed, since principles of biological oxidation of FFA have been discovered by Knoop with "phenyl-labelled" free fatty acids (27), this tracer proved to be very promising for investigation of cardiac lipid metabolism (28).

Recently ^{123m}Te or stable tellurium has been incorporated into the aliphatic chain of various long chain FFA or phenyl-pentadecanoic acid (10,29,30). These types of FFA analogs, labelled at the terminal C-atom of the aliphatic chain or in para-position of the terminal benzene ring, exhibit pronounced cardiac uptake in comparable amounts as other I-FFA but are retained in the heart muscle (10,29,30). Retention of these tracers is probably due to inhibited oxidation or intracellular complexation of the tracer with cytosolic proteins (31) Where-as 17-iodo-9- tellura-heptadecanoic acid was rapidly deiodized in the rat heart, introduction of the iodine label at the terminal benzene- or vinyl group resulted in stable iodine binding at the FFA-molecule and in tracer retention in the heart muscle (31). Similar to other FFA-analogs, tellurium fatty acids are taken up by the heart in close relation to rMBF (10). Since metabolic degradation of these tracers is inhibited, tellurium-FFA, radioiodinated at a terminal phenyl- or venyl-group, may have potential for non-invasive assess-ment or rMBF. Similarly, branched chain radiolabelled fatty acids like β-methyl-FFA, which are taken up but are not degraded in heart muscle (32), may be promising for non-invasive assessment of rMBF in conjunction with SPECT (fig 3).

In the following chapters biokinetics of various radio-iodinated FFA will be discussed in more detail. Results will be grouped according to the metabolic sequence of cardiac FFA-metabolism, i.e.

1) Cardiac uptake and flow dependence of I-FFA accumulation in the heart
2) Tracer turnover in the heart muscle
   a) hydrophilic metabolites
   b) lipophilic metabolites
      and
3) SPECT studies of I-FFA-metabolism as well as
4) principal clearance patterns of cardiac I-FFA-turnover in patients.

1. Cardiac uptake of I-FFA and flow-dependence of I-FFA
   accumulation in the heart

First experiments of Poe et al indicated a very close
relation of cardiac IHA-uptake to regional tissue perfusion in
normal and acutely ischemic myocardium. Recent studies in our
laboratory - using I-PPA as FFA-tracer - confirmed these
observations (21). In addition, at increasing pacing-induced
cardiac demand and consequently increased regional myocardial
blood-flow (rMBF), only a moderate increase of I-PPA-uptake
was found indicating limitations in the use of long chain
I-FFA as flow tracers at increased rMBF. Transmural distribution of I-PPA uptake was grossly homogeneous despite significantly higher subendocardial rMBF, supporting the hypothesis
of inhomogeneous substrate-utilization in the heart muscle with
preferential glucose utilization in subendocardium (33).
Dependence of cardiac I-FFA uptake on important modulating
factors of the heart's FFA utilization as albumin/FFA-ratio,
alternate substrate utilization, hormonal control, intracellular
binding proteins or availability of free HS-CoA has not been
established as yet.

2. I-FFA-turnover in the heart

Kinetics of I-FFA in the murine heart has been the subject
of extensive investigations. After i.v. tracer injection, IHA
and other radioiodinated aliphatic FFA, as well as I-PPA are
rapidly taken up by the heart muscle (fig 4). After maximal
heart uptake at 1-2 min p.i., a subsequent two component
elimination pattern was found (6). Velocity of IHA elimination
is comparable to that of ^{11}C-palmitic acid. In contrast, I-PPA
elimination seems to be somewhat delayed (34). Bimodal time
course of IHA-elimination has been explained by the combined
effect of immediate β-oxidation and subsequent washout of the
"final" catabolite ^{123}I-iodide (35); the second cardiac clearance component might be related to the fractional tracer turnover in cardiac lipids. I-PPA-clearance from the heart was
found to be governed by velocity of ^{123}I-benzoic acid product-
tion rate - the final catabolite of I-PPA degradation - and

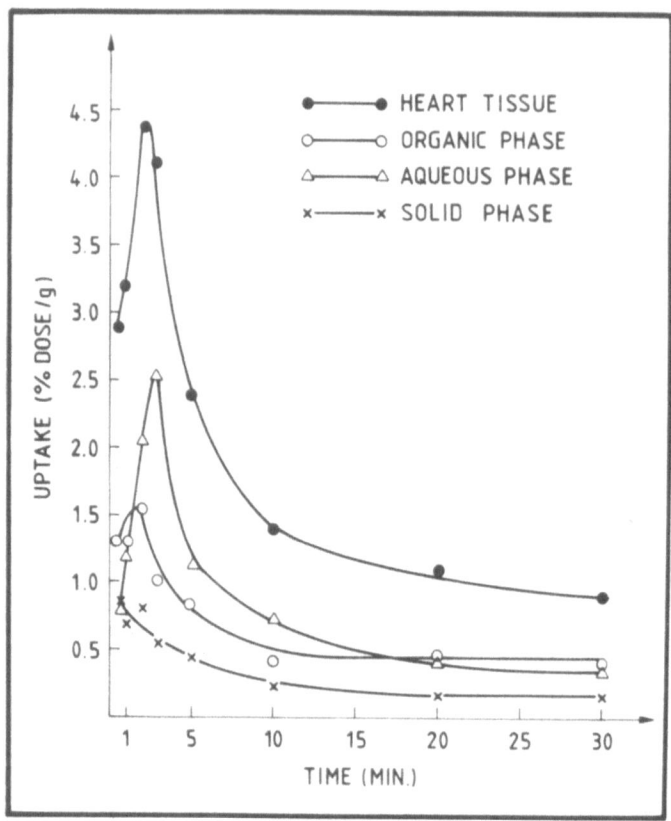

Fig. 4. Kinetics of cardiac radioactivity after i.v. I-PPA injection.
Fast metabolic incorporation into cardiac lipids and degradation to
hydrophilic catabolites can be seen. Mean value of six determinations
per time point.

from turnover in cardiac lipids (36,37).

2a. Turnover of hydrophilic metabolites in the heart
muscle

The complex cardiac kinetics of I-FFA led to the investigation of the intracellular tracer distribution in myocardium.
After injection of radioiodinated aliphatic FFA the main
radiolabelled fraction in heart muscle was a hydrophilic
catabolite, which turned out to be I123-iodide (24,38).
This finding, confirmed by several authors in several experimental models in vivo and in the isolated perfused

Langendorff rat heart (24,25,39), introduced considerable
controversy and doubt in the applicability of aliphatic I-FFA
as metabolic tracer for cardiac FFA metabolism (35). However,
the metabolic step of aliphatic I-FFA deiodination and the
rate limiting step for metabolic degradation and/or deiodination and subsequent wash-out of the iodide (or conceivably
short chain labelled metabolites) from the heart have not yet
been determined exactly. More confusing, in clinical studies
of patients with congestive cardiomyopathies - most in advanced
stage - inhomogeneous tracer wash-out was observed in a clinical situation of at least at the level amenable to coronary
angiography-homogeneous and undisturbed tissue perfusion.
These findings leave--to the authors opinion - the applicability of aliphatic I-FFA as metabolic tracer of certain steps
of cardiac FFA-metabolism open for discussion by now.

Intracardiac turnover of terminal phenyl-substituted
[123]I-labelled pentadecanoic acid (I-PPA) has been extensively
studied by our group (21,23,34,36,37,40). It was found that
I-PPA is rapidly oxidized to a hydrophilic catabolite comigrating in TLC with ^{123}I-benzoic acid indicating rapid oxidation
of I-PPA in the heart muscle (36). A recent gaschromatographic/
mass spectrometric (GCMS) study in isolated Langendorf-perfused
rat hearts proved cardiac oxidation of I-PPA to ^{123}I-benzoic
acid (28). Moreover no significant tissue retention of the
terminal catabolite(s) was found in this study (28). In keeping
with these results we found - despite a transitory high production of hydrophilic catabolites in heart muscle - no significant catabolite retention in vivo (23) (fig 4).

In Langendorf-perfused rat hearts a close correlation of
the production rate of ^{123}I-benzoic acid and $^{14}CO_2$ was found
indicating a high relation of I-PPA and ^{14}C-palmitic acid
oxidation under control conditions, as well as during stimulated or partially inhibited cardiac lipolysis (36). Precordial
registered radioactivity clearance, assessed in Langendorff
rat hearts after intra-aortic bolus injection of ^{14}C-palmitic
acid and I-PPA simultaneously, was closely related to [123]I-
benzoic acid and $^{14}CO_2$-production, i.e. cardiac FFA oxidation

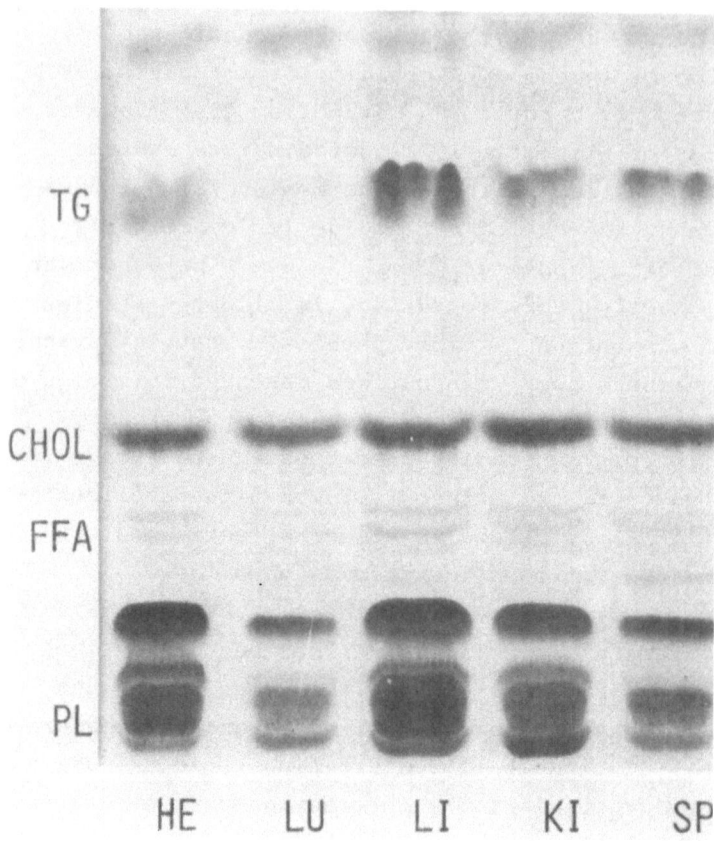

·Fig. 5. TLC of lipids extracted from heart (HE), lung (LU), Liver (LI),
kidney (KI) and spleen (SP) of rats (fig 5a) and autoradiographs of
I-PPA (fig 5b) or ^{14}C-palmitic (fig 5c) acid labelled lipids. Note very
simular radioactivity uptake into main lipid fractions. Increased
intensity of labelled lipids on ^{14}C autoradiograph is due to the much
longer exposure time. TG: Triglycerides, CHOL: cholesterin comigrating
fraction, FFA: free fatty acids, PL: phospholipids.

(36). Therefore it is suggested that quantitative parameters
of cardiac lipid metabolism may be derived from cardiac radioactivity clearance after i.v. I-PPA injection.

2b. Kinetics of in vivo I-FFA labelled cardiac lipids
    Kinetics of in vivo labelled cardiac lipids after i.v.
injection of aliphatic or phenylated radioiodinated fatty
acids has been studied by several authors. Results presented
by Daus et al and others indicated IHA-uptake into main cardiac

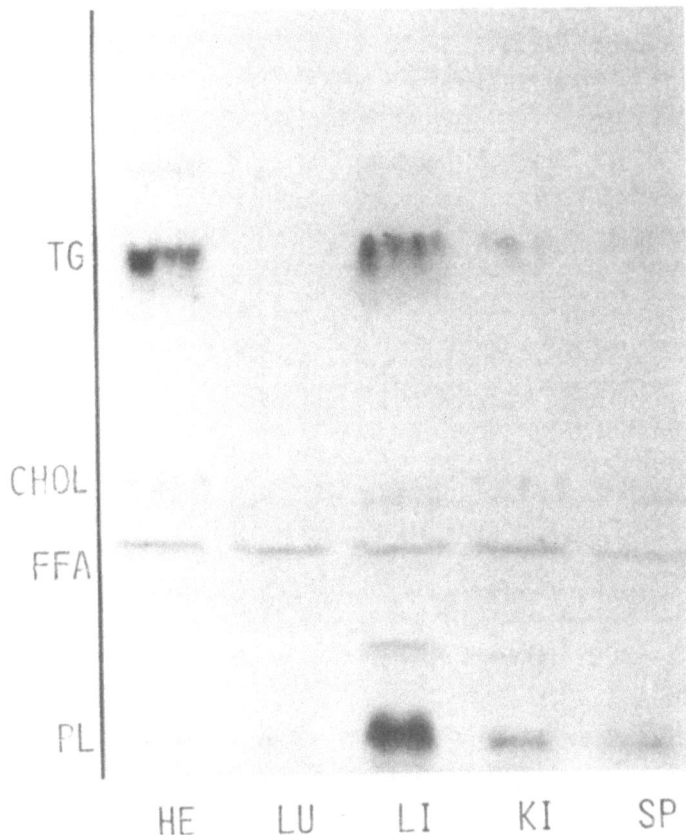

TG

CHOL

FFA

PL

HE   LU   LI   KI   SP

Fig. 5b.

lipid fraction (phospholipids, triglycerides, FFA) (34).
Interestingly a recent study performed in our laboratory showed -
compared to distribution of ^{14}C palmitic acid labelled lipids
in heart muscle (24), an atypical tissue distribution of IHA-
labelled cardiac lipids with relative high uptake in the phospholipid fraction (PL) and relative slow uptake in cardiac
triglycerides.

In contrast I-PPA labelled cardiac lipids showed in vivo
labelling of the main myocardial lipid fractions (fig 5) in
nearly identical amounts as values reported for ^{14}C-palmitic
acid (23,41) (fig 5). A double tracer study, where ^{14}C-palmitic
and ^{131}I-PPA were used, showed a significant correlation of
relative radioactivity uptake in main cardiac lipid fractions

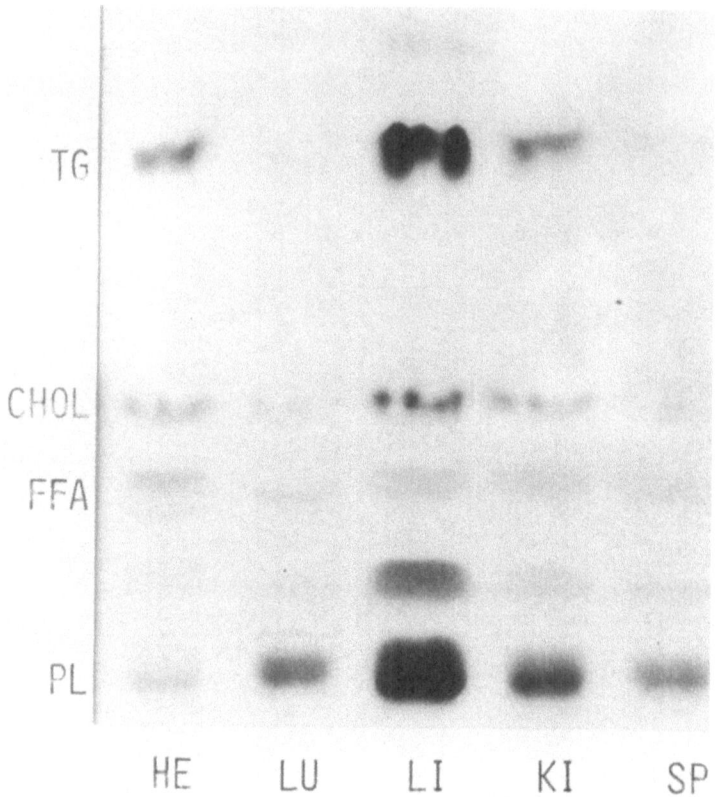

TG

CHOL

FFA

PL

HE   LU   LI   KI   SP

Fig. 5c

(R = 0.7 - 0.88 for TG-, PL-, DG- and FFA-fraction (23). I-PPA
was identified in [127]I-PPA labelled cardiac lipids by GC/MS.
Uptake of I-PPA, determined by GC/MS ([127]I-PPA or radioactivity (^{123}I-PPA) was identical over a range of carrier free
tracer delivery to about 0.5 mg/min I-PPA-supply to the heart
(28).

Kinetics of in vivo labelled cardiac lipids showed - after
an initial tracer clearance period - low levels of "free"
I-PPA, diglycerides and phospholipids (23). In contrast, predominant fast tracer uptake and bicomponent tracer elimination was found in cardiac triglycerides, indicating a metabolic heterogeneity of myocardial triglyceride-pools. Similar
results have been reported for ^{14}C-palmitic or ^{3}H-oleic acid

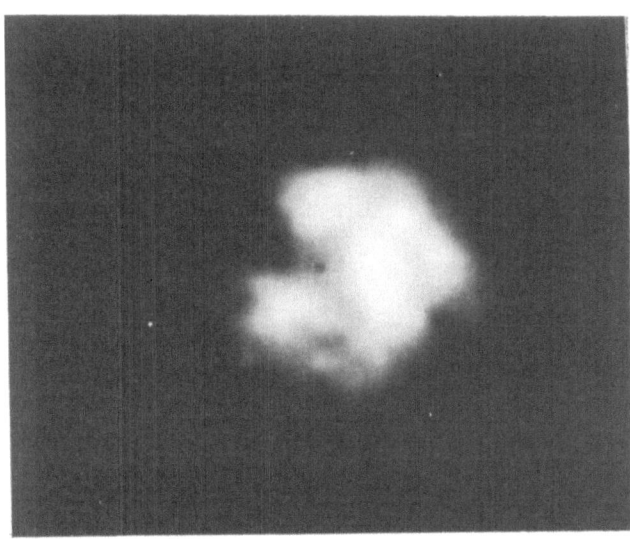

Fig. 6a. SPECT of a dog's heart with an acute myocardial infarct in anterolateral wall ; cardio-CT after contrast infusion of the same dog (fig 5b) shows excellent correspondence of location and extent of ischemic myocardium, visualized with both methods. Note side-inverted display of cardio-CT due to different reconstruction algorithm.

labelled cardiac triglycerides (41,42). Although far from a complete understanding of metabolic turnover of radiolabelled iodofatty acids in heart muscle, data reported for cardiac kinetics of certain fatty acids deliver a framework for interpretation of relative metabolic flow rates of overall cardiac lipid metabolism through externally recorded myocardial tracer turnover curves.

3. SPECT studied of cardiac I-FFA turnover

Single photon emission computed tomography (SPECT) bears a great potential for evaluation of regional tissue integrity and function. There are a few recent studies, where cardiac I-PPA metabolism has been studied by means of this new imaging modality. Rellas and co-workers were able to evaluate myocardial clearance of I-PPA in control dogs and animals with acute myocardial infarct with quantitative SPECT (43). These

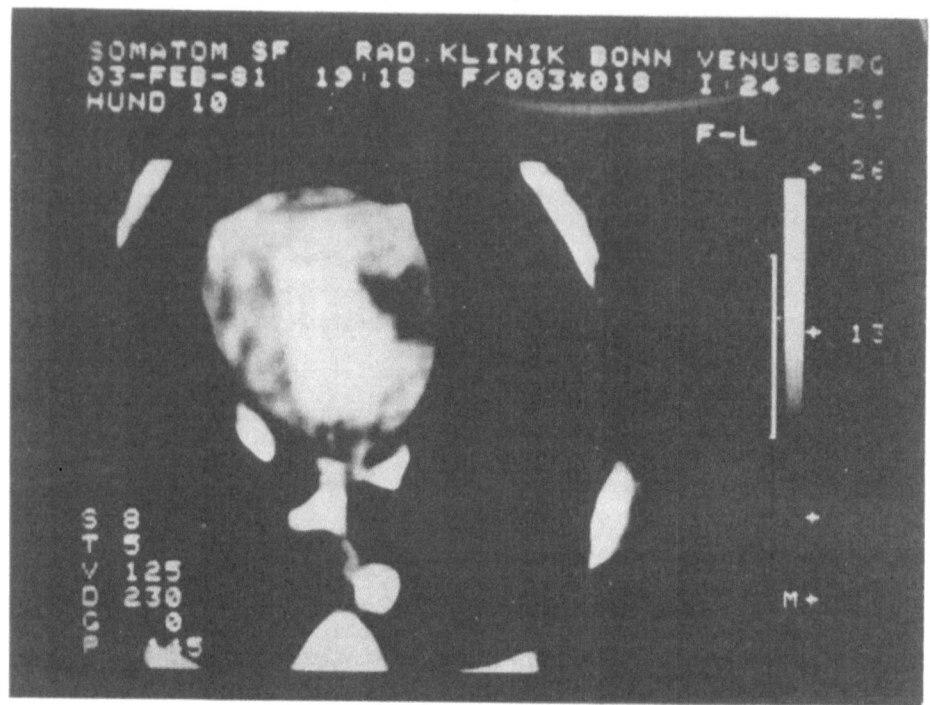

Fig. 6b.

authors reported encouraging results for non-invasive assessment of regional myocardial fatty acid metabolism during
evolving myocardial infarction. Their results indicated prospects of this investigation modality for prediction of cell
viability and control of therapeutic interventions.

Using I-PPA as tracer and quantitative sequential SPECT
acutely ischemic myocardium could be localized in dogs by our
group (44). Good image quality of the tomograms, acquired at
rest, indicated the great potential of this investigation
modality for myocardial infarct detection and quantitation
(fig 6). With serial SPECT we could show highly reduced tracer
turnover in animals with acute ischemic myocardium and reduced
cardiac mechanical function (30% reduction of left ventricular
ejection fraction compared to control animals). In control

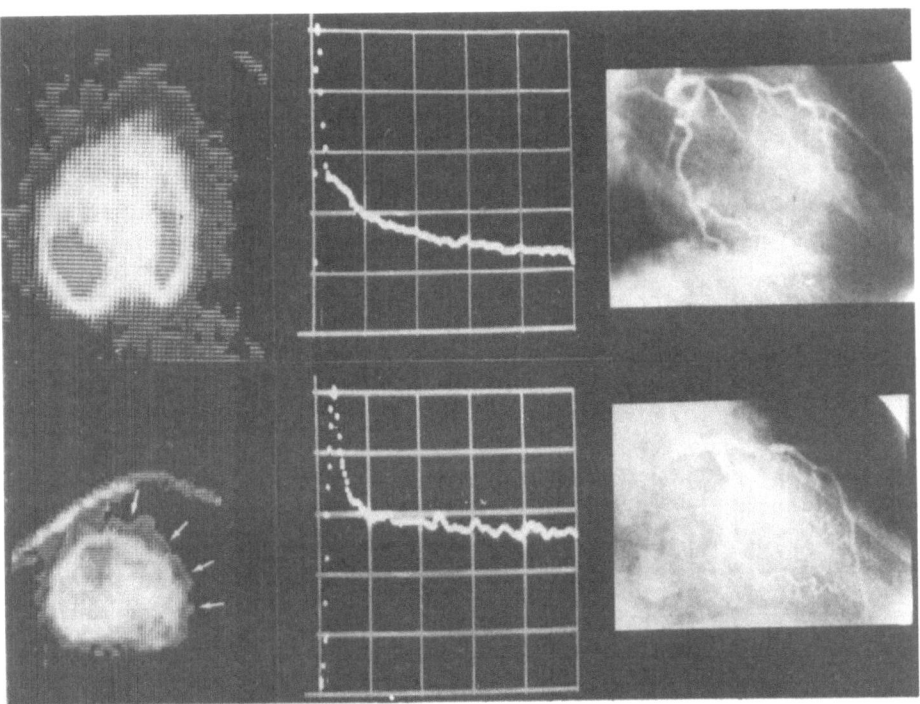

Fig. 7. Myocardial scintigram, cardiac tracer-clearance curves (0-10 min p.i.) and coronary angiogram in a control patient (upper row) and a patient with 90% LAD stenosis (lower row). I-PPA injection into left coronary artery. Note reduced tracer uptake and slower monocomponent tracer clearance in CAD patient after first vascular spike.

animals, I-PPA turnover showed a bicomponent radioactivity clearance (44) very similar to cardiac clearance determined by means of ^{11}C-palmitate clearance and PET (11). These results have been confirmed by I-PPA-turnover studies in comparable experimental models with tissue counting techniques by Kulkarni and co-workers (45).

A recent study reported by Rösler and co-workers tried to assess regional cardiac IHA uptake and metabolism in patients by repeated 7-pinhole tomoscintigraphy. Myocardial infarcts (up to 4 weeks post event) and scars (with a history of more than 4 weeks post event) were detected with 80-85% sensitivity. These authors however were not able to extract relevant information from "radioactivity elimination rates" of normal

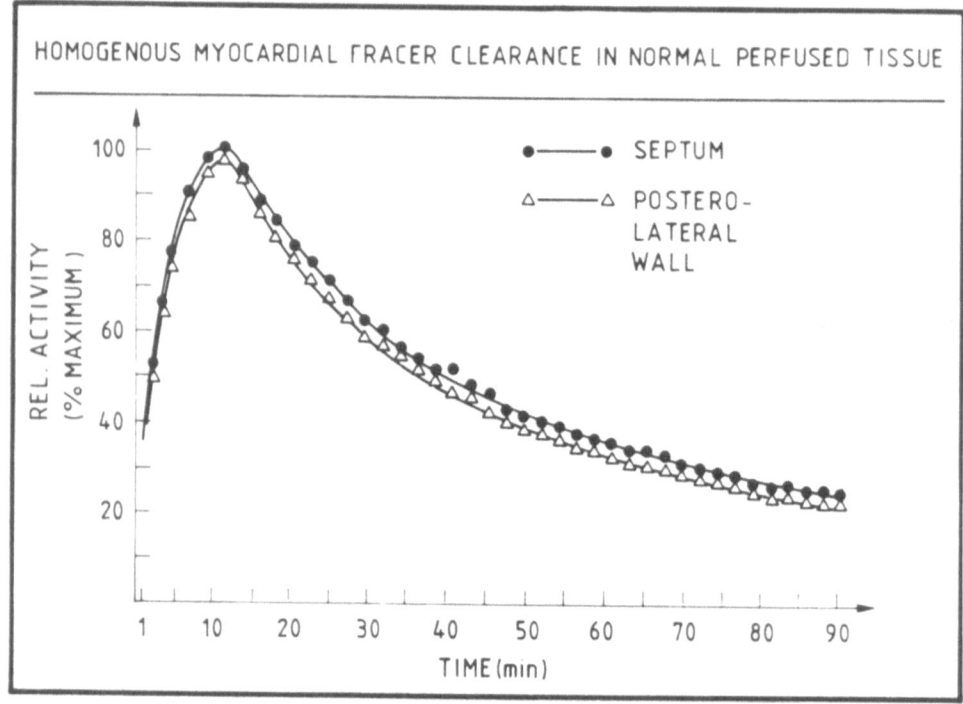

Fig. 8. Homogeneous cardiac tracer clearance in a control patient with normal coronary arteries after i.v. I-PPA injection. Back-ground corrected time activity curves.

myocardium. They found, however, certain types of cardiac lesions with prolonged tracer clearance, which might be associated to the patient's prognosis (46).

4. Principle clearance patterns of cardiac I-FFA turnover in patients

In patients IHA and related compounds as well as I-PPA are rapidly cleared from peripheral blood after i.v. injection (47). Only after 10 min p.i. is a slowly increasing amount of blood radioactivity observed, necessitating back-ground correction procedures if cardiac tracer clearance is to be determined (40). "Background" radioactivity is due to I[123]-iodide after application of aliphatic I-FFA or [123]I- benzoic- and ^{123}I-hippuric acid as well as probably ^{123}I-benzoic acid-glucuronide (40) if I-PPA is used.

Cardiac uptake of I-FFA is rapid and in the normal heart, homogeneous (47) (fig 7). Maximal heart uptake is achieved 5-10 min p.i. at studies performed at rest. In studies performed immediately after ergometric exercise maximal heart uptake is earlier due to increased HMV, increased MBF and reduced circulation time of the tracer.

Cardiac radioactivity clearance is homogeneous in the normal heart (47((fig 8) after i.v. injection of I-FFA. If data are acquired sufficiently long - usually 70-90 min - a bicomponent tracer clearance is found in normal myocardium (40,47). Half times of 20 to 35 min have been reported, if tracer clearance is followed for only 40 min and cardiac clearance is fitted with a monoexponential function (17). Dudczak reported values of 9.55 ± 1.43 min ($\bar{x} \pm$ SD, N = 22) and 54.9 ± 18.2 min ($\bar{x}$ SD, N = 20) for IHA elimination from normal myocardium (9). Using I-PPA, elimination half-times of 11.2 ± 1.41 min and 75.8 ± 31.6 min ($\bar{x}$ SD, N = 40) have been found for tracer clearance from normal myocardium of patients (47).

After bicycle exercise several authors failed to demonstrate an enhanced cardiac tracer elimination of control patients after IHA injection (8,48). It is unclear, if these observations are due to the properties of the tracer itself, if cardiac lipolysis, which is expected to raise with increasing demand (1) was not sufficiently (long?) stimulated or if alternate substrates (i.e. lactate and glucose) exerted a partial inhibitory effect on myocardial lipolysis, thus preventing the expected increase of the heart's lipid metabolism. Preliminary results obtained with I-PPA in patients with severe CAD and symptom-limited exercise revealed an increase of cardiac radioactivity clearance from normal perfused segments (49). Half times of 6.3 ± 1.3 min ($\bar{x} \pm$ SD, N = 9) after exercise versus 11.2 ± 1.41 at rest ($\bar{x} \pm$ SD, N = 40) were reported for the first elimination component (49). Thus, similar to increased cardiac tracer clearance after Isoproterenol-stimulation of myocardial lipolysis, observed in the isolated Langendorff rat heart, increased cardiac demand is

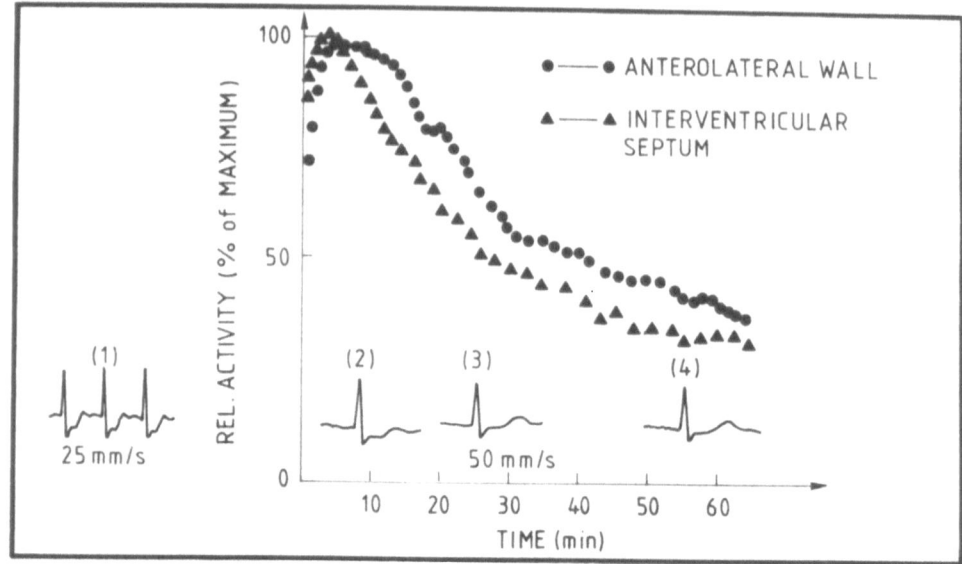

Fig. 9. Initial ischemia-induced delay of myocardial tracer clearance in the territory of a severe coronary stenosis, compared to normal clearance pattern in normal perfused area. ECG findings are shown in the insert (lead 4) at peak exercise (1), 15 min p.i. (2), 40 min p.i. (3) and 60 min p.i.

probably associated with increased cardiac lipolysis resulting in increased turnover of I-PPA. However, it is unclear, to what extent this demand-induced stimulation of cardiac lipid metabolism is counter-balanced by increasing utilization of competitive substrates in normal and diseased heart muscle.

In the territory of significantly obstructed coronary arteries, two different metabolic patterns of I-FFA turnover have been observed: 1) using IHA or I-PPA as tracer, I-FFA turnover can be markedly prolonged (17,8,47) (fig 10). This finding may be interpreted as metabolic sequelae of reduced oxygen delivery and consequently reduced FFA-oxidation (1,2). Biochemically the metabolic fate of I-FFA might be shifted from predominant primary oxidation and/or turnover via a fast turnover fraction of cardiac triglycerides to turnover in the slow turnover fraction of cardiac lipids (phospholipids and a pool of cardiac triglycerides with delayed turnover).

Preliminary results reported from our laboratory established an association of exercise-induced myocardial ischemia –

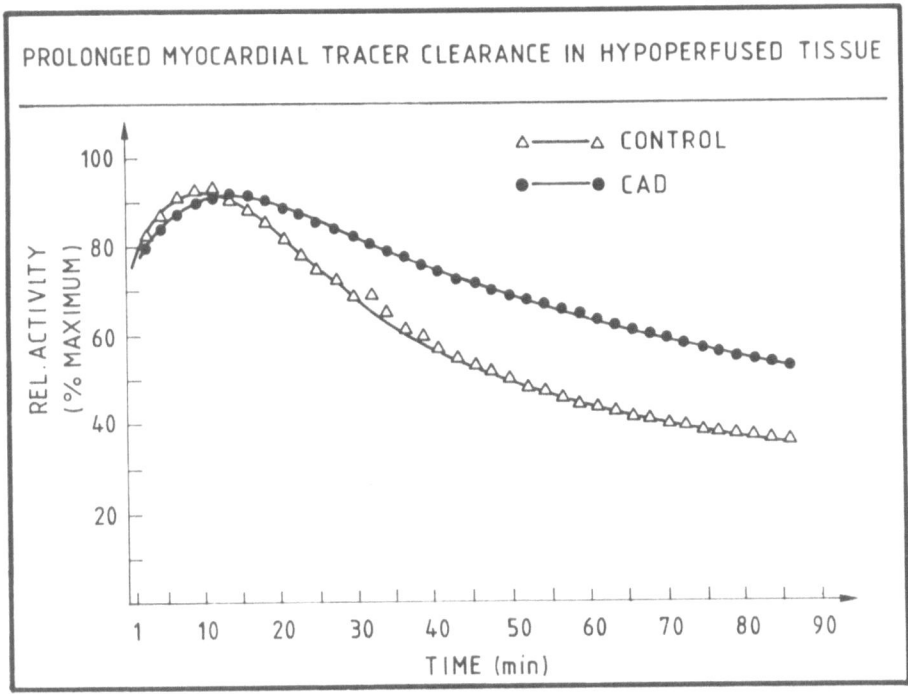

PROLONGED MYOCARDIAL TRACER CLEARANCE IN HYPOPERFUSED TISSUE

Fig. 10 a, b. Common I-PPA clearance pattern in the territory of highly
(>75%) stenosed coronary arteries; (fig 10a): delayed cardiac tracer
clearance; (fig 10b): enhanced cardiac tracer clearance; back-ground
corrected-time activity curves; investigations performed at rest without
clinical or ECG-findings of myocardial ischemia.

documented by stress-induced ECG abnormalities and significant
angina - and a delay of regional cardiac I-PPA turnover (49)
(fig 9). For a comprehensive discussion of the clinical results,
the reader is refered to Dudczak's contribution in this book
(50).

2) Markedly accelerated turnover of I-PPA in the territory of
some highly stenosed coronary arteries has been described in
studies performed at rest or after maximal exercise (47,49)
(fig 10). This metabolic pattern has been occasionally observed as well if ^{11}C-palmitic acid is used as tracer of cardiac
FFA-metabolism (51). The interpretation of these findings is
still unclear, since cardiac lipid turnover is expected to
be rather slow in these segments. Interestingly, however,
severe ultrastructural disturbances of cardiac tissues with

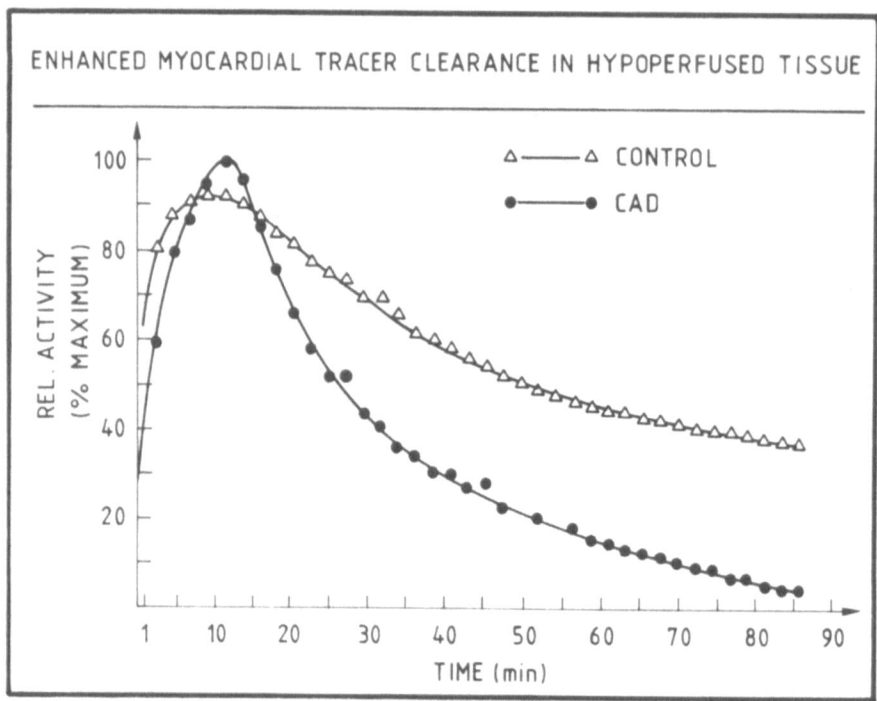

Fig. 10b.

increased amounts of functionally incompletely decoupled mitochondria have been observed in heart muscle specimens of
patients with severe CAD (52,53). Thus increased cardiac lipid
turnover might be related to the amount and functional integrity
of cardiac mitochondria and may be indicative of an adaption
of the myocardium to repetitive ischemic events. In addition,
incomplete I-FFA oxidation (54) or increased lipid washout
documented in acutely ischemic myocardium (36,55) has to be
taken into consideration. Further studies are needed to eluci-
date this very interesting metabolic pattern. These studies
are not only of theoretical interest, but are also beyond any
doubt, clinically important since increased cardiac turnover
of I-FFA has been observed in our laboratory exclusively in
severe CAD, indicating a poor prognosis of this special
metabolic pattern.

In conclusion, there are promising new tracers for evaluation of cardiac lipid metabolism. Evaluation of tissue perfu-

sion should be possible by the use of these tracers - at least
in relative terms. Localization and quantitation of acute
myocardial infarction, especially in conjunction with quantitative SPECT-imaging, has great potential by means of I-FFA.
Qualitative or semiquantitative assessment of parameters of
overall cardiac lipid metabolism seems to be possible on a
regional basis using at least certain radioiodinated fatty
acids with stable iodine-binding in vivo.

Ischemic inhibition of cardiac lipid metabolism is probably
associated with a delay of cardiac turnover of phenylated
I-FFA and can be regionally displayed in clinical examinations.
Conceivably the use of these tracers in conjunction with a
dedicated imaging modality may deliver a clue to the quantitation of myocardial ischemia and evaluation of reversibility
of ischemic tissue injury. In patients with CAD certain metabolic patterns of cardiac phenyl-fatty acid turnover seem to
imply a relation to the patients prognosis. Although far from
a complete understanding of cardiac I-FFA metabolism, a new
diagnostic tool for clinical, non-invasive assessment of one
important metabolic branch of the heart's energy producing
capacity is emerging, thus expanding our diagnostic armamem-
tarium in completion of the well established procedures for
assessment of perfusion and mechanical function of the heart.

REFERENCES

1. Neely, JR, Morgan HE, Relationship between carbohydrate and lipid metabolism and the energy balance of heart muscle. Ann. Rev. Physiol. 34:413, 1974.

2. Gilbertson, JR, Cardiac muscle. In: Lipid metabolism in mammals, 1. Snyder F (ed), Plenum Press, New York, pp 367-397, 1977.

3. Bing JR, Cardiac metabolism. Physiol. Rev. 45:171, 1965.

4. Evans JR, Gunton RW, Baker RG, Beanlands DS, Spears JC, Use of radio-iodinated fatty acid for photoscans of the heart. Circulation Res. 16:1, 1965.

5. Robinson CA, Lee AW, Radioiodinated fatty acids for heart imaging: Iodine monochloride addition compared to iodine replacement labelling. J. nucl. Med. 16:17, 1975.

6. Maculla HJ, Stöcklin G, Kupfernagel Ch, Freundlieb Ch, Höck A, Vyska K, Feinendegen E, Comparative evaluation of fatty acids labelled with C-11, Cl-34m, Br-77 and I-123 for metabolic studies of the myocardium: Concise communication. J. nucl. Med. 19:298, 1978.

7. Feinendegen LE, Vyska K, Freundlieb Ch, Höck A, Machulla HJ, Kloster G, Stöcklin G, Non-invasive analysis of metabolic reaction in body tissue. The case of myocardial fatty acids. Eur. J. Nucl. Med. 6:191, 1981.

8. Van der Wall EE, Heidendahl GAK, Den Hollander W, Westera G, Roos JP, Metabolic myocardial imaging with I-123 labelled heptadecanoic acid in patients with angina pectoris. Eur. J. Nucl. Med. 6:391, 1981.

9. Dudczak R, Schmoliner R, Kletter K, Dufler DK, Frischauf H, Angelberger P, Losert U, Myocardial turnover rates of I-123 heptadecanoic acid. In: Nuclear Medicine and Biology III, IIIrd World Congress of Nucl. Med. Biol. Raynaud C (ed), Pergamon Press, pp 2518-2521, 1982.

10. Okada RD, Knapp F, Elmaleh DR, Yasuda T, Boucher CA, Strauss HW, Tellurium-123m-labelled-9-Talluraheptadecanoic acid: Possible cardiac imaging agent, Circulation 65:305, 1982.

11. Schelbert HR, Henze E, Phelps ME, Emission tomography of the heart. Sem. Nucl. Med. 4:355, 1980.

12. Knust EJ, Kupfernagel Ch, Stöcklin G, Long chain F-18 fatty acids for the study of regional metabolism in heart and liver; odd-even effects of metabolism in mice. J. nucl. Med. 20:1170, 1979.

13. Schelbert HR, Imaging metabolism and biochemistry - a new look at the heart. Amer. Heart J. 105:522, 1983.

14. Sobel BE, Diagnostic promise of positron tomography. Amer. Heart J. 103:673, 1982.

15. Gunton RW, Evans JR, Baker RG, Beanlands DS, Spears JC, Demonstration of myocardial infarction by photoscans of the heart. Amer. J. Cardiol. 16:482, 1965.

16. Poe ND, Robinson GD, Graham LS, McDonald NS, Experimental basis for myocardial imaging with I-123-labelled hexadecanoic acid. J. nucl. Med. 17-1077, 1976.

17. Freundlieb Ch, Höck A, Vyska K, Feinendegen LE, Machulla HJ, Stöcklin G, Myocardial imaging and metabolic studies with (17-J-123)-iodohepta-

decanoic acid. J. nucl. Med. 21:1043, 1980.

18. Vyska K, Höck A, Freundlieb Ch, Profant M, Feinendegen LE, Machulla HJ, Stöcklin G, Myocardial imaging and measurement of myocardial fatty acid metabolism using w-I-123-heptadecanoic acid. J. nucl. Med. 20:650, 1979 (abstract).

19. Höck A, Freundlieb Ch, Vyska K, Lösse B, Erbel R, Feinendegen LE, Myocardial imaging and metabolic studies in patients with idiopathic congestive cardiomyopathy. J. nucl. Med. 24:22, 1983.

20. Van der Wall EE, Den Hollander W, Heidendahl GAK, Westera G, Majid PA, Roos JP, Dynamic myocardial scintigraphy with I-123-labeled free fatty acids in patients with myocardial infarction. Eur. J. Nucl. Med. 6:383, 1981.

21. Reske SN, Schön S, Eichelkraut W, Hahn N, Machulla HJ, Flow-dependance of uptake of (^{123}I-Phenyl)-pentadecanoic acid in the canine heart. J. nucl. Med. 24:12, 1983 (abstract).

22. Feinendegen LE, Personal communication.

23. Reske SN, Sauer W, Machulla HJ, Winkler C, Metabolism of 15(p^{123}I-phenyl)-pentadecanoic acid in heart muscle and in non-cardiac tissues. (Submitted for publication).

24. Reske SN, Auner G, Winkler C, Kinetics of 17(^{123}I) iodoheptadecanoic acid in myocardium of rats. J. Radioanal. Chem. 79:355, 1983.

25. Opatley SJ, Halama JR, Holden JE, DeGrado T, Shug AL, On the rate-limiting step in myocardial clearance of label from 16-Iodohexadecanoic acid. J. nucl. Med. 24:12, 1983 (abstract).

26. Maculla HJ, Marsmann M, Dutschka K, Biochemical concept and synthesis of a radioiodinated phenyl fatty acid for in vivo metabolic studies of the myocardium. Eur. J. Nucl. Med. 5:171, 1980.

27. Knoop F, Der Abbau aromatischer Fettsäuren im Tierkörper. Beitr. chem. Physiol. Path. Braunschweig p 150, 1905.

28. Schmitz B, Reske SN, Machulla HJ, Egge H, Winkler C, Cardiac metabolism of ω (p-iodo-phenyl)-pentadecanoic acid: a gas-chromatographic mass spectrometric analysis. (Submitted for publication).

29. Knapp FF, Ambrose KR, Callahan AP, Ferren LA, Grigsby A, Irgolic KJ, Effects of chain length and tellurium position on the myocardial uptake of Tc-123m fatty acids. J. nucl. Med. 22:988, 1981.

30. Goodman MM, Knapp FF, Callahan AP, Ferren LA, A new, well-retained myocardial imaging agent: radioiodinated 15(p-iodophenyl)-6-tellura pentadecanoic acid. J. nucl. Med. 23:904, 1982.

31. Knapp FF, Personal communication.

32. Lioni E, Elmaleh, DR, Levy S, Brownell GL, Strauss WH, Beta-Methyl (1-^{11}C) heptadecanoic acid: a new myocardial metabolic tracer for positron emission tomography. J. nucl. Med. 23:169, 1982.

33. Breull W, Flohr H, Schuhardt S, Dohm H, Transmural gradients in myocardial metabolic rate. Basic Res. Cardiol. 76:399, 1981.

34. Daus HJ, Reske SN, Vyska K, Feinendegen LE, Pharmacokinetics of p(^{131}I-phenyl)-pentadecanoic acid in the heart. In: Nuklearmedizin, Proc. 13th Congr. Eur. Soc. Nucl. Med. Schmidt HAE, Wolf F (eds),

Schatauer, pp 108-111, 1981.

35. Stöcklin G, Kloster G, Metabolic analogue tracers. In: Computed emission tompgraphy, Ell P, Holman BL, (eds), Oxford Med. Publ. New York, Toronto, pp 318-324, 1982.

36. Reske SN, Knust EJ, Machulla HJ, Breull W, Winkler C, Comparison of cardiac ^{14}C-palmitic- and (^{123}I-phenyl)-pentadecanoic acid oxidation. J. nucl. Med. 24:118, 1983 (abstract).

37. Reske SN, Machulla HJ, Winkler C, Metabolism of 15(p^{123}I)-phenyl-pentadecanoic acid in hearts of rats. J. nucl. Med. 25:1982 (abstracts).

38. Visscher FG, Personal communication.

39. Kloster G, Stöcklin G, Wuitz W, Smith EF, III, Schrör K, Radioiodinated ω-halofatty acids: Biochemical investigations in normal and ischemic isolated perfused hearts. Proc. 21st. Int. Ann. Meeting, Soc. Nucl. Med. Eur. Adam WE (ed). (in press).

40. Reske SN, Jod-123-Phenyl-Pentadecansäure - Ein neuer tracer zur Untersuchung des myokardialen Metabolismus freier Fettsäuren. Nuklearmediz. 1:25, 1983.

41. Crass MF, III, McCaskill ES, Shipp JC, Marthy VK, Metabolism of endogenous lipids of cardiac muscle: Effect of pressure development. Amer. J. Physiol. 220:428, 1972.

42. Stein O, Stein Y, Lipid synthesis, intracellular transport and storage. J. Cell Biology, 36:63, 1968.

43. Rellas JS, Morgan CG, Corbett JR, Kulkarni PV, Bush L, Devous MD, Parkey RW, Willerson JT, Lewis SE, Quantitative tomographic imaging of myocardial clearance of I-123 phenyl-pentadecanoic acid in acute myocardial infarction. J. nucl. Med. 24:12, 1983 (abstract).

44. Reske SN, Biersack HJ, Lackner K, Machulla HJ, Knopp R, Hahn N, Winkler C, Assessment of regional myocardial uptake and metabolism of ω (p-I-123 phenyl) pentadecanoic acid with serial single photon emission tomography. Nuklearmedizin, Vol. XXI, 6:249, 1982.

45. Kulkarni PV, Parkey R, Bonte F, Buja M, Lewis S, Willerson J, Radioiodine labelled phenylpentadecanoic acid uptake as a metabolic indicator during experimental canine myocardial ischemia. Circulation 64, suppl. IV, p 152, 1981 (abstract).

46. Rösler H, Hess T, Weiss M, Noelpp U, Müller G, Hoeflin F, Kinser J, Tomoscintigraphic assessment of myocardial metabolic heterogenity. J. nucl. Med. 24:285, 1983.

47. Reske SN, Simon H, Machulla HJ, Biersack HJ, Knopp R, Winkler C, Myocardial turnover of p(^{123}I-phenyl)- pentadecanoic acid in patients with CAD. J. nucl. Med. 23:34, 1982 (abstract).

48. Höck A, Raffenbeul D, Freundlieb Ch, Vyska K, Lösse B, Feinendegen LE, Left ventricular dysfunction and myocardial fatty acid metabolism in patients with coronary artery disease. Proc. 21st Int. Ann. Meeting, Soc. Nucl. Med. Eur. Adam WE (ed). (in press).

49. Reske SN, Nitsch J, Grube E, Luderitz B, Winkler C, Ischemia-induced inhibition of myocardial 15(p-^{123}I-phenyl-pentadecanoic acid turnover in CAD. Circulation, (abstract) (in press).

50. Dudczak R, Imaging with ^{123}I fatty acids. In: Developments in nuclear cardiology. Biersack HJ, Cox PH (eds), Martinus Nijhoff Publ. The Hague, Boston, London, (in press).

51. Schelbert HR, Personal communication.

52. Flameng W, Suy R, Schwarz F, Borgers M, Piessens J, Thone F, Van Ermen H, De Geest H, Ultrastructural correlates of left ventricular contraction abnormalities in patients with chronic ischemic heart disease: Determinants of reversible segmental asynergy postrevascularization surgery. Amer. Heart J. 102:846, 1981.

53. Schaper W, Personal communication.

54. Moore KH, Radloff JR, Hull FE, Sweely CC, Incomplete fatty acid oxidation by ischemic heart: β-hydroxy fatty acid production. Amer. J. Physiol. 239:257, 1980.

55. Schön HR, Schelbert HR, Najafi A, Hansen H, Huang SC, Barrio J, Phelps ME, C-11 labeled palmitic acid for the non-invasive evaluation of regional myocardial fatty acid metabolism with positron computed tomography II. Kinetics of C-11 palmitic acid in acutely ischemic myocardium. Amer. Heart J. 103:548, 1982.

II. GATED BLOOD-POOL IMAGING

ASSESSMENT OF LEFT VENTRICULAR GLOBAL FUNCTION

H.-P. BREUEL, M. BÄHRE

INTRODUCTION

Radionuclide Ventriculography (RNV), i.e. the noninvasive
evaluation of left ventricular performance following the application of radionuclides has had a major impact on many aspects of
cardiology and has proven its clinical value and reliability in the
last few years. Nowadays it is an accepted method in clinical
practice and permits the assessment of both regional and global
cardiac function. Although the following deals mainly with the
changes in global left ventricular function, this cannot be regarded
separately from changes in regional function (1-6), in terms of
describing impaired left ventricular performance; they are both
complementary and interrelated aspects of the same problem.

Method

There are two principal approaches, Gated Equilibrium Blood
Pool Scintigraphy and First Pass Radionuclide Angiocardiography
(7,8).

Clinically, the most frequently performed procedure is Gated
Equilibrium Blood Pool Scintigraphy. In this approach, the entire
equilibrium blood pool, which is homogenously mixed with an intra-
vascular tracer (almost exclusively autologous red cells labelled
with Tc^{99m}-pertechnetate), is imaged. Because externally detected
counts are proportional to left ventricular volumes, evaluation of
changes in counts permits the noninvasive evaluation of changes of
left ventricular volumes during the cardiac cycle by synchronizing
the collection of scintillation data with a physiological marker
suitable for temporally identifying the sequence of the cardiac
cycle, i.e. the R-wave of the ECG. Repetitive sampling of the

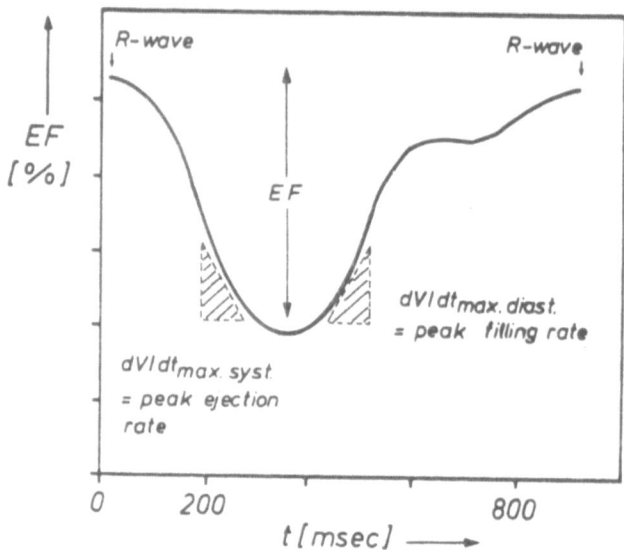

Fig. 1. Left ventricular volume curve.

cardiac cycle thus can be performed until an adequate count density is achieved.

The "gating" technique, first described by Hoffmann and Kleine (9) was developed because there are too few counts recorded within an individual cardiac cycle to give sufficient quantitative data. These data of the volume change during the heart cycle are stored in a computer memory. During or after data acquisition is finished, the recorded data of the volume changes of the left ventricle are sorted for a defined R-R-interval of the same length and a left ventricular volume curve is created which can be analysed (fig. 1).

The conventional method of gated equilibrium blood pool scintigraphy employs a simple frame mode data acquisition (10-12). The cardiac cycle is divided into constant time segments, usually 16 to 64, each represented by an image. Space for the images is reserved in the memory of the computer, which simply adds the particular images. The advantages of this frame mode technique include the modest amount of the required computer data storage and the fact that the data are formatted in real time during acquisition and thus are immediately available for creating the left ventricular volume curve. The important disadvantages of the frame mode technique are the limited time resolution, which only

permits the calculation of the ejection fraction, and the need
for a uniform heart rate, because in the presence of a slight
arrhythmia - even the respiratory arrhythmia of normal subjects -,
the variations in R-R-intervals cause inaccurate temporal positioning of events in the diastolic portion of the cardiac cycle (12,13),
preventing calculation of peak filling rates of the ventricle.

These shortcomings of the frame mode data acquisition can be
overcome by the list mode data acquisition (10,11,12,86). In this
acquisition technique, the computer memory stores individual
scintillations as separate events together with time markers and
R-wave markers, instead of complete images of the left ventricle
as in the frame mode technique. These time markers may be spaced
by very short intervals (usually 10 msec), thus providing temporal
resolution equal to 100 frames per sec. After the data acquisition is complete, the data are sorted and reformatted by means
of the time and R-wave markers into image sequences representing a "representative" cardiac cycle, which is not influenced by
cardiac arrhythmias. However, list mode acquisition of radionuclide
data calls for significant storage space in computer memory and
requires a time consuming (10 to 20 min) reformatting before
analysis.

First Pass Radionuclide Angiocardiography is completely
different from gated blood pool scintigraphy. In this approach to
describing left ventricular function, only the initial transit of
a radioactive bolus through the central circulation is analysed.
The analysis of these first pass data is derived with indicator
dilution principles (14-16). The main assumption of the first pass
radionuclide angiocardiography is the homogenous mixing of the
intravenously injected bolus with blood in the left ventricle. On
the other hand, an important pre-requisite to be met for quantitative analysis of indicator dilution methods is the immediate entry
of the indicator in the compartment to be measured (delta function).
That is true regardless whether the indicator is labelled or not
and whether the indicator concentration is measured invasively
within the compartment or noninvasively above the compartment as
in radionuclide angiocardiography. Of course these two requirements
(homogenous mixing and rapid entry of the indicator bolus in the

compartment) cannot both be fullfilled simultaneously but, in
clinical practice, first pass radionuclide ventriculography has
proven to be of identical value as gated equilibrium blood pool
scintigraphy with frame mode acquisition provided that the tracer
is really injected as a compact bolus. Injection of the tracer
into the femoral vein instead of an antecubital vein can reduce
the number of patients whose results cannot be analysed because
of technical reasons (17). For analysis, a representative cardiac
cycle can be created with either the R-wave of the electrocardiogram or the peak of the volume curve to align end-diastoles of
several consecutive beats (usually three to six cycles). Alter-
natively, in the gated first pass technique, data are stored
directly in a series of equal frames starting immediately after
the R-wave. The picture file is identical to that obtained in
equilibrium blood pool imaging with frame mode data acquisition,
except that only a few cardiac cycles are used.

Parameters

The most important parameters for the assessment of left ventricular global performance derived from the left and right ventricular volume curve by RNV are the ejection fraction (EF) under
resting and exercise conditions and the peak filling rate of the
left ventricle at rest.

The left ventricular ejection fraction (LVEF) describes the
percentage of left ventricular end-diastolic volume (EDV), which
leaves the heart during systole:

$$(1) \qquad EF = \frac{EDV - ESV}{EDV} \times 100 \quad (\%)$$

Left ventricular ejection fraction can be directly obtained withou
further calculation from the RNV-left ventricular volume curve and
has proven to be a reliable parameter of left ventricular systolic
function. A decreased resting left ventricular ejection fraction
indicates an impaired left ventricular performance, whereas a
diminished LVEF at exercise generally does not. This is because
left ventricular ejection fraction is a complex parameter which is

influenced not only by intrinsic myocardial performance but also
by preload and afterload changes (18,19), heart rate (19-21) and
other factors. Left ventricular ejection fraction measured by RNV
may also be influenced by the method of background correction
(22-26) and to a smaller extent by the time resolution of data
acquisition (27,28). In innumerable studies the accuracy (25,26,
29,30,31,32) and high reproducibility (30,33,34,35,36,37,38,39,40)
of both resting and exercise LVEF measurements by radionuclide
ventriculography, as a prerequisite for widespread clinical application and serial measurements, has been demonstrated. The variability of RNV-ejection fraction calculations between two independent
observers is less than 2% and the absolute difference between two
sequential studies is about the same (39), so that a change in
LVEF of 5% or more (absolute percentage) can be considered as a
significant change (3,41,42), whether due to exercise or pharmacological interventions.

Usually, LVEF is determined both at rest and during exercise.
Since patients with heart diseases are mainly symptomatic only
during exercise, it is logical that the hemodynamic evaluation
also should be performed during exercise. Exercise is at present
the safest and most convenient means of stimulating the myocardium
to demand maximal or near maximal blood flow and is the only way
of stimulating such a high demand for oxygen delivery that even
moderate impairment of coronary blood flow capacity becomes detectable (43). Even when the diagnosis is certain, stress testing is
used to determine the approach to therapy, i.e. to evaluate the
degree of benefit from vasodilator, beta-blocker or surgical
therapy.

The stress testing most commonly employed in RNV is the upright
or supine bicycle exercise. Even if there are some differences in
the hemodynamic responses to exercise in the upright and supine
position (43,44,45,46,47), the increase in LVEF in both methods
is comparable (but more pronounced in the upright position). In
patients, who cannot achieve maximal exercise levels (limited
exercise capacity because of peripheral vascular diseases or inadequate heart rate to exercise because of disorders associated
with chronotropic incompetence), some other methods of stress

testing have been recommended: cold pressor test (1,48,49) isometric handgrip stress (1,45,50,51) and atrial pacing (21,52,53).

The cold pressor stimulus is a sympathomimetic response
associated with a reflex increase in blood pressure (49). Its
sensitivity and specificity for detecting patients with left
ventricular dysfunction is reported to be similar to bicycle
exercise testing (48,50).

Isometric handgrip exercise has the advantage that it
requires minimal movement of the patient thus reducing the
potential problem of motion artefacts. The **normal** left ventricle
responds to stress of isometric exercise with little change in
its filling pressure but with an increase in stroke work. In
contrast, the ventricle whose function is impaired displays an
increase in filling pressure but little increase, or even a fall,
in stroke work (54,55). Isometric handgrip testing is safer for
patients with coronary artery disease and might be superior to
bicycle exercise or the cold pressor test in examining patients
by RNV, but the data available so far are insufficient to permit
a final decision on the value of this technique.

In recent years, a technique for the determination of right
ventricular EF has been developed that corrects for the contribution of right atrial activity to right ventricular activity and
thus permits the RVEF calculations (8,56,57,58,59).

The left ventricular peak filling rate is another sensitive
indicator of abnormal left ventricular function, being reduced
even at rest in many patients with only slightly impaired left
ventricular performance and a normal LVEF at rest (60,61,62,
63,64,65).

Usually the peak filling rate is normalized to the end diasto-
ic counts. Reliable and reproducible results necessitate considerable computing facilities; left ventricular filling rate should
only be evaluated if the following prerequisites are met:
a)   time resolution of at least 50 Hz (28,66);
b)   averaging of the volume curve by Fourier analysis (4,6,27);
c)   calculation only by means of heart cycles of the same length
     to avoid image shift in the diastolic part of the volume curve
     which influences the peak filling rates (11,12,13,66).

In practice, calculation of left ventricular peak filling rates therefore requires data acquisition in list mode (12). First pass radionuclide angiography and frame mode gated equilibrium blood pool scintigraphy generally cannot be used to estimate this parameter accurately.

Up to now it is unclear whether the response of the filling rate to exercise provides information of additional diagnostic importance. The calculation of left ventricular peak ejection rate as an index of left ventricular systolic function as well as the calculation of the times of the end-systole, of the peak filling rate and of the peak ejection rate is much easier but usually adds no further information to that obtained from left ventricular ejection fraction.

Whereas the estimation of relative left ventricular volumes during systole and diastole is, by definition, easy to perform (changes of counts in the left ventricle are identical to changes in volume), the calculation of absolute left ventricular volumes involves serious problems. The application of the area-to-length method (as used in echocardiography and ventriculography) to RNV does not provide reliable results in individual patients (67). However, in the last few years RNV-methods have been published which are independent of geometric assumptions (68,69,70,71,72) and which may result in an accurate estimation of end-systolic and end diastolic left ventricular volumes. If these results are confirmed by other groups, the noninvasive determination of left ventricular volumes might add information of tremendous importance to single ejection fraction evaluations, since changes of loading conditions can be recognized which influence the ejection fraction and thus may conceal left ventricular impairment by RNV-exercise testing.

Coronary artery disease

In patients with CAD the resting LVEF (table 1) is often decreased (5,63,76,80), but is in most cases not significantly different from normal subjects (61,62,73,75,77,78,81), even if some groups have demonstrated a strong connection between the amount of LVEF decrease and the number of vessels which are

Table 1. Resting EF, peak ejection rate and peak filling rate in normal subjects and patients with CAD

	normal subjects			patients with CAD		
	EF	peak ejektion rate	peak filling rate	EF	peak ejektion rate	peak filling rate
Borer, 1978 (73)	57 ± 1	-	-	48	-	-
Breuel, 1978 (63)	69.3±3.8	4.2±0.5	4.3±0.6	44.2±12.3	2.5±0.9	2.0±0.8
Maddox, 1979 (5)	65 ± 8	-	-	43 ± 17	-	-
Breuel, 1979 (74)	69.3±3.8	4.2±0.5	4.3±0.6	pts. with one vessel CAD: 51.2±13.2 pts. with two vessel CAD: 43.6±14.4	3.1±0.9 2.5±0.8	2.6±0.9 1.9±0.8
Lindsay, 1980 (75)	65 ± 2	-	-	pts. with one vessel CAD: 62 ± 2 pts. with two vessel CAD: 54 ± 3 pts. with three vessel CAD: 52 ± 2	-	-
Bähre, 1980 (76)	71.3±5.8	4.2±0.5	4.3±0.6	44.2±11.7	2.5±1.0	2.0±0.7
Dehmer, 1981 (77)	72 ± 2	-	-	pts. with one vessel CAD: 68 ± 4 pts. with two- ore three-vessel CAD: 56 ± 3	-	-
Bonow, 1981 (60)	55 ± 6	2.7±0.5	3.3±0.6	pts. with normal resting EF: 54 ± 7 pts. with decreased resting EF: 32 ± 7	2.8±0.6 1.9±0.5	2.1±0.5 1.3±0.4
Reduto, 1981 (61) ·	67 ± 9	-	3.1±0.8	57±13	-	pts. with normal EF at rest: 2.7±0.7 pts. with abnormal EF at rest: 1.7±0.5
Hecht, 1981 (78)	68 ± 8	-	-	59±10	-	-
Simon, 1981 (79)	66.5±5.1	3.6±0.7	4.1±0.3	42.5±17.8	2.6±1.1	2.3±0.9
Bonow, 1982 (62)	-	-	-	55±6	-	2.3±0.6

Table 2. Left ventricular performance in patients with CAD at rest and during exercise.

	EF at rest	EF during exercise	peak ejection rate at rest	peak ejection rate during exercise	peak filling rate at rest	peak filling rate during exercise
Borer, 1978 (73)	48	36	-	-	-	-
Kent, 1978 (83)	51 ± 3	39 ± 2	-	-	-	-
Lindsay, 1980 (75)	1-vessel-CAD: 62 ± 2 / 2-vessel-CAD: 54 ± 3 / 3-vessel-CAD: 52 ± 2	59 ± 2 / 50 ± 3 / 48 ± 3	-	-	-	-
Nechwatal, 1980 (84)	59 ± 12	50 ± 16	-	-	-	-
Upton, 1980 (85)	61 ± 8	52 ± 8	-	-	-	-
Simon, 1981 (80)	34 ± 14	33 ± 11	1.6 ± 0.6	1.5 ± 0.5	1.2 ± 0.4	1.5 ± 0.6
Schwaiger, 1981 (40)	60 ± 10	58 ± 14	3.6 ± 0.8	3.9 ± 13.1	2.6 ± 0.9	4.3 ± 16.9
Dehmer, 1981 (77)	1-vessel-CAD: 68 ± 4 / 2-and-3-vessel CAD: 56 ± 3	78 ± 2 / 52 ± 3	-	-	-	-
Reduto, 1981 (61)	57 ± 13	57 ± 16	-	-	1.8 ± 0.7	2.5 ± 0.9
Ratib, 1982 (3)	54 ± 12	50 ± 13	-	-	-	-
Tan, 1982 (87)	40 ± 9	35 ± 11	-	-	-	-
Hecht, 1982 (39)	56 ± 14	51 ± 18	-	-	-	-

involved (74,75,77,82). Nevertheless, the sensitivity of RNV
to detect a CAD by means of the resting left ventricular ejection fraction is only about 20 to 30%.

At exercise however, typical changes can be demonstrated which
permit the diagnosis of CAD even in patients with normal resting
LVEF. Left ventricular ejection fraction at exercise fails to
increase, or may even decrease (table 2), and/or new regional
wall motion abnormalities appear (2,3,39,49,61,73,75,77,80,84,85,
86,87,88). In normal subjects however, LVEF increases at exercise
more than 5% (EF units) and wall motion abnormalities and regional
disturbances can never be demonstrated. This typically different
behaviour of the EF-exercise response results from an increase in
end diastolic volume (EDV) and a decrease in end systolic volume
(ESV) during exercise stress in normal subjects (87), whereas
patients with CAD are characterized by a more pronounced increase
in the already enlarged end diastolic volume (77,85). The different
EF-exercise response pattern between patients with CAD and normal
subjects was first described by Borer et al (73,81) and has subsequently been confirmed in principle by other groups. False positive
results, i.e. an increase in EF-response to exercise in patients
with CAD, are mainly caused by inadequate exercise stress (88), by
a treatment with beta-blocking drugs or by technical errors due to
underestimating the resting EF or calculating the maximal (=exer-
cise) value (41). False negative results (i.e. no change in exercise EF-response in normal patients) is mainly due to the presence
of beta-blockade (89), which has been shown to reduce the resting
EF slightly and to blunt (but not to eliminate) the normal increase
in EF during exercise (90,91,92).

If adequate exercise is maintained (developing of chest pain or
depression of at least 1 mm or a pressure-rate product greater than
250), the sensitivity of RNV in detecting patients with CAD is
about 94% but this falls to only 62% with inadequate exercise testing (88).

All studies dealing with the diagnosis of CAD by exercise
RNV have concluded that this method is a sensitive tool for the
noninvasive detection of patients with CAD (1,3,39,41,73,77,78,81,
93-99,164). Its overall sensitivity is about 80 to 90% and its

Table 3. EF in patients with cardiomyopathy or congestive heart failure

	EF at rest	EF during exercise	
Schoolmeester, 1981 (100)	Group I: 22.3±6.1 Group II: 19.3±4.7	16.7±6.8 24.6±6.4	chronic congestive eardiomyopathy Group I: ischemic cardiomyopathy Group II: primary cardiomyopathy
Francis, 1982 (103)	20 ± 2	-	congestive heart failure
Ricci, 1982 (104)	29.7±7.5	-	congestive heart failure
Franciosa, 1982 (105)	25 ± 6	-	chronic heart failure
Massie, 1982 (106)	19 ± 6	-	chronic congestive heart failure
Firth, 1982 (107)	19 ± 5	-	congestive heart failure
Hecht, 1982 (101)	19.8±9.6	18.8±11.4	chronic congestive cardiomyopathy

specificity about 90 to 100%, but only if other heart diseases with a similar exercise ejection fraction response as seen in patients with CAD (e.g. valvular heart disease, cardiomyopathy (100-102) can be excluded (e.g. by echocardiography), if truly maximal exercise testing is performed and if a therapy with beta-blockers has been stopped before RNV.

As has already been observed in 1978 by Breuel et al (63,64), peak filling rate is a more sensitive parameter of left ventricular performance than is the left ventricular ejection fraction, even under resting conditions. Subsequently these findings have been confirmed by others, who demonstrated that the peak filling rate is altered, even at rest, in up to 90% of patients with CAD and impaired left ventricular systolic function (4,60,61,62).

The abnormalities of left ventricular diastolic filling are not specific for CAD and may appear in patients with valvular heart disease and hypertrophic cardiomyopathy. However, that is also true for the lack of LVEF-increase in these patients (table 3) and for the appearance of regional wall motion abnormalities, as was demonstrated by Hecht (78). The cause of abnormal left ventricular diastolic filling in the absence of abnormal systolic function and/or evidence of active ischemia is unexplained (62). The reduced peak filling rate at rest in patients with CAD and normal systolic function may be caused by an asymptomatic decrease in myocardial perfusion. During active myocardial ischemia diastolic dysfunction develops from impaired early diastolic left ventricular relaxation or increased diastolic tone, thus decreasing the peak filling rate; myocardial relaxation during early diastole is an active, energy dependent, process and previous investigations have shown that hypoxia may impair the rate of myocardial relaxation by reducing available substrate for ATP-dependent dissociation of actin and myosin. Additionally, acidosis appears to increase the affinity of sarcoplasmic reticulum for calcium, thereby resulting in prolongation of relaxation time (61).

Reduction of peak filling rate in patients after myocardial infarction results from myocardial fibrosis with alterations in the distensibility characteristics of the left ventricle.

The volume ejected early in systole has also been proposed as an indicator of abnormal left ventricular function at rest in patients with CAD, a normal EF and normal wall motion (108). However, it could be demonstrated (109) that resting left ventricular emptying curves are identical in normal subjects and patients with CAD who have a normal EF and no wall motion disturbances. Therefore, not only is the "first third" ejection fraction unable to detect patients with CAD but also the entire resting left ventricular emptying curve obtained with RNV can probably not be used to distinguish between patients with CAD and normal subjects.

Further to the diagnostic evaluation of patients with suspected CAD, the functional assessment of known disease is an important indication for the use of RNV. Several studies have dealt with patients who have had an acute myocardial infarction (MI) (table 4). Resting LVEF is reduced in about 70% of all patients with acute myocardial infarction (112). The type and degree of ventricular dysfunction depends on the localization of the acute infarction.

A depressed ejection fraction is more common in patients with anterior (90 to 100% of all patients) than in those with inferior infarction (about 60%). In patients with inferior infarction the mean EF is lower in patients who have concomitant ST-segment depression in the precordial leads (104,120). In patients with anterior infarction, regional EF as a quantitative measure of regional left ventricular performance is uniformly depressed in the infarcted zone, whereas in patients with inferior infarction abnormalities of regional performance are less severe and can only be demonstrated in 70% of patients.

Only 30% of patients with inferior infarction but 69% of those with anterior infarction also have an abnormal regional performance in noninfarcted zones (111). These findings demonstrate a close dependance of global on regional function in noninfarcted as well as infarcted zones. Furthermore the mean resting LVEF is significantly lower in patients with higher clinical classification (112, 116), but the clinical classification as well as the X-ray-findings fail to correlate with EF in individual cases. Thus early radio-nuclide ventriculography adds significantly to the discriminant power of clinical and radiographic characterization of ventricular function in patients with acute myocardial infarction. Furthermore, from the clinical point of view it is important that RNV allows an assessment of the prognosis of patients with acute myocardial infarction. Several recent studies have stressed the prognostic importance of the resting LVEF as a predictor of early mortality and the subsequent development of congestive heart failure (CHF) or sudden death.

Death due to pump failure occurred in 55% of patients with an EF of 30% or less but only in about 5-10% of the remainder (110, 113). A scintigraphic LVEF equal to or less than 52% measured early after the event is seen in 93% of patients who die; but is also seen in 58% of patients who survive and provides a positive predictive accuracy for death of only 35% (118). The negative predictive accuracy of LVEF measurements is generally greater than the positive predictive accuracy - i.e. it is more certain that a

Table 4. Radionuclide ventriculography after myocardial infarction (MI)

	time after MI	EF
Pichler, 1979 (110)	24 hours	anterior infarction: 34 ± 10 inferior infarction: 61 ± 8
Wynne, 1980 (111)	40 hours	anterior infarction: 31 ± 3 inferior infarction: 51 ± 3
Battler, 1980 (112)	day 1 to 4 after ad- mission	MIRU Class I : 48 ± 10 Class II : 45 ± 18 Class III: 36 ± 10
Shah, 1980 (113)	24 hours	anterior infarction: 34 ± 9 inferior infarction: 50 ± 14
Corbett, 1981 (114)	19 days	no cardiac event in the 6 month follow-up: rest EF: 66 Ex EF : 76 minor cardiac event: rest EF: 51 Ex EF : 47 major cardiac event: rest EF: 44 Ex EF : 37
Wackers, 1982 (115)	soon after admission	anterior infarction: 36 ± 6 inferior infarction: 45 ± 15
Sanford, 1982 (116)	day 1 to 4 after ad- mission	Killip Class I : 50 ± 14 Class II : 42 ± 17 Class III: 27 ± 7
Upton, 1982 (117)	3 weeks/ 8 weeks	3 weeks: anterior infarction: rest EF : 35 ± 10 submax. Ex. EF: 36 ± 13 inferior infarction: rest EF : 51 ± 11 submax. Ex. EF: 50 ± 15 previous infarction: rest EF : 23 ± 8 submax. Ex. EF: 26 ± 10 8 weeks: anterior infarction: rest EF : 36 ± 10 max. Ex. EF: 37 ± 13 inferior infarction: rest EF : 53 ± 11 max. Ex. EF: 50 ± 13 previous infarction: rest EF : 23 ± 9 max. Ex. EF: 28 ± 10
Perez-Gonsales, 1982 (118)	4 days	EF related to the late prognosis: asymptomatic patients : 54.1 patients with angina : 52.5 patients with CHF : 42.7 patients who died of cardic causes: 40.2
Wasserman, 1982 (119)	at least 8 weeks	anterior infarction: single vessel disease: rest EF : 45 ± 3; Ex EF: 43 ± 3 multi vessel disease : rest EF : 40 ± 2; Ex EF: 34 ± 2 inferior infarction: single vessel disease: rest EF : 53 ± 2; Ex EF: 57 ± 3 multi vessel disease : rest EF : 50 ± 2; Ex EF: 45 ± 2

patient will not develop CHF or die if LVEF is less abnormal.

Nemerowski et al (121) demonstrated that LVEF (and RVEF) changes variably during the hospital course of acute myocardial infarction. Early determination of LVEF has prognostic implications whereas its subsequent changes are less closely related to short-term prognosis. These changes tend to occur mostly within the first few days after the acute event and appear to be unpredictable according to the demographic, clinical and hemodynamic status on admission. These LVEF changes typically occur without concurrent change in regional wall motion, suggesting changes in ventricular loading rather than changes in intrinsic myocardial performance.

The evaluation of left ventricular function at rest and during submaximal exercise in the convalescent phase at 3 and 8 weeks following acute myocardial infarction appears to be more sensitive and specific than stress ECG in detecting exercise induced myocardial ischemia and permits the identification of patients with depressed resting ventricular function or exercise induced myocardial ischemia who may benefit from intensive medical or surgical therapy (117). Furthermore, patients at risk of future cardiac events during the ensuing 6 months can be identified by exercise RNV; in 88% of patients without important cardiac events (death, recurrent myocardial function, unstable angina) during the 6 months follow-ups there was no abnormality in the response of LVEF to submaximal exercise (114).

RNV has also been used to evaluate the effects of several potential therapies for CAD, including coronary bypass surgery, aneurysmectomy (122) and coronary angioplasty (62). 3 to 6 months after successful coronary artery bypass graft surgery, LVEF levels after maximal exercise are significantly higher than preoperatively whereas in patients with blocked or stenosed grafts LVEF decreases significantly during exercise (79,83,123,124,125). The improved LV-functional reserve postoperatively is associated with clinical improvement.

Important observations have been made by Freeman et al (126) and Bähre et al (79) that patients with normal left ventricular function preoperatively frequently demonstrate an abnormal left ventricular reserve postoperatively. Even in patients with success-

ful coronary artery bypass surgery and normalized EF response
postoperatively, the peak filling rate at rest shows unchanged
pathological values. A preoperatively reduced peak filling rate
(equal to or less than 2.0) is associated with a worse prognosis
as far as the postoperative improvement of left ventricular
performance is concerned, regardless the preoperative LVEF-exer-
cise response (79).

Bonow (62) recently demonstrated that, in patients with one-
vessel CAD, no evidence of previous myocardial infarction, normal
resting left ventricular ejection fraction but abnormal LV diastolic filling peak (peak filling rate >2.5), the LV diastolic
filling improved after Percutaneous Transluminal Coronary Angioplasty and became normal in the majority of patients. These data
suggest, that in this subgroup of patients with abnormalities
of LV diastolic filling as the earliest parameter of impaired lef
ventricular function, these abnormalities are not fixed but appea
to be reversible manifestations of reduced coronary flow.

Furthermore RNV permits an assessment of the results of drug
therapy in patients with CAD.

During the last decade beta adrenoceptor blocking drugs have
become widely accepted for treatment of patients with angina
pectoris. Their effectiveness is attributed primarily to a decrea
in myocardial oxygen consumption requirements, indirectly reflect
by a reduction in heart rate and systolic blood pressure during
exercise.

Propranolol has either no effect on the basal left ventricula
function in normal subjects (92), improves resting left ventricul
ejection fraction (91) or even reduces left ventricular performan
(90).

During exercise, a dose-related negative inotropic effect
produces a decline in exercise left ventricular ejection fraction
(90,91,92) in normal subjects, thus reducing EF-response to exercise during treatment with beta blocking drugs. In patients with
CAD, the effect of propranolol on exercise ventricular performanc
depends on the presence or absence of ischemic dysfunction during
exercise (92). In patients with an ischemic functional response t
exercise (unchanged or decreased delta EF), propranolol signific-

antly improves regional and global performance during and after exercise and prevents exercise-induced left ventricular dysfunction (41,84,91,92,127,128,129). In CAD patients with a normal response to exercise, propranolol has no significant effect on exercise and post-exercise ventricular function (92). This implies that the ischemic myocardium is more sensitive to the effects of beta-blockade. Whilst therapy with beta-blocking drugs usually improves left ventricular regional function, acute beta-blockade may, however, result in an impairment of regional wall movement despite improvement of ischemic signs (ST-lowering and anginal symptoms) (84).

RNV following the administration of nitroglycerin may be useful in evaluating the variability of abnormally contracting ventricular segments in patients with CAD (130,131), thus detecting abnormally contracting ischemic segments by improvement or non-improvement respectively of dyssynergies resulting from nitrates. In patients with CAD, nitroglycerin reduces exercise-induced regional wall motion abnormalities (73), which can be mitigated by prophylactic nitroglycerin.

In normal subjects, as well as in patients with CAD, both resting and exercise EF increase (73,80,130,131,132,133,134) but the improvement is more striking in the normals. However, the most important effect of nitroglycerin is the improvement of the exercise EF-response in patients with CAD, which might be explained by a reduced myocardial oxygen demand (preload and afterload reduction) or by a reduction in ischemia due to improving myocardial oxygen supply.

Valvular heart disease

RNV does not permit the detection of patients with valvular heart disease (as opposed to CAD) but resting and exercise ventricular performance studies are uniquely suited for defining functional status in these patients.

Most studies have dealt with the evaluation of patients with aortic regurgitation (table 5). The severity of valvular regurgitation is conventionally assessed by contrast ventriculography. However, this approach is highly invasive and does not allow

128

Table 5. Left ventricular performance in patients with aortic
regurgitation

	EF at rest	EF exercise during	peak filling rate at rest	
Borer et al, 1978 (135)	47 62	38 57	- -	symptomatic pts., asymptomatic pts.
Borer et al, 1979 (136)	46	37	-	symptomatic pts.
Manyari et al, 1981 (137)	61	54	-	asymptomatic pts.
Dehmer et al, 1981 (138)	59 73	50 72	- -	symptomatic pts., asymptomatic pts.
Henze et al, 1982 (139)	56	45	-	symptomatic pts.
Schuler et al, 1982 (18)	62	63	-	asymptomatic pts.
Lewis et al, 1982 (140)	50 57	49 64	- -	symptomatic pts. asymptomatic pts.
Breuel et al, 1983 (141)	56	-	2.3	symptomatic pts.

serial measurements of left ventricular performance for evaluating
effects of therapeutic interventions, i.e. valve replacement or
drug therapy. Additional problems may arise in the accurate determination of left ventricular volumes from altered left ventricular
geometry in valvular heart diseases. These shortcomings can be
overcome by radionuclide methods.

At rest, mean LVEF in aortic insufficiency, even in symptomatic patients, is usually not significantly different from that

of normal subjects (18,56,78,135,137,138,139,140,142,143) but, in some patients, may be slightly decreased (136,138,140,141,142,144). The average resting LVEF is higher in asymptomatic than in symptomatic ones (135,138,140).

During exercise, the mean left ventricular EF is unchanged in up to 50% of all asymptomatic patients (135,136,138,139) and declines in the majority of symptomatic patients (18,135,138). Whereas during exercise EDV increases and ESV decreases in normal subjects, patients with symptomatic aortic insufficiency show an increase in EDV and ESV, which are both already increased in the resting state (138,139). These changes in left ventricular volumes during exercise may be helpful in the characterization of left ventricular performance in patients with chronic aortic regurgitation. Resting RVEF is unaltered but increases significantly with exercise (56).

An abnormal resting LVEF is not necessarily predictive of abnormal LV exercise reserve (140). Therefore only exercise testing permits evaluation of the left ventricular performance of patients with aortic regurgitation. The response of EF during exercise is a sensitive and useful clinical index of the functional reserve of the left ventricle in patients with aortic regurgitation (135). Subnormal EF during exercise generally appears before the manifestation of left ventricular dysfunction, commonly assessed non-invasively or at cardiac catheterization. Therefore a depressed EF at rest implies diminished left ventricular performance but a "normal" resting EF does not necessarily imply normal left ventricular function.

The presence of left ventricular dysfunction induced only by stress probably represents an intermediate point between normal left ventricular function and the development of left ventricular dysfunction at rest, which is associated with a poor long-term prognosis (135, 136).

Furthermore, exercise induced regional wall motion abnormalities (which have been thought a reliable indicator of CAD only) were found in 42% of patients with aortic insufficiency without CAD, predominantly in the infero-apical segment of the left ventricle (78). The mechanism of these wall motion abnormalities is unclear. They may be produced by the relative reduction in both minor and major axis shortening with exercise. On the other hand the ventricular hypertrophy of patients with chronic aortic regurgitation produces uneven gradients of regional myocardial perfusion, so that a disparity between oxygen demand and supply during exercise might result in regional changes in those areas with relatively poor perfusion (78).

These abnormalities in the EF during exercise in patients with chronic aortic regurgitation do not generally indicate impairment in the intrinsic contractile state of the myocardium, because EF is also affected by alterations in preload and after-load (18). The development of an acute pressure load during exercise might preclude an increase in EF even if ventricular function is normal.

However, the presence of important intrinsic left ventricula dysfunction in patients with aortic regurgitation and an abnorma ejection fraction response to exercise is suggested by studies indicating that EF during exercise, although improved, most often does not revert to normal after aortic valve replacement i patients with preoperatively depressed EF (136,142). Only in asymptomatic patients with normal resting LVEF and a decreased ejection fraction response (137), the EF at exercise increases after valve replacement and cannot be distinguished postoperativ ely from that of normal subjects. The lack of adequate ejection fraction response during exercise in patients with chronic aorti regurgitation as an early indicator of impairment of intrinsic contractile state of the left ventricle is also indicated by the observation that, in patients with chronic aortic valve insuff-iciency, both maximal ejection rate and maximal filling rate are markedly decreased, even under resting conditions, but are not altered in patients with aortic stenosis or mitral valve insuff-iciency (141). That is consistent with the finding (18), that the slope of the end systolic pressure-volume relation, a sen-sitive indicator of myocardial contractility (145), is within the normal range in patients with a normal left ventricular exercise reserve but significantly lower in patients who experience left ventricular dysfunction during exercise. In any

Table 6. Left ventricular performance in patients with other types of
valvular heart disease than aortic regurgitation

	Type of valvular disease	EF at rest	EF during exercise
Henze at al, 1981 (56)	mitral valve insufficiency	52	42
Henze et al, 1982 (139)	mitral valve insufficiency	56	43
Boucher et al, 1981 (144)	mitral valve insufficiency	66	-
Newman et al, 1981 (146)	mitral valve prolapse	61	71
Gottdiener et al, 1981 (147)	mitral valve prolapse	57	64
Borer et al, 1981 (148)	aortic stenosis	68	57
Hofman et al, 1981 (142)	aortic stenosis	69	-

event, the potential usefulness of radionuclide ventriculography
during exercise in the evaluation of left ventricular performance
of patients with chronic aortic regurgitation does not depend on
whether an abnormal ejection fraction always indicates intrinsic
myocardial dysfunction (135). LVEF during exercise has proven
valuable emperically as an early indicator of diminished left
ventricular functional reserve and can help to assess the appropriate timing of operative interventions.

Only a few studies have dealt with other types of valvular
heart disease (table 6).

In patients with severe aortic stenosis, a normal (141,142,148) or a slightly decreased ejection fraction (142) is present at rest. Whilst aortic valve replacement does not change the EF at rest, it significantly improves the EF response during exercise (142, 148).

In patients with mitral valve regurgitation or mitral valve prolapse, the resting EF is either slightly decreased (56), or within the normal range (139,144). With exercise, LVEF as well as RVEF decrease rapidly in patients with mitral valve regurgitation, thus behaving differently from patients with chronic aortic regurgitation, in whom the RVEF increases (56,139).

After mitral valve replacement, EF decreases early in the postoperative period because of loading changes but remains slightly depressed at late postoperative follow-up (144).

Thus, further studies are needed to assess the clinical usefulness of RNV in patients with aortic valve stenosis, mitral valve insufficiency and other valvular heart diseases.

RNV in clinical pharmacology and drug therapy monitoring

Assessment of the global left ventricular function by radionuclide techniques can be used not only to design and optimize therapy in a specific patient (7) but is an accepted part of the methodological approach for evaluation new drugs and a suitable tool for noninvasive sequential drug therapy monitoring.

The application of RNV can be recommended for the study of two different problems.

a) To exclude adverse drug effects on left ventricular performance in the process of drug safety evaluation. To answer that important question, mainly the left ventricular peak filling rate should be used, since isolated assessments of LVEF provide only limited evidence because of dependence on preload and afterload changes. The demonstration of an unchanged peak filling rate during or after drug therapy excludes a harmfull effect on left ventricular myocardial performance.

b) To demonstrate hemodynamic effects of new drugs particularly after long-term medication (106,149,150). Although the demonstration of a drug-induced cardiovascular effect is not equivalent to therapeutic efficacy (which principally has to be demonstrate(

by its clinical benefits), RNV
type of hemodynamic changes to be expected, as well as information
on the mode of action and the onset and duration of the pharmacological effects.

Noninvasive RNV in this indication has not only the advantage
of a lacking risk for the patient but, above all, in contrast to
classical cardiac catheterization, does not itself cause hemodynamic changes. Compared with echocardiography, RNV is superior
in two respects:

in 30 to 40% of all patients (32,151) and, furthermore, the calculation of LVEF and volumes is afflicted with unpredictable errors in
patients with non-uniformly enlarged or dyskinetic left ventricular
such as occur in patients with CAD and/or congestive heart failure.

From the great number of studies conducted in this field a few
examples have been selected to demonstrate the capabilities and
limitations of RNV for the assessment of global left
function:

The traditional role of digoxin and other cardiac glycosides
in the management of ventricular dysfunction has recently come
under scrutiny. In the absence of overt cardiac failure, the
administration of glycosides has been variously reported as having
a deleterious, beneficial or no effect on ventricular dysfunction.
Firth et al (152) thus performed a study to assess the effects of
chronic oral digoxin therapy on left ventricular ejection fraction,
end diastolic and end systolic volumes, stroke volume and cardiac
output at rest and during supine exercise with multigated blood
pool imaging. They could demonstrate that chronic digoxin therapy
in patients with stable ischemic heart disease provides improved
ventricular function at peak exercise in patients with well
preserved left ventricular function at rest.

The afterload-reducing agent prazosin, an alpha-1 blocking
agent, improves left ventricular function and increases performance,
with decreased left ventricular end systolic volume and increased
EF and cardiac output in patients with heart failure refractory
to other treatments (153). In patients with chronic stable heart
failure, long-term therapy with prazosin does not influence the

resting EF during treatment but the exercise EF increases significantly (154).

In terms of the application of RNV to assessment of the hemodynamic effect of vasodilators the reports of Haq (155) and of Firth (107) provide the important information that the changes in ventricular size produced by these drugs might be too small for detection with echocardiography of RNV in patients with severe left ventricular dilatation and an EF of less than 30%. However, it is probable that, in these particular patients, the estimation of pulmonary transit times (MPTT) by simple radiocardiography (156) might add diagnostically important information for the monitoring of patients with vasodilator therapy (151).

Terbutaline is a member of another group of pharmacological agents that has been studied in relation to the effects on left heart function. Terbutaline, a beta agonist, was shown in several studies to increase right heart as well as left heart performance in patients with chronic obstructive pulmonary disease (8,157, 158), patients with congestive heart failure (159) and patients with previous myocardial function (160), especially those with depressed global cardiac function.

Oral theophylline, a widely used bronchodilator in chronic obstructive pulmonary disease, produces a sustained modest enhancement of resting biventricular performance (161).

Furthermore the cardiotoxic effect of the highly efficacious therapeutic agent doxorubicin (Adriamycin) has been evaluated in several clinical studies (162,163). Serial assessment of left ventricular EF by radionuclide ventriculography allows identification of patients at risk for the development of congestive heart failure before clinical signs of left ventricular dysfunction occur and predicts the onset of doxorubicin cardiotoxicity.

Conclusions

Radionuclide ventriculography (RNV) is a simple noninvasive method for evaluating regional and global cardiac performance at rest and during exercise and is useful in a wide variety of clinical settings. RNV is indicated:

<u>in suspected CAD</u>:
- to exclude a CAD: normal regional and global left ventricular function both at rest and during maximal exercise.
- to identify left ventricular contractility abnormalities.
- to detect a myocardial ischemia: no change or decrease in EF at maximal exercise (often a reduced peak filling rate will already exist at rest), evidence of wall motion abnormalities and/or appearance of new regional function disturbances at maximal exercise (only if a valvular heart disease can be excluded).

<u>in known CAD</u>:
- to assess the functional status of a coronary artery stenosis.
- to evaluate a therapeutic effect.
- to provide information on prognosis of patients following myocardial infarction.

<u>in diseases other than coronary artery disease</u>
- to assess the left ventricular function in a known valvular heart disease, particularly after surgical therapy (aortic valve replacement).
- to assess the left ventricular performance in patients with idiopathic cardiomyopathy.

Because sequential studies can be easily performed, RNV appears ideally suited for studying the natural course of heart disease and determining the effects of medical and surgical interventions. At the present time, patient categorization should involve both resting echocardiographic indices and the RNV exercise left ventricular response, since they appear to provide complementary information.

REFERENCES

1. Bodenheimer MM, Banka VS, Fooshee CM et al, Detection of coronary heart disease using radionuclide determined regional ejection fraction at rest and during handgrip exercise: correlation with coronary arteriography. Circulation 58:640, 1978.

2. Adam WE, Bitter F, Nechwatal et al, Functional imaging of gated blood pool investigations for quantification of regional wall motion abnormalities. J. nucl. Med. 22:47, 1981.

3. Ratid O, Henze E, Schön H et al, Phase analysis of radionuclide ventriculograms for the detection of coronary artery disease. Amer. Heart J. 104:1, 1982.

4. Miller TR, Goldman KJ, Sampathkumaran KS et al, Analysis of cardiac diastolic function: Application in coronary artery disease. J. nucl. Med. 24:2, 1983.

5. Maddox DE, Wyne J, Uren R et al, Regional ejection fraction: a quantitative radionuclide index of regional left ventricular performance. Circulation 59:1001, 1979.

6. Links JM, Douglass KH, Wagner HN, Patterns of ventricular emptying by fourier analysis of gated blood pool studies. J. nucl. Med. 21: 978, 1980.

7. Berger HJ, Zaret BL, Nuclear Cardiology: Cardiovascular performance. N. Eng. J. Med. 305:855, 1981.

8. Berger HJ, Matthay RA, Noninvasive radiographic assessment of cardiovascular function in acute and chronic respiratory failure. Amer. J. Cardiol. 47:950, 1981.

9. Hoffmann G, Kleine N, Die Methode der radio-kardiografischen Funktionsanalyse. Nuklearmedizin 7:350, 1968.

10. Knopp R, Datenverarbeitung in der klinischen Nuklearmedizin. Nucl. Med. Stuttg. 18:160, 1979.

11. Knopp R, Bähre M, Breuel HP et al, Die Methoden der Datenakquisition bei der Herzfunktionsszintigraphie. Vor- und Nachteile, diagnostische Wertigkeit. Nucl. Med. Stuttg. 19:155, 1980.

12. Knopp R, Breuel HP, Bähre M et al, Herzfunktionsszintigraphie – List Mode oder Frame Mode? In: Nuklearmedizin, Nuklearmedizin im interdisziplinären Bezug. Schmidt HAE, Wolf F, Mahlstedt J (eds), Stuttgart, New York, pp 63-66, 1981.

13. Bauer R, Sauer E, Langhammer H et al, Radionuklidventrikulographie bei Herzrhytmusstörungen. In: Nuklearmedizin, Nuklearmedizin im interdisziplinären Bezug. Schmidt HAE, Wolf F, Mahlstedt J (eds), Stuttgart, New York, pp 224-228, 1981.

14. Breuel HP, Emrich D, Kardiologie und Angiologie. In: Nuklearmedizin, Funktionsdiagnostik und Therapie. Emrich D (ed), Stuttgart, pp 224-225, 1979.

15. Meier P, Zierler KL, On the theory of the indicator dilution method for measurement of blood flow and volume. J. appl. Physiol. 6:731, 1954.

16. Zierler KL, Circulation times and the theory of indicator-dilution methods for determination blood flow and volume. In: Handbook of

Physiol. Circulation 1, Washington , p. 585, 1962.

17. Breuel HP, Emrich D, Heimburg P et al, Optimierung der Funktions-szintigraphie durch Injektion in die Vena femoralis. Fortschr. Röntgen-str. 121:378, 1974.

18. Schuler G, Von Olshausen K, Schwarz F et al, Noninvasive assessment of myocardial contractility in asymptomatic patients with severe aortic regurgitation and normal left ventricular ejection fraction at rest. Amer. J. Cardiol. 50:45, 1982.

19. Slutsky R, Watkins J, Peterson K, et al, The response of left vent-ricular size and function to atrial pacing, volume loading and after-load stress in CAD patients. Circulation 62:III, 1980.

20. Ricci DR, Orlick AE, Alderman EL et al, Influence of heart rate on left ventricular ejection fraction in human beings. Amer. J. Cardiol. 44:447, 1979.

21. Swiryn S, Pavel D, Byrom E et al, Assessment of left ventricular function by radionuclide angiography during induced supraventricular tachycardia. Amer. J. Cardiol. 47:555, 1981.

22. Breuel HP, Knopp R, Winkler C, Backgroundkorrektur bei der Funktions-szintigraphie des linken Ventrikels. NucComp. 8:77, 1977.

23. Slutsky R, Pfisterer M, Verba J et al, Influence of different background and left-ventricular assignments on the ejection fraction in equilibrium radionuclide angiography. Radiology 135:725, 1980.

24. Schicha H, Karsch KR, Rentrop P et al, Vergleich verschiedener gated-blood-pool-Verfahren zur Bestimmung der linksventrikulären Ejektions-fraktion mit dem Angiogram. In: Radioaktive Isotope in Klinik und Forschung. Vol. 14:75, 1980.

25. Folland ED, Hamilton GW, Larson SM et al, The radionuclide ejection fraction: A comparison of three radionuclide techniques with contrast angiography. J. nucl. Med. 18:1159, 1977.

26. Green MV, Brody WR, Douglas MA et al, Ejection fraction by count rate from gated images. J. nucl. Med. 19:880, 1978.

27. Fischer P, Knopp R, Breuel HP, Zur Anwendung der harmonischen Analyse bei der Funktionsszintigraphie des Herzens. Nucl. Med. Stuttg. 18: 167, 1979.

28. Breuel HP, Fischer P, Knopp R, Nuklearmedizinisch bestimmte Volumen-kurven des linken Ventrikels. Untersuchungen zur zeitlichen Auflösung. Nucl. Med. Stuttg. 18:172, 1979.

29. Secker-Walker RH, Resnick L, Kunz H et al, Measurement of left ventricular ejection fraction. J. nucl. Med. 14:798, 1976.

30. Starling MR, Crawford MH, Sorensen SG et al, Comparative accuracy of apical biplane cross-sectional echocardiography and gated equilibrium radionuclide angiography for estimating left ventricular size and performance. Circulation 63:1075, 1981.

31. Klein Chr, Brill G, Oberhausen E et al, Radiokardiographische Bestimmung des Herzminutenvolumens und der Ejektionsfraktion. Ein Vergleich mit konventionellen kardiologischen Untersuchungsverfahren. Z. Kardiol. 67:92, 1978.

32. Bähre M, Grube E, Knopp R et al, Vergleichende Untersuchungen zur Bestimmung der globalen und regionalen linksventrikulären Funktion durch Laevokardiographie, Funktionsszintigraphie und zweidimensionale Echokardiographie. In: Nuklearmedizin, Nuklearmedizin im interdisziplinären Bezug. Schmidt HAE, Rössler H (eds), Stuttgart, New York, pp 422-425, 1982.

33. Okada RD, Kirschenbaum HD, Kushner FG et al, Observer variance in the qualitative evaluation of left ventricular wall motion and the quantitation of left ventricular ejection fraction using rest and exercise multigated blood pool imaging. Circulation 61:128, 1980.

34. Upton MT, Rerych SK, Newman GE et al, The reproducibility of radionuclide angiographic measurements of left ventricular function in normal subjects at rest and during exercise. Circulation 62:126, 1980.

35. Sorensen SG, Ritchie JL, Caldwell JH et al, Serial exercise radionuclide angiography. Circulation 61:600, 1980.

36. Slutsky R, Hooper W, Gerber K et al, Assessment of right ventricular function at rest and during exercise in patients with coronary heart disease: A new approach using equilibrium radionuclide angiography. Amer. J. Cardiol. 45:63, 1980.

37. Slutsky R, Karliner J, Battler A et al, Reproducibility of ejection fraction and ventricular volume by gated radionuclide angiography after myocardial infarction. Radiology 132:155, 1979.

38. Pfisterer ME, Battler A, Swanson SM et al, Reproducibility of ejection fraction determinations by equilibrium radionuclide angiography in response to supine bicycle exercise: concise communication. J. nucl. Med. 20:491, 1979.

39. Hecht HS, Josephson MA, Hopkins JM et al, Reproducibility of equilibrium radionuclide ventriculography in patients with coronary artery disease: Response of left ventricular ejection fraction and regional wall motion to supine bicycle exercise. Amer. Heart J. 104:567, 1982.

40. Schwaiger M, Silber S, Klein U et al, Reproduzierbarkeit szintigraphisch bestimmter linksventrikulärer Funktionsparameter in Ruhe und während Belastung.
Z. Kardiol. 70:262, 1981.

41. Caldwell JH, Hamilton GW, Sorensen SG et al, The detection of coronary artery disease with radionuclide techniques: a comparison of rest-exercise thallium imaging and ejection fraction response. Circulation 61:610, 1980.

42. Pfisterer ME, Ricci DR, Schuler G et al, Validity of left-ventricular ejection fractions measured at rest and peak exercise by equilibrium radionuclide angiography using short acquisition times. J. nucl. Med. 20:484, 1979.

43. Sheffield L Th, Exercise stress testing. In: Heart disease. Braunwald E (ed), Philadelphia, pp 253-277, 1980.

44. Poliner LR, Dehmer GJ, Lewis SE et al, Left ventricular performance in normal subjects: A comparison of the response to exercise in the upright and supine positions. Circulation 62:528, 1980.

45. Freeman M, Berman D, Maddahi J et al, Upright or supine - which position is better for exercise scintigraphic ventriculography? J. nucl. Med. 21:6, 1981.

46. Kramer B, Massie B, Topic N, Hemodynamic differences between supine and upright exercise in patients with congestive heart failure. Circulation 66:820, 1982.

47. Freemann MR, Berman DS, Staniloff H et al, Comparison of upright and supine bicycle exercise. Amer. Heart J. 102:182, 1981.

48. Kurtz RG, Besozzi MC, Brady TJ et al, Cold pressor radionuclide ventriculography. J. nucl. Med. 21:4, 1981.

49. Giles RW, Marx P, Berger HJ et al, Importance of rapid sequential sampling of left ventricular function during the cold pressor test by beat-to-beat assessment with the computerized nuclear probe. J. nucl. Med. 22:47, 1981.

50. Brennand-Roper DA, Wainwright RJ, Hilson AJW et al, Which stress test should be performed during technetium-99m gated cardiac blood pool scintigraphy to detect coronary artery disease (CAD)? J. nucl. Med. 21:4, 1981.

51. DePuey EG, Sung C, Sonnemaker RE et al, Exercise radionuclide ventriculography in patients with chest pain and no prior infarction. J. nucl. Med. 21:5, 1981.

52. Hecht HS, Chew CY, Burnam M et al, Radionuclide ejection fraction and regional wall motion during atrial pacing in stable angina pectoris: Comparison with metabolic and hemodynamic parameters. Amer. Heart J. 101:726, 1981.

53. Stone D, Dymond D, Elliot AT et al, Use of first-pass radionuclide ventriculography in assessment of wall motion abnormalities induced by incremental atrial pacing in patients with coronary artery disease. Brit. Heart J. 43:369, 1980.

54. Helfant RH, deVilla M, Meister SG, Effect of sustained isometric handgrip exercise on left ventricular performance. Circulation 44:982, 1971.

55. Kivowitz C, Parmley WW, Donoso R et al, Effects of isometric exercise on left cardiac performance: The grip-test. Circulation 44:994, 1971.

56. Henze E, Wisenberg G, Schelbert HR, Effects of exercise on regurgitant fraction and right and left ventricular function in aortic and mitral insufficiency. J. nucl. Med. 21:49, 1981.

57. Maddahi J, Berman DS, Matsuoka DT et al, Right ventricular ejection fraction during exercise in normal subjects and in coronary artery disease patients: Assessment by multiple-gated equilibrium scintigraphy. Circulation 62:133, 1980.

58. Korr KS, Gandsman EJ, Winkler ML et al, Hemodynamic correlation of right ventricular ejection fraction measured with gated radionuclide angiography. Amer. J. Cardiol. 49:71, 1982.

59. Friedman BJ, Holman BL, Scintigraphic prediction of pulmonary arterial systolic pressure by regional right ventricular ejection fraction during the second half of systole. Amer. J. Cardiol. 50: 1114, 1982.

60. Bonow RO, Bacharach SL, Green MV et al, Impaired left ventricular diastolic filling in patients with coronary artery disease: Assessment with radionuclide angiography. Circulation 64:315, 1981.

61. Reduto LA, Wickemeyer WJ, Young JB et al, Left ventricular diastolic performance at rest and during exercise in patients with coronary artery disease. Circulation 63:1228, 1981.

62. Bonow RO, Kent KM, Rosing DR et al, Improved left ventricular diastolic filling in patients with coronary artery disease after percutaneous transluminal coronary angioplasty. Circulation 66:1159, 1982.

63. Breuel HP, Felix R, Knopp R et al, Funktionsszintigraphie der Kontraktion des linken Ventrikels. III. Ergebnisse bei Patienten mit koronärer Herzerkrankung. Fortschr. Röntgenstr. 128:317, 1978.

64. Breuel HP, Knopp R, Felix R et al, Funktionsszintigraphie der Kontraktion des linken Ventrikels. II. Methodische Untersuchungen zur Background-Korrektur. Fortschr. Röntgenstr. 129:18, 1978.

65. Reduto LA, Wickemeyer WJ, Young JB et al, Left ventricular diastolic performance at rest and during exercise in patients with coronary artery disease. Circulation 63:1228, 1981.

66. Knopp R, Breuel HP, Schmidt H et al, Funktionsszintigraphie des Herzens. I. Datentechnische Grundlagen und Methodik. Fortschr. Röntgenstr. 128:44, 1978.

67. Massie BM, Kramer BL, Gertz EW et al, Radionuclide measurement of left ventricular volume: Comparison of geometric and counts-based methods. Circulation 65:725, 1982.

68. Slutsky R, Karliner J, Ricci D et al, Left ventricular volumes by gated equilibrium radionuclide angiography: A new method. Circulation 60:556, 1982.

69. Dehmer GJ, Firth BG, Hillis LD et al, Nongeometric determination of right ventricular volumes from equilibrium blood pool scans. Amer. J. Cardiol. 49:78, 1982.

70. Dehmer GJ, Lewis SE, Hillis LD et al, Nongeometric determination of left ventricular volumes from equilibrium blood pool scans. Amer. J. Cardiol. 45:293, 1980.

71. Johnson St M, Mauritson DR, Corbett J et al, Effects to verapamil and nifedipine of left ventricular function at rest and during exercise in patients with prinzmetal's variant angina pectoris. Amer. J. Cardiol. 47:1289, 1981.

72. Slutsky R, Karliner J, Ricci D et al, Left ventricular volumes by gated equilibrium radionuclide angiography: a new method. Circulation 60:556, 1979.

73. Borer JS, Bacharach SL, Green MV et al, Effect of nitroglycerin in exercise-induced abnormalities of left ventricular regional function and ejection fraction in coronary artery disease. Circulation 57:314, 1978.

74. Breuel HP, Simon H, Bähre M et al, Die Funktionsszintigraphie des Herzens nach Indikatorgleichverteilung zur nichtinvasiven Beurteilung der links-ventrikulären Funktion. Klin. Wochenschr. 57:839, 1979.

75. Lindsay J, Nolan NG, Goldstein SA et al, The usefulness of radionuclide ventriculography for the identification and assessment of patients with coronary heart disease. Amer. Heart J. 99:310, 1980.

76. Bähre M, Simon HS, Breuel HP et al, Noninvasive examination of left ventricular function in coronary artery disease: A modified gated blood pool technique. In: Advances in Clinical Cardiology, quantification of myocardial ischemia I. Heiss HW (ed), G. Witzstrock Publishing House, Inc, New York, pp 161-169, 1980.

77. Dehmer GJ, Lewis SE, Hillis LD et al, Exercise-induced alterations in left ventricular volumes and the pressure-volume relationship: A sensitive indicator of left ventricular dysfunction in patients with coronary artery disease. Circulation 63:1008, 1981.

78. Hecht HS, Hopkins JM, Exercise-induced regional wall motion abnormalities on radionuclide angiography. Amer. J. Cardiol. 47:861, 1981.

79. Bähre M, Simon H, Knopp R et al, Herzfunktionsszintigraphie bei Patienten mit koronärer Herzkrankheit vor und nach bypass-operation. In: Nuklearmedizin, Nuklearmedizin im interdisziplinären Bezug. Schmidt HAE, Wolf F. Mahlstedt J (eds), Stuttgart, New York, pp 280-283, 1981.

80. Simon H, Bähre M, Schuppan U et al, Assessment of the effect of isosorbide dinitrate on left ventricular hemodynamics at rest and under exercise in patients with CHD blood pool scintigraphy. In: Nitrates III. Lichtlen PR et al (eds), Berlin, Heidelberg, New York, pp 387-395, 1981.

81. Borer JS, Bacharach SL, Green MV et al, Real-time radionuclide cineangiography in the noninvasive evaluation of global and regional left ventricular function at rest and during exercise in patients with coronary-artery disease. New Engl. J. Med. 296:839, 1977.

82. McEwan P, Newman GE, Portwood J et al, Correlation of rest and exercise radionuclide angiocardiographic ventricular function with the number of significantly stenosed vessels in 230 patients with coronary artery disease. J. nucl. Med. 20:687, 1980.

83. Kent KM, Borer JS, Green MV et al, Effects of coronary-artery bypass on global and regional left ventricular function during exercise. New Engl. J. Med. 298:1434, 1978.

84. Nechwatal W, Sigel II, Bitter F et al, Die globale und regionale Funktion des linken Ventrikels bei koronärer Herzerkrankung nach Betablockade und Furosemid. Dtsch. med. Wschr. 105:1687, 1980.

85. Upton MT, Rerych SK, Newman GE et al, Detecting abnormalities in left ventricular function during exercise before angina and ST-segment. Circulation 62:341, 1980.

86. Knopp R, Breuel HP, Bähre M et al, Herzfunktionsszintigraphie - list mode oder frame mode? In: Nuklearmedizin, Nuklearmedizin im interdisziplinären Bezug. Schmidt HAE, Wolf F, Mahlstedt J, (eds), Stuttgart, New York, pp 63-66, 1981.

87. Tan ATH, Sadick N, Kelly DT et al, Verapamil in stable effort angina: Effects on left ventricular function evaluated with exercise radionuclide ventriculography. Amer. J. Cardiol. 49:425, 1982.

88. Brady TJ, Thrall JH, Lo K et al, The importance of adequate exercise in the detection of coronary heart disease by radionuclide ventriculography. J. nucl. Med. 21:1125, 1980.

89. Sorensen SG, Caldwell J, Ritchie J et al, "Abnormal" response of ejection fraction to exercise in healthy subjects, caused by region-of-interest selection. J. nucl. Med. 22:1, 1981.

90. Sorensen SG, Ritchie JL, Caldwell JH et al, Serial exercise radionuclide angiography: Validation of count-derived changes in cardiac output and quantitation of maximal exercise ventricular volume change after nitroglycerin and propranolol in normal men. Circulation 61:600, 1980.

91. Wisenberg G, Marshall R, Schelbert H et al, The effect of oral propranolol on left ventricular function at rest and during exercise in normals and in patients with coronary artery disease as determined by radionuclide angiography. J. nucl. Med. 20:639, 1979.

92. Marshall RC, Wisenberg G, Schelbert HR et al, Effect of oral propranolol on rest, exercise and postexercise left ventricular performance in normal subjects and patients with coronary artery disease. Circulation 63:572, 1981.

93. Baron J, Miller H, Braun S et al, An accurate method for the detection of coronary heart disease (CHD) using equilibrium radionuclide ventriculography (ERV) and the regional ejection fraction image (REFI) at rest and during handgrip stress (HGS). J. nucl. Med. 21:4, 1981.

94. Berger HJ, Reduto LA, Johnstone DE et al, Global and regional left ventricular response to bicycle exercise in coronary artery disease. Amer. J. Cardiol. 66:13, 1979.

95. Cardwell HH, Ritchie JL, Hamilton GW et al Comparative sensitivity and specificity of exercise radionuclide ventriculography and rest exercise thallium imaging in the detection of coronary artery disease. J. nucl. Med. 20:687, 1980.

96. Brady TJ, Thrall JH, Lo K et al, Sensitivity of exercise radionuclide ventriculography in coronary artery disease detection: Importance of adequate exercise. J. nucl. Med. 20:687, 1980.

97. McEwan P, Newman GE, Port S et al, Sensitivity and Specificity of exercise radionuclide angiography in detecting coronary disease. Amer. J. Cardiol. 45:408, 1980.

98. Austin EH, Cobb FR, Coleman RE et al, Prospective evaluation of radionuclide angiocardiography for the diagnosis of coronary artery disease. Amer. J. Cardiol. 50:1212, 1982.

99. Newman GF, Rerych SK, Upton MT et al, Comparison of electrocardiographic and left ventricular functional changes during exercise. Circulation 62:1204, 1980.

100. Schoolmeester WL, Simpson AG, Sauerbrunn BJ et al, Radionuclide angiographic assessment of left ventricular function during exercise in patients with a severe reduced ejection fraction. Amer. J. Cardiol. 47:804, 1981.

101. Hecht HS, Karahalios SE, Ormiston JA et al, Patterns of exercise response in patients with severe left ventricular dysfunction: Radionuclide ejection fraction and hemodynamic cardiac performance evaluations. Amer. Heart J. 104:718, 1982.

102. Manyari DE, Paulsen W, Boughner DR et al, Resting and stress left ventricular function in patients with hypertrophic cardiomyopathy. J. nucl. Med. 22:22, 1981.

103. Francis GS, Goldsmith St R, Cohn JN, Relationship of exercise capacity to resting left ventricular performance and basal plasma norepinephrine levels in patients with congestive heart failure. Amer. Heart J. 104:725, 1982.

104. Ricci S, Zaniol P, Teglio V et al, Sustained haemodynamic and clinical effects of captopril in long-term treatment of severe chronic congestive heart failure. Brit. J. clin. Pharmac. 14:2095, 1982.

105. Franciosa JA, Weber KT, Levine TB et al, Hydralazine in the long-term treatment of chronic heart failure: Lack of difference from placebo. Amer. Heart J. 104:587, 1982.

106. Massie BM, Kramer BL, Topic N, Acute and long-term effects of captopril on left and right ventricular volumes and function in chronic heart failure. Amer. Heart J. 104:1197, 1982.

107. Firth BG, Dehmer GJ, Markham RV et al, Assessment of vasodilator therapy in patients with severe congestive heart failure: Limitations of measurements of left ventricular ejection fraction and volumes. Amer. J. Cardiol. 50:954, 1982.

108. Holman BL, Wynne J, Idoine J et al, Disruption in the temporal sequence of regional ventricular contraction. Circulation 61:1075, 1980.

109. Denenberg BS, Makler PT, Bove AA et al, Normal left ventricular emptying in coronary artery disease at rest: Analysis by radiographic and equilibrium radionuclide ventriculography. Amer. J. Cardiol. 48:311, 1981.

110. Pichler M, Shah PK, Swan HJC, Globale und regionale Myokardfunktion in der Frühphase des akuten Myokardinfarktes. Dtsch. med. Wschr. 104:577, 1979.

111. Wynne J, Sayres M, Maddox DE et al, Regional left ventricular function in acute myocardial infarction: Evaluation with quantitative radionuclide ventriculography. Amer. J. Cardiol. 45:203, 1980.

112. Battler A, Slutsky R, Karliner J et al, Left ventricular ejection fraction and first third ejection fraction early after acute myocardial infarction: Value for predicting mortality and morbidity. Amer. J. Cardiol. 45:197, 1980.

113. Shah PK, Pichler M, Berman DS et al, Left ventricular ejection fraction determined by radionuclide ventriculography in early stages of first transmural myocardial infarction. Amer. J. Cardiol. 45:542, 1980.

114. Corbett JR, Dehmer GJ, Lewis SE et al, The prognostic value of submaximal exercise testing with radionuclide ventriculography before hospital discharge in patients with recent myocardial infarction. Circulation 64:535, 1981.

115. Wackers FJ, Berger HJ, Weinberg MA et al, Spontaneous changes in left ventricular function over the first 24 hours of acute myocardial infarction: Implications for evaluating early therapeutic interventions. Circulation 66:748, 1982.

144

116. Sanford CF, Corbett J, Nicod P et al, Value of radionuclide ventriculography in the immediate characterization of patients with acute myocardial infarction. Amer. J. Cardiol. 49:637, 1982.

117. Upton MT, Palermi ST, Jones RH et al, Assessment of left ventricular function by resting and exercise radionuclide angiography following acute myocardial infarction. Amer. Heart J. 104:1232, 1982.

118. Perez-Gonzalez J, Botvinick EH, Dunn R et al, The late prognostic value of acute scintigraphic measurement of myocardial infarction size. Circulation 66:960, 1982.

119. Wasserman AG, Katz RJ, Cleary P et al, Noninvasive detection of multivessel disease after myocardial infarction by exercise radionuclide ventriculography. Amer. J. Cardiol. 50:1242, 1982.

120. Gibson RS, Crampton RS, Watson DD et al, Precordial ST-segment depression during acute inferior myocardial infarction; clinical, scintigraphic and angiographic correlations. Circulation 66:732, 1982.

121. Nemerovski M, Shah PK, Pichler M et al, Radionuclide assessment of sequential changes in left and right ventricular function following first acute transmural myocardial infarction. Amer. Heart J. 104:709, 1982.

122. Dymond DS, Stephens JD, Stone DL et al, Combined exercise radionuclide and hemodynamic evaluation of left ventricular aneurysmectomy. Amer. Heart J. 104:977, 1982.

123. Lim YL, Kalff V, Kelly MJ et al, Radionuclide angiographic assessment of global and segmental left ventricular function at rest and during exercise after coronary artery bypass graft surgery. Circulation 66:972, 1982.

124. Bähre M, Simon H, Knopp R et al, Herzfunktionsszintigraphie bei Patienten mit koronärer Herzkrankheit vor und nach Bypass OP. Z. Kardiol. 70:262, 1981.

125. Newman GE, Rerych SK, Jones RH et al, Noninvasive assessment of the effects of aorta-coronary bypass grafting on ventricular function during rest and exercise. J. thorac.cardiovasc. Surg. 79:617, 1980.

126. Freeman M, Gray R, Berman D et al, Does coronary bypass surgery improve global and regional left and right ventricular response to exercise? J. nucl. Med. 21:49, 1981.

127. Borer JS, Bacharach SL, Green MV et al, Effects of propranolol on left ventricular function during exercise in patients with coronary artery disease. Circulation 58, II:61, 1978.

128. Battler A, Ross J, Slutsky R et al, Improvement of exercise-induced left ventricular dysfunction with oral propranolol in patients with coronary heart disease. Amer. J. Cardiol. 44:318, 1979.

129. Berger HJ, Lachman A, Giles RW et al, Effects of high dose oral propranolol on exercise left ventricular performance in coronary artery disease. J. nucl. Med. 22:16, 1981.

130. Breuel HP, Simon H, Bähre M et al, Funktionsszintigraphie des Herzens nach sublingualer Nitrogabe bei Patienten mit koronarer Herzerkrankung. Z. Kardiol. 68:821, 1979.

131. Salel AF, Berman DS, DeNardo GL et al, Radionuclide assessment of nitroglycerin influence on abnormal left ventricular segmental contraction in patients with coronary heart disease. Circulation 53:975, 1976.

132. Stauch M, Kress P, Geffers H et al, Influence of isosorbide dinitrate and mononitrate on the ejection fraction and wall motion parameters at rest and under exercise in patients with coronary heart disease. In: Nitrates III, Lichtlen PR et al (ed), Berlin, Heidelberg, New York, pp 396-400, 1981.

133. Ritchie JL, Sorensen SG, Kennedy JW et al, Radionuclide angiography: Noninvasive assessment of hemodynamic changes after administration of nitroglycerin. Amer. J. Cardiol. 43:278, 1979.

134. Slutsky R, Battler A, Gerber K et al, Effect of nitrates on left ventricular size and function during exercise: Comparison of sublingual nitroglycerin and nitroglycerin paste. Amer. J. Cardiol. 45:831, 1980.

135. Borer JS, Bacharach SL, Green MV et al, Exercise-induced left ventricular dysfunction in symptomatic and asymptomatic patients with aortic regurgitation: Assessment with radionuclide cineangiography. Amer. J. Cardiol. 42:351, 1978.

136. Borer JS, Rosing DR, Kent KM et al, Left ventricular function at rest and during exercise after aortic valve replacement in patients with aortic regurgitation. Amer. J. Cardiol. 44:1297, 1979.

137. Manyari DE, Purves P, Kostuk WJ, Effect of valve replacement of left ventricular function at rest and during exercise in aortic valvular insufficiency. J. nucl. Med. 22:23, 1981.

138. Dehmer GJ, Firth BG, Hillis LD et al, Alterations in left ventricular volumes and ejection fraction at rest and during exercise in patients with aortic regurgitation. Amer. J. Cardiol. 48:17, 1981.

139. Henze E, Schelbert HR, Wisenberg G et al, Assessment of regurgitation fraction and right and left ventricular function at rest and during exercise: A new technique for determination of right ventricular stroke counts from equilibrium blood pool studies. Amer. Heart J. 104:953, 1982.

140. Lewis SM, Riba AL, Berger HJ et al, Radionuclide angiographic exercise left ventricular performance in chronic aortic regurgitation: Relationship to resting echographic ventricular dimensions and systolic wall stress index. Amer. Heart J. 103:498, 1982.

141. Breuel HP, Heusinger JH, Hanisch K, Funktionsszintigraphie des Herzens bei Patienten mit Herzklappenerkrankungen. Nucl. Med. 23:221, 1984.

142. Hofmann M, Schwarz F, Schuler G et al, The effect of arotic valve replacement on left ventricular function at rest and during exercise. J. nucl. Med. 21:4, 1981.

143. Iskandrian AS, Hakki A, Kane SA et al, Quantitative radionuclide angiography in assessment of hemodynamic changes during upright exercise: Observations in normal subjects, patients with coronary artery disease and patients with patients with aortic regurgitation. Cardiol. 48:239, 1981.

144. Boucher CA, Bingham JB, Osbakken MD et al, Early changes in left ventricular size and function after correction of left ventricular volume overload. Amer. J. Cardiol. 47:991, 1981.

145. Sagawa K, Editorial: The end-systolic pressure-volume relation of the ventricle: Definition, modifications and clinical use. Circulation 63:1223, 1981.

146. Newman GE, Gibbsons RJ, Jones RH, Cardiac function during rest and exercise in patients with mitral valve prolapse. Amer. J. Cardiol. 47:14, 1981.

147. Gottdiener JS, Borer JS, Bacharach SL et al, Left ventricular function in mitral valve prolapse: Assessment with radionuclide cineangiography. Amer. J. Cardiol. 47:7, 1981.

148. Borer JS, Bacharach SL, Jeffrey MV et al, Left ventricular function in aortic stenosis: Response to exercise and effects of operation. Amer. J. Cardiol. 41:382, 1978.

149. Nakashima Y, Fouad FM, Tarazi RC, Long-term captopril therapy in congestive heart failure: Serial hemodynamic and echocardiography changes. Amer. Heart J. 104:827, 1982.

150. Mason DT, Hermanovich J, Evensen M et al, Oral captopril in ambulatory management of severe congestive heart failure: Sustained beneficial effects on ventricular function with 6 month therapy shown by cardiac catheterization, nuclear scintigraphy, echography, treadmill exercise and symptomatology. Amer. J. Cardiol. 45:411, 1980.

151. Leinberger H, Invasive und nichtinvasive Funktionsparameter zur Kontrolle der Therapie mit vasodilatatorischen Substanzen. In: Vasodilatatoren. Westermann W, Witzstrock (eds), Baden-Baden, pp 81-92, 1980.

152. Firth BG, Dehmer GJ, Corbett JR et al, Effect of chronic oral digoxin therapy on ventricular function at rest and peak exercise in patients with ischemic heart disease. Amer. J. Cardiol. 46:481, 1980.

153. Poliner L, Twieg D, Parkey R et al, Radionuclide angiography and hemodynamic assessment of prazosin in patients with medically refractory heart failure. Amer. J. Cardiol. 43:103, 1979.

154. Goldman SA, Jahnson LL, Escala E et al, Improved exercise ejection fraction with long-term prazosin therapy in patients with heart failure. Amer. J. Med. 68:36, 1980.

155. Hag A, Rakowski H, Baigrie R et al, Vasodilator therapy in refractory congestive heart failure: A comparative analysis of hemodynamic and noninvasive studies. Amer. J. Cardiol. 49:439, 1982.

156. Feinendegen LE, Minimal transit time. Nucl. Med. Stuttgart, 17:185, 1978.

157. Hooper WW, Slutsky RA, Kocienski DE et al, Right and left ventricular response to subcutaneous terbutaline in patients with chronic obstructive pulmonary disease: Radionuclide angiographic assessment of cardiac size and function. Amer. Heart J. 104:1027, 1982.

158. Brent BN, Mahler D, Berger HJ et al, Augmentation of right ventricular performance in chronic obstructive pulmonary disease by terbutaline: A combined radionuclide and hemodynamic study. Amer. J. Cardiol. 50:313, 1982.

159. Slutsky R, Hemodynamic effects of inhaled terbutaline in congestive heart failure patients without lung disease: Beneficial cardiotonic and vasodilator beta-agonist properties evaluated by ventricular catheterization and radionuclide angiography. Amer. Heart J. 101:556, 1981.

160. Slutsky R, Hooper W, Gerber K et al, Left ventricular size and function after subcutaneous administraton of terbutaline. Chest 79:501, 1981.

161. Matthay RA, Berger HJ, Davies R et al, Improvement in cardiac performance by oral long-acting theophylline in chronic obstructive pulmonary disease. Amer. Heart J. 104:1022, 1982.

162. Alexander J, Dainiak N, Berger HJ et al, Serial assessment of doxorubicin cardiotoxicity with quantitative radionuclide angio-cardiography. New Engl. J. Med. 300:278, 1979.

163. Ritchie JL, Sorensen SG, Narahara KA et al, Radionuclide ejection fraction: Prediction of adriamycin cardiotoxicity. J. nucl. Med. 19:671, 1978.

164. Borer JS, Kent KM, Bacharach SL et al, Sensitivity, specificity and predictive accuracy of radionuclide cineangiography during exercise in patients with coronary artery disease. Circulation 60: 572, 1979.

INVESTIGATION OF REGIONAL WALL MOTION OF THE HEART BY
MEANS OF RADIONUCLIDE VENTRICULOGRAPHY (RNV)

R. BAUER, H.W. PABST, H. LANGHAMMER

INTRODUCTION

Various heart diseases result in global and/or regional
wall motion disorders, causing changes and reduction in heart
function. The most common of these is coronary artery disease
(CAD), in which stenoses of coronary arteries result in an
insufficient blood and oxygen supply to the myocardium involved.
In the early stages of the disease, this hypoperfusion only
becomes significant during exercise, but as the disease
progresses, hypoperfusion will also cause symptoms when the
patients are at rest. This hypoperfusion at first produces
reversible wall motion disorders, which may, however, develop
into irreversible myocardial infarctions, as has been shown
by Tennant and Wiggers in 1935 (1).

Other heart disorders such as hypertensive heart disease,
incompetent valves, peri- and myocarditis, irregularities of
the conductive system or primary myocardial diseases (COCM,
HCM) may also result in a reduction of global and regional
heart function, although in these cases, however, the manifestation of the contraction disorders and the heart function at
rest and during exercise will differ according to the disease.
If the disease is known, global parameters of heart volume
such as ventricular volume, ejection fraction (EF) and rates
of volume will indicate the severity of the disease to the
clinician and he will be able to assess the reduction of the
heart function (2-5). However, when a diagnosis or differential
diagnosis is to be made, or during follow-up after surgery or
control after the intervention by pharmaceuticals, the assessment of regional wall motion is of decisive help to the

clinician (7-12).

Method

The regional motility of both the left and right ventricles can best be assessed if the areas of interest are viewed tangentially. Consequently, it is necessary to take recordings from different views. Usually in anterior views the antero-basal, antero-lateral, apical and inferior parts of the left ventricle form the lateral contour, as can be seen in fig 1.

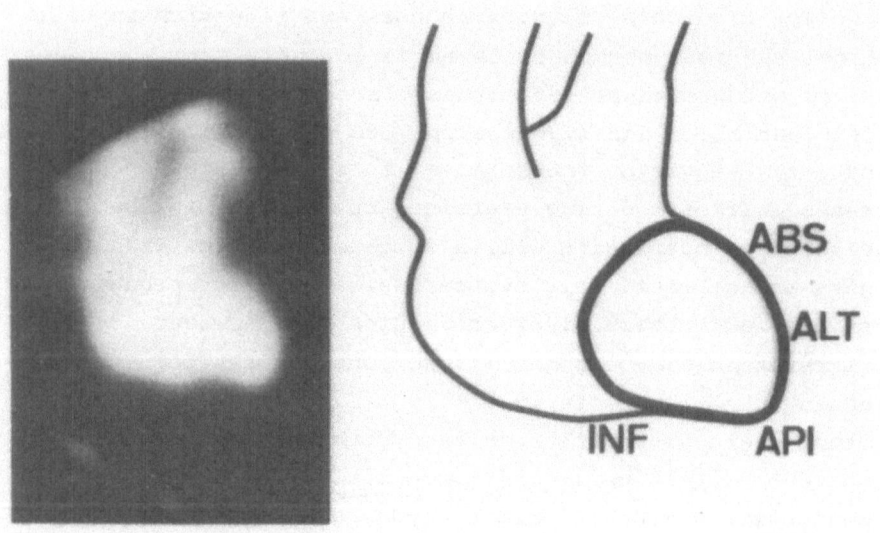

Fig. 1. Enddiastolic image of the heart in an anterior view and schematic representation of the contour with the antero-basal (ABS), antero-lateral (ALT), apical (API) and inferior (INF) wall.

Another recording is usually performed in the left anterior oblique view, LAO-35 to LAO-45. In this position, the septum interventriculare which lies parallel to the recorded gamma rays can be discerned and the apex of the heart and the postero-lateral and postero-basal wall of the left ventricle form the lateral contours, as is shown in fig 2.

Additional recordings are performed in the case of special queries. The motility of the anterior wall can be assessed in

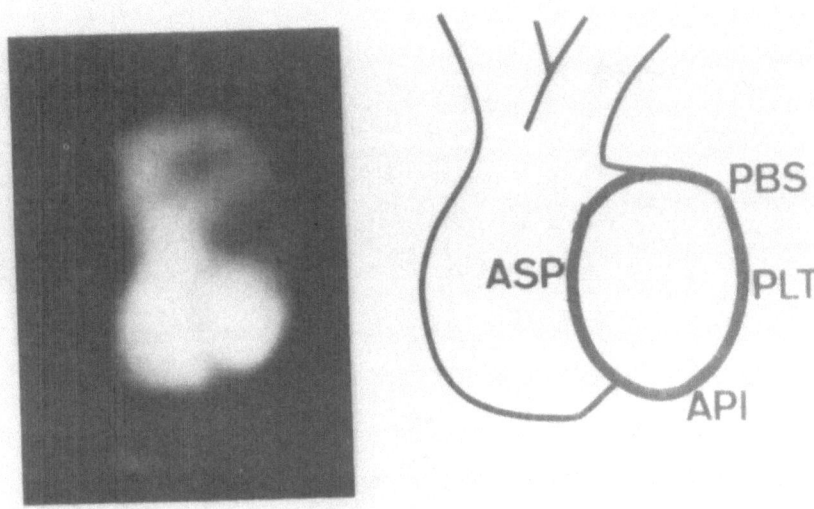

Fig. 2. Enddiastolic image and schematic contour of the heart in LAO-40 view, showing the postero-basal (PBS), postero-lateral (PLT), apical (API) and antero-septal (ASP) wall.

the right anterior oblique view, RAO-30, whereas the LAO-70 and left lateral views (LL) are particularly useful for the examination of the postero-basal wall of the left ventricle.

Two prerequisites for the correct assessment of regional wall motion using RNV are both the reliable acquisition of data and reconstruction of representative cycles using EKG-gating after equilibration of the tracer. It takes a recording time of 200 to 300 s after injection of 15 - 25 mCi of an intravasal tracer to reproduce statistically significant representative heart cycles. During this period of time the heart rate will change according to respiration, the changing activity of the vegetative nervous system or in response to ergometric stress.

According to which recording techniques are used, varia-tions in heart rate will lead to a significant decrease in the acquisition time of the last images of the representative heart cycle. On account of this, the visual assessment of the heart function using the "cine-mode" is rendered more difficult and a correct computation of amplitude and phase images is

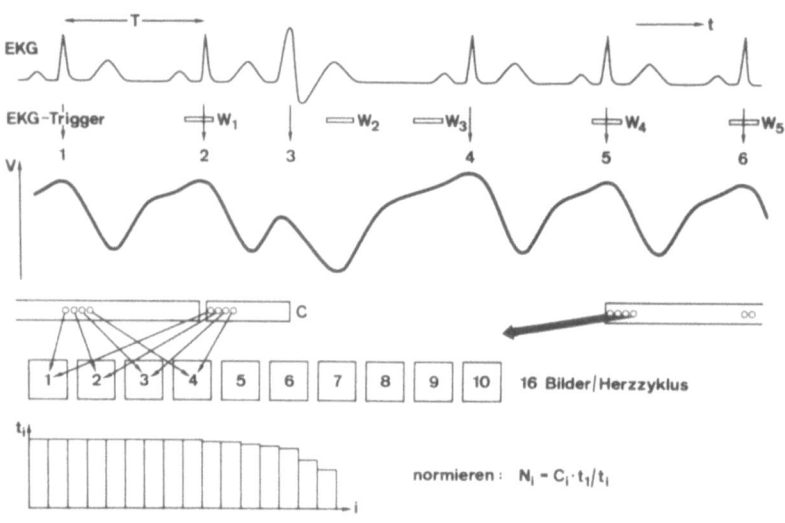

Fig. 3. Data acquisition in arrhythmia: A trigger signal (1-6) and a time window (w_1 - w_5) are generated from the QRS-complex of the EKG. V depicts the time-volume-curve of the left ventricle. Data acquisition is only performed if the trigger i falls within the time window w_{i-1} of the preceeding beat. Data are stored in frame mode in 16 frames of time length T/16 each. At the end of the acquisition, all the frames are normalized to the total acquisition time t_1 of the first frame.

made impossible. Whereas only the first two thirds of the heart cycle are necessary to calculate most of the global parameters of the heart function, an exact analysis of the regional motility necessitates an accurate recording of the whole of the heart cycle.

We have developed an acquisition program which makes acquisition and reconstruction of a significant representative heart cycle possible, even when patients are suffering from severe arrhythmias (13). A schematic reproduction of this type of data acquisition is depected in fig 3. The essential characteristics of this program are as follows:

1) recordings are only made following heart beats of a well defined length and
2) the individual frames are all normalized according to an

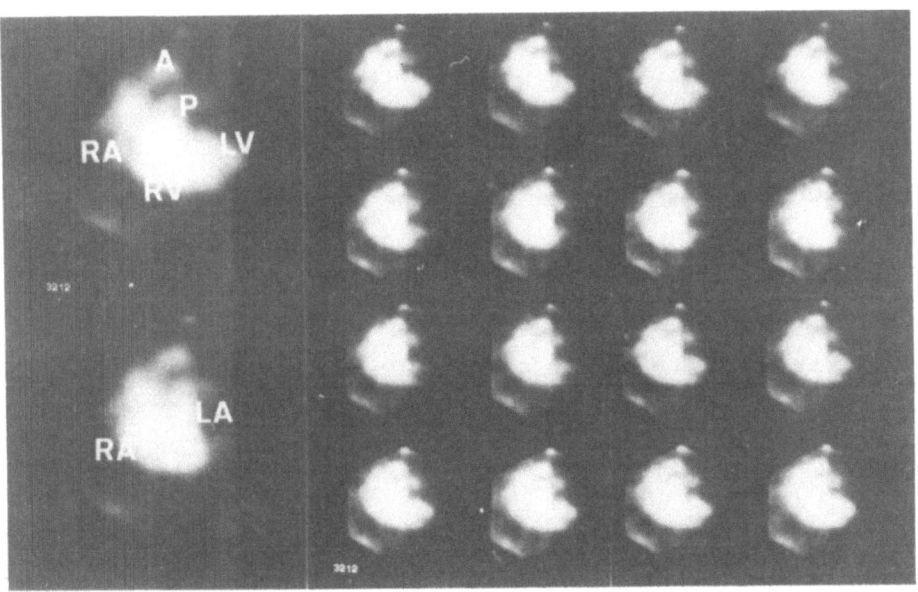

Fig. 4. The 16 images of a representative heart cycle in an anterior view and the enddiastolic (1st) and endsystolic (7th) image with aorta (A), a.pulmonalis (P), right and left atrium (RA, LA) and right and left ventricle (RV, LV) (from 6).

equal acquisition time.

This program can be easily implemented in any computer. Since the recording is performed in "frame-mode", there is no necessity for special, expensive hardware.

The regional wall motion can be assessed both after equilibration of the tracer with the RNV or during the first pass, radionuclide-angiocardiography (RNA). When the RNA is employed, a multicrystal camera should be used, because only this special device can guarantee a high enough count rate to yield sufficient statistics (14-16). Nevertheless, first pass techniques always afford two injections of tracer when two different views of the heart have to be obtained. Therefore, we only apply the RNV for the assessment of regional wall motion, which in addition allows for recording heart function over

154

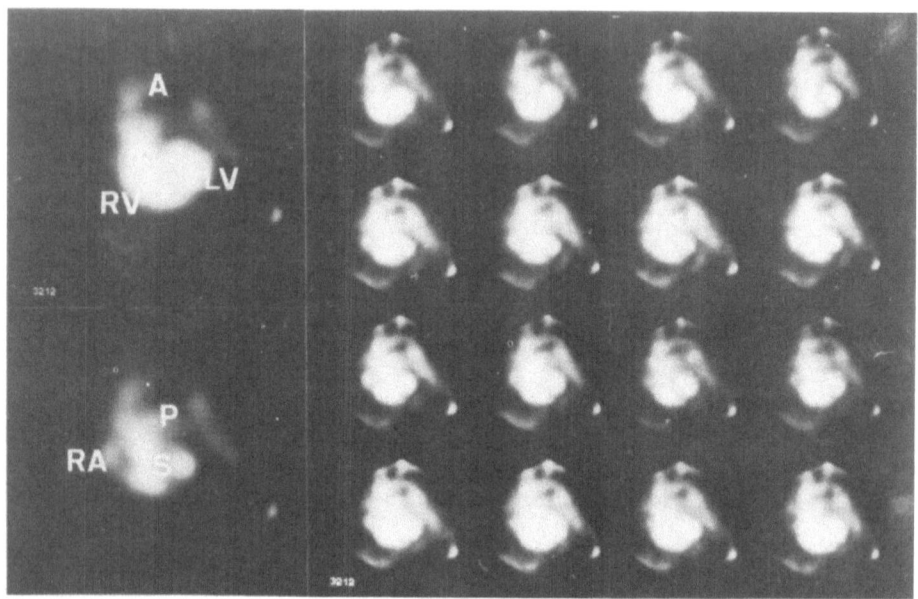

Fig. 5. The 16 images of a representative heart cycle in LAO-40 view, and in addition the enddiastolic and endsystolic images with aorta (A), a.pulmonalis (P), right atrium (RA), right and left ventricle (RV, LV) and septum interventriculare (S) (from 6).

several hours in different views and functional states.

Regional wall motion can be assessed from the images of the representative heart cycle in 5 different ways:

1) visually by means of the "cine-mode", which is a film-like sequential representation of the frames of the heart cycle on a television monitor,

2) by means of isocontours, which allow for a quantification of the degree of contraction during systole,

3) by quantitative analysis of regional ejection fraction,

4) by means of ejection fraction images and

5) by the parametric images of the amplitudes and phases as obtained from Fourier analysis.

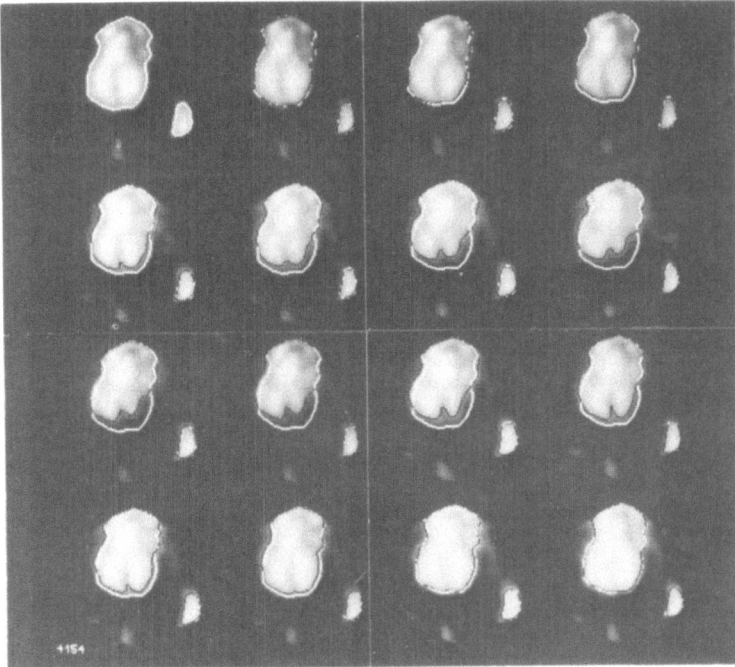

Fig. 6. 16 images of a representative heart cycle of a healthy patient with isocontours of the enddiastolic image (white) and of all the respective images (black), showing normal regional contraction.

Visual assessment of regional heart function.

Figs 4 and 5 depict the frames of a representative heart cycle of a healthy patient at rest in the anterior and LAO-40 view. The first image on the upper left represents the heart at the beginning of the QRS complex. At this point in time, both atria are contracted and both ventricles are filled to a maximum. Consequently, this image is known as the "enddiastolic image", since it represents the ventricles recorded at end-diastole with respect to the hemodynamic situation.

During systole, both ventricles contract, reaching their maximal contraction in the 7th or 8th frame at rest. At this time, both atria are filled to a maximum. Afterwards, the atria empty themselves into the ventricles, which in turn enlarge continuously. At the end of the heart cycle, i.e. in approximately the 15th or 16th frame of the LAO-40 view, the contraction of the atria in response to the P-wave of the EKG

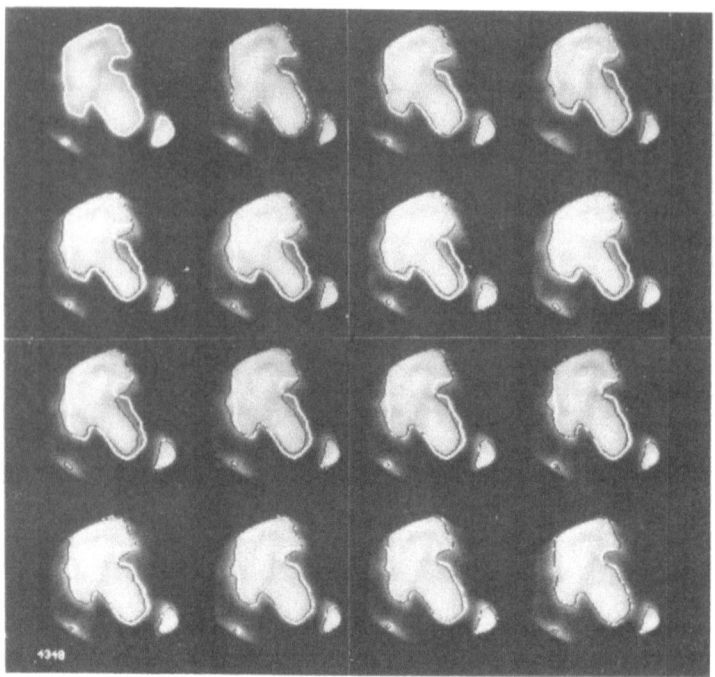

Fig. 7. 16 images and isocontours (as in fig. 6) of a patient who had an extended transmural myocardial infarction. The antero-septal and apical wall is hypo- to akinetic.

can be observed. This presentation of the 16 individual frames of the representative heart cycle demonstrates that all the lateral parts of the left ventricle contract simultaneously and equally well.

The contraction and relaxation process can be much better evaluated visually by means of the "cine-mode". Here, all the individual images of the representative heart cycle are projected sequentially on to a TV monitor. This projection takes the form of a continuous cycle, with the first image following immediately on again from the last.

This technique permits a very detailed assessment of regional wall motility. Usually, wall motion is defined as normo-, hypo-, hypo- to a- and a- to dyskinetic. Occasionally, in patients suffering from aortic or mitral regurgitation at an early compensated state or who have had some small myocardial infarction, a hyperkinesis of the vital myocardium can be observed (17).

When using the cine mode to investigate heart function, a
monochrome representation of the scintigrams is necessary
which is capable of differentiating between at least 50 different tones of grey. The images should be normalized, so that
the brightest grey tone corresponds to the maximal intensity
of the brightest image. Enhancing the contrast by substracting
the background can also facilitate the investigation.

However, the original recordings should always be taken
into consideration prior to any manipulation of the images
(such as back-ground subtraction, for example). If Tc^{99m}
labelled red cells are used as tracer and a good labelling is
achieved with a negligible concentration of Tc^{99m}, the para-
cardial background must be low (18). If an elevation of the
background is encountered, a left heart insufficiency must be
assumed.

Various authors have been able to obtain a very good
correspondence between the scintigraphic and contrast-angio-
graphic obtained results of regional heart function using
cine-mode techniques described above, or even simpler, only
enddiastolic and endsystolic images, differentiating between
normo-, hypo-, a- and dyskinetic areas (4,8,9,12,14).

Isocontours

Regional wall motion can be quantified by computation of
isocontours. This method is presented in the figs 6 and 7.
The isocontour of the enddiastolic image is projected onto
all 16 frames of the representative cycle. In addition, from
the 2nd to the 16th frame the isocontours at the same level
are computed and displayed concurrently for each respective
frame.

The isocontours of a patient with normal global and regional heart function demonstrate a regular, even contraction of
all the tangentially recorded walls of the ventricle during
systole. In contrast to this, however, the apex of the heart
and the antero-septal wall of the patient shown in fig 7 are
akinetic, following a large transmural myocardial infarction.

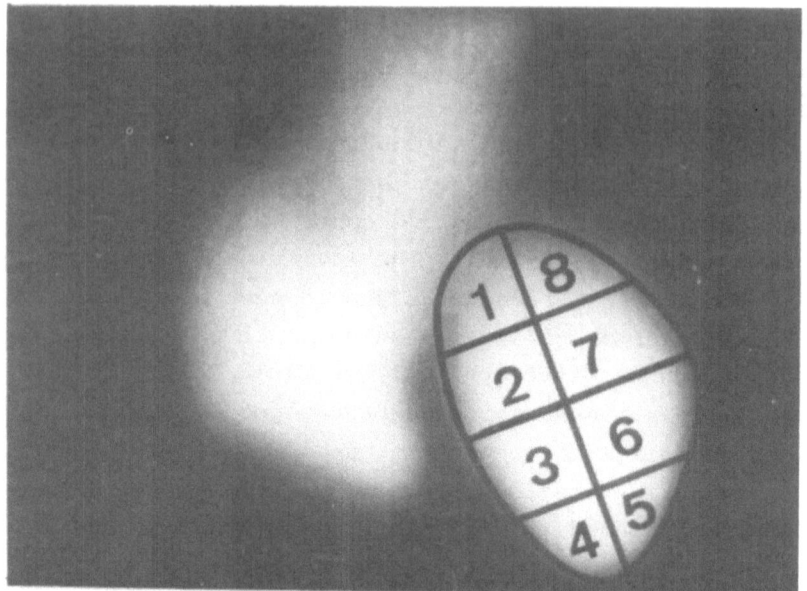

Fig. 8. Segmentation of the left ventricle into 8 segments for computing
regional (segmental) ejection fraction (REF): Segments ≠ 2 and 3 represent the antero-septal, ≠4 and 5 the apical and ≠ 6 and 7 the postero-
lateral wall.

Using isocontours, normal values of percentual contraction
of the different sectorial parts of the left ventricle can
be computed. These values can be used for comparison with
regional motility disorder values, thus quantifying them.
However, one essential limitation of the procedure should be
mentioned, which is that an isocontour does not represent the
exact lateral edge: for example, if an isocontour provides a
clear depiction of the antero-lateral wall, this means normally
that the apex of the heart will be cut out, whereas if the
apex is delineated clearly, the rest of the ventricle will be
out of proportion and too large. In addition, large vessels
behind the ventricle distort every isocontour and the septum
can never be depicted by means of an isocontour. Consequently,
isocontours only have a limited usefulness in the quantification of regional wall motion, which is why they are not very
often used for this purpose.

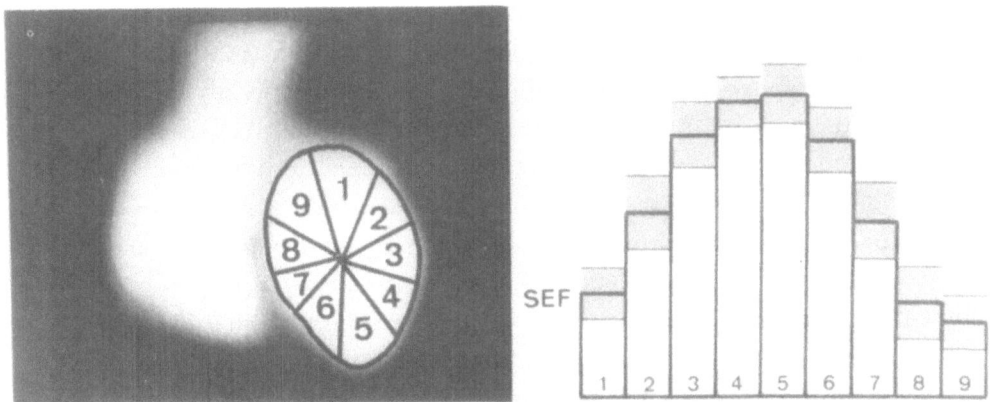

Fig. 9. Subdivision of the left ventricle into 9 sectors in computation
of sectorial ejection fraction (SEF) and representation of a sectorial
EF-profile.

Regional ejection fraction

Some investigators have computed regional ejection fractions,
using segmental or sectorial subdivisions of the left ventricle.
In the segmental analysis, the largest hemiaxis of the ventricle
is sought - a procedure similar to the computation of EF in
contrast angiography. Some short axes are then drawn perpendicular to this axis, which subdivide the ventricle into a certain
number of segments. The EF can then be regionally computed
within these segments (REF).

As can be seen from fig 8, Maddox et al (19) subdivided
the ventricle in this way into 8 segments. Using a parallel
slant-hole collimator, they recorded the left ventricle in a
modified LAO-40 view. The antero-septal REF was computed in
segments 2 and 3, the apical REF in segments 4 and 5 and the
postero-lateral REF in segments 6 and 7. They also computed
the normal values of REF in a group of 10 healthy patients:
66 ± 13% antero-septal, 85 ± 12% apical and 74 ± 16% postero-
lateral. In 33 patients, motility disorders were found using
contrast angiography, which in 27 regions were hypokinetic and

in 17 regions akinetic. The mean REF of hypokinetic segments was 44% and the mean value of the akinetic segments as low as 24%.

Standtke et al (20) computed a sectorial EF (SEF) using an almost fully-automated computer program. As shown in fig 9, nine sectors are drawn around the center of gravity of the left ventricle and the resulting SEF's are displayed as EF profile. In a group of 42 healthy patients, the highest SEF of about 80% was determined at the apex of the heart, whereas the lowest SEF of about 45% was found at the basis of the heart. This normal SEF profile can be used as a point of reference when examining the SEF of patients with various different heart diseases. The results of these analyses are highly reproducible, since they are performed with minimal operator intervention. For this reason, it is particularly easy to investigate relatively slight changes in regional motility, e.g. induced by drug treatment or ergometric exercise, via intra-individual comparison.

Since, in scintigraphy, contours and edges are not very clearly discernable, this means that the various hemiaxes can not be very well defined. This results in a certain amount of uncertainty and variability of segmental regional EF (REF). On the other hand, however, the centre of gravity of the left ventricle can be easily computed and sectorial regional EF (SEF) is highly reproducible. Consequently, we consider SEF to be an appropriate method for the evaluation of regional wall motion disorders, and superior to REF for this particular purpose.

Ejection fraction images

Maddox et al (21) computed images of regional ejection fraction in order to assess regional wall motility. Firstly, stroke volume images were computed as the difference between the enddiastolic (I_{ED}) and the endsystolic image (I_{ES}). Afterwards, these volume changes were normalized according to the local enddiastolic volume. The ejection fraction image (I_{EF}) is defined as:

$$I_{EF} = (I_{ED} - I_{ES}) \; / \; I_{ED} \tag{1}$$

In equation 1, the operations '-' and '/' denote matrix operators, which must be applied for each individual pixel on the image matrix.

Using this technique, it is possible to display some essential aspects of regional ventricular dynamics during systole. Maddox et al (21) were able to achieve a satisfactory correspondence between scintigraphical and contrast angiographical results. The I_{EF} images are operator-independent except for the determination of the background. Using this technique of ejection fraction images, it was possible to distinguish a number of wall motion abnormalities located not only tangentially but also in the middle of the ventricle. However, in spite of these advantages, this technique has not been widely used by investigators for the following reasons. The I_{EF} is computed as the difference between two individual images, and the result is divided by the pixel value of another individual image. As a consequence, the single pixel values are subject to considerable statistical variations. Secondly, if the maximal and minimal volumes in different pixels are not obtained at the same time, disorders in the conductive system can lead to incorrect results and the I_{EF} values will be too low. These advantages are overcome in the Fourier analysis method, which in addition to an amplitude image that is comparable to the I_{EF} image, also provides information on the time course of contraction and relaxation by means of the phase image. Consequently, with the introduction of the Fourier method, the computation of regional ejection fraction images was abandoned.

Fourier analysis

The principles of Fourier analysis are demonstrated in fig 10. The time activity curves of both the atria or the ventricles can be approximated in first order by a single sine wave.

A sine function is given mathematically by:

162

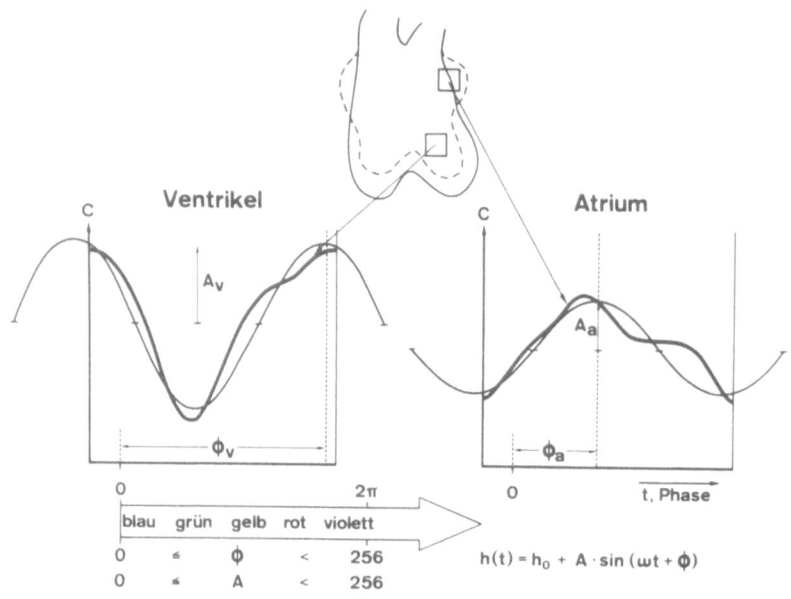

Fig. 10. Principles of Fourier analysis: Approaximation of a time-volume curve by a sine wave h (t), which is completely determined by the amplitude A and the phase Φ. The parameters A and Φ are normalized to values between 0 and 255 which can be represented by a suitable color scale.

$$h(t) = h_0 + A \cdot \sin (\omega t + \phi) \tag{2}$$

A sine wave is completely defined by two parameters, the amplitude A and the phase Φ. ω is the frequency which is related to the cycle time T by:

$$\omega = 2 \pi / T \tag{3}$$

The amplitude gives the amount of change in activity relating to the volume change during a heart cycle. The phase correlates to the time dependence of contraction and relaxation relative to the maximum of the time activity curve. Computation of amplitudes and phases is performed by the usual equations, which are to be found in every mathematical textbook.

$$A= (s^2 + c^2)^{1/2} \qquad \text{and} \quad \Phi = \text{arc tan } (c/s) \text{ with} \qquad (4)$$

$$s= 2/n \sum_{i=1}^{n} c_i \cdot \sin (2\pi i/n) \text{ and } c=2/n \sum_{i=1}^{n} c_i \cdot \cos (2\pi i/n) \quad (5)$$

n means the number of images per representative cycle (which is 16 in our acquisition program, c_i means the counts in the region of interest of image number i.

Not only can this analysis be used to approximate the time activity curve obtained from a large ROI, but it can also be extended and refined so as to produce the time activity curve of every individual pixel of the image matrices. Thus, amplitude and phases can be computed regionally for every pixel, yielding the two images of amplitude and phases. This application of the Fourier analysis was first performed by Adam and Bitter in 1977 (22) for the assessment of regional wall motion. The Fourier analysis is particularly important because an essential part of the dynamic information contained in the time sequence of the individual images within the representative cycle can be displayed in just two parametric images - the amplitude and the phase image.

The amplitude image provide a good representation of the maximal volume change and the phase image displays the time course and the synchronicity of regional contraction. Fourier analysis employs the information from all the corresponding pixels of the n images of the complete representative heart cycle. Therefore, the resulting amplitudes and phases are statistically well defined. Since neither the contours of the heart nor the back-ground have to be computed, reproducibility is 100%. As a result, amplitude and phase images provide a reliable, operator-independent and exactly reproducible method of assessing regional wall motion with maximally high resolution.

In order to obtain a better insight into amplitudes and

164

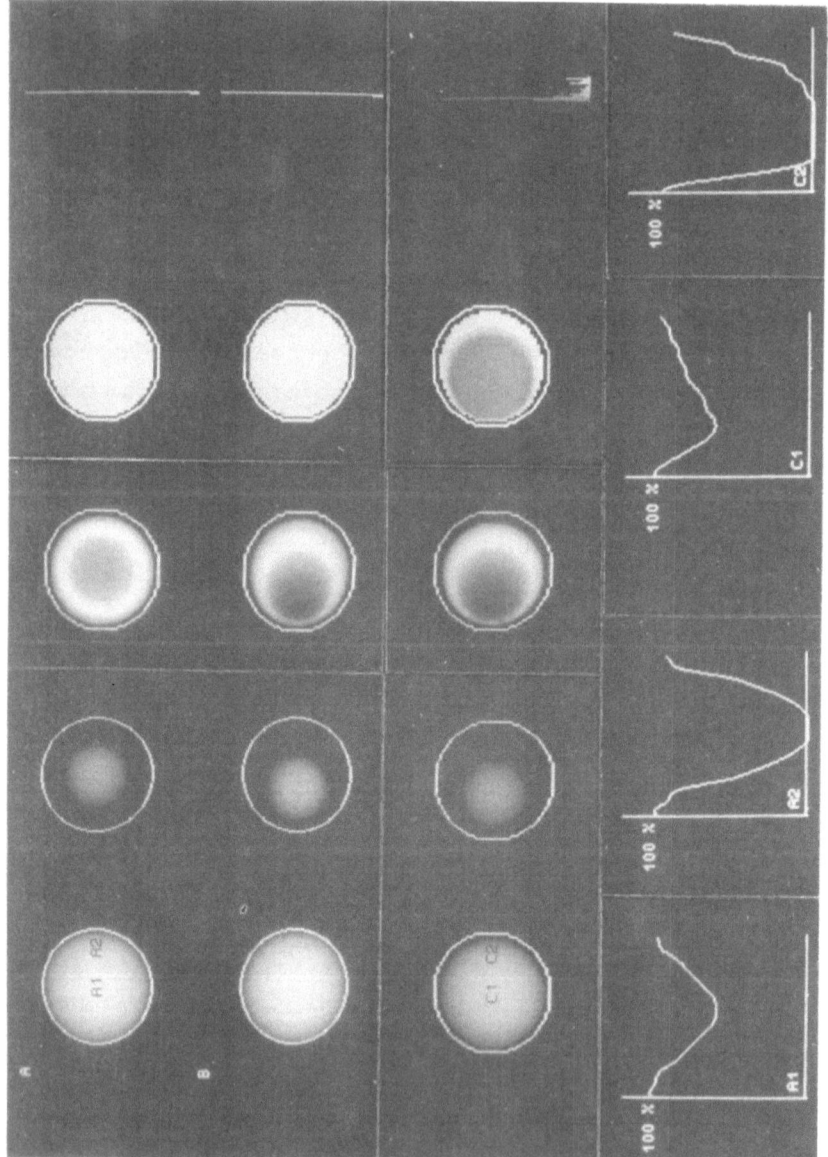

Fig. 11. Legend: see next page.

Fig. 11. Results of a sphere model with different patterns of contraction and filling, showing "diastolic", "systolic", amplitude and phase images with phase histograms (from left to right) and time activity curves from distinct regions (A1, A2, C1 and C2):
Upper line (A): concentric, sinusoidal volume change.
Middel line (B): excentric, sinusoidal volume change and
Lower line (C): excentric, saw-tooth shaped volume change.

phases, the behaviour of the left ventricle was simulated using a simple sphere model (23,24). 16 images were computed of a sphere which was filled homogeneously with activity. Its volume was periodically altered. The resulting images simulate a "representative cycle". Amplitudes and phases were computed according to equations 4 and 5. Fig. 11 shows the images when the sphere was filled maximally, corresponding to the "end-diastolic image", the "systolic image" of minimal filling, the amplitude and the phase image and a phase histogram and below time activity curve obtained from different parts of the pulsating sphere.

The upper line shows the result of a concentric, sinusoidal decrease and increase in volume. The phases of all parts of the sphere are exactly the same and the phase histogram only shows a single line. The amplitude of the border zones is higher than that in the center of the sphere. This can be explained by means of the time activity curves. Whereas the activity in the center falls from 100% at "diastole" to only 55% at "systole", activity near the lateral wall drops from 100 to 0%.

The middle line shows the result of another sinusoidal change in volume, although here the movement is not concentric. The center of gravity of the sphere moves during contraction, simulating the behaviour of the left ventricle. Accordingly, the amplitude of the contralateral side is higher than that of the side the sphere is moving to. Nevertheless, the phase is exactly the same for all the parts of the sphere.

The lower line shows the results of an excentric movement, which was not sinusoidal but shaped like a saw-tooth with a rapid contraction and a retarded filling. In this case, the phases of the outer contra-lateral side of the sphere are retarded with respect to the phases of the rest of the sphere. This result becomes comprehensible if one compares the time activity curves from the center of the ventricle (C1) with those of the lateral wall (C2). When approximating the curve C1 by a sine wave, the pixels of the images at the middle of the representative cycle influence the result as much as the images of the beginning and end of the cycle. Because the minimum appears early, the minimum of the approximating sinus curve is shifted from the middle of the cycle to the beginning. In contrast, the phase of the approximated sine wave of the curve C2 is determined mainly by the information from the very first and last images of the representative cycle, where-as the images in the middle of the cycle have no activity and therefore cannot influence the phases. For these reasons, the minimum is computed at a point in time near the middle of the representative cycle.

A correct interpretation of the results of the lower line would therefore be as follows: the phases of the middle parts of the sphere and of the parts near the basis (the ipsi-lateral side of the movement of the center of gravity) are premature. However, the number of pixels with a premature phase is much larger than that with a normal phase. Since all the phases are relative and since it is tempting to assume that the majority is "normal" and the minority "pathological", the phase image is interpreted as a retardation of the phases of the lateral part of the sphere with respect to the rest of the phases.

Clinical relevance of regional wall disorders

Fig 12 shows diastole, systole, amplitudes and phases as well as a ^{201}Tl myocardial scintigram of a patient with severe CAD and previous myocardial function. The left ventricle is enlarged, the antero-lateral wall is akinetic and the apex is even dyskinetic. As is to be expected, the myocardial scinti-gram shows a hypoperfusion or a complete perfusion deficiency of the walls with contraction disorders. The combination of all these findings is typical for a large transmural myocardial infarction.

167

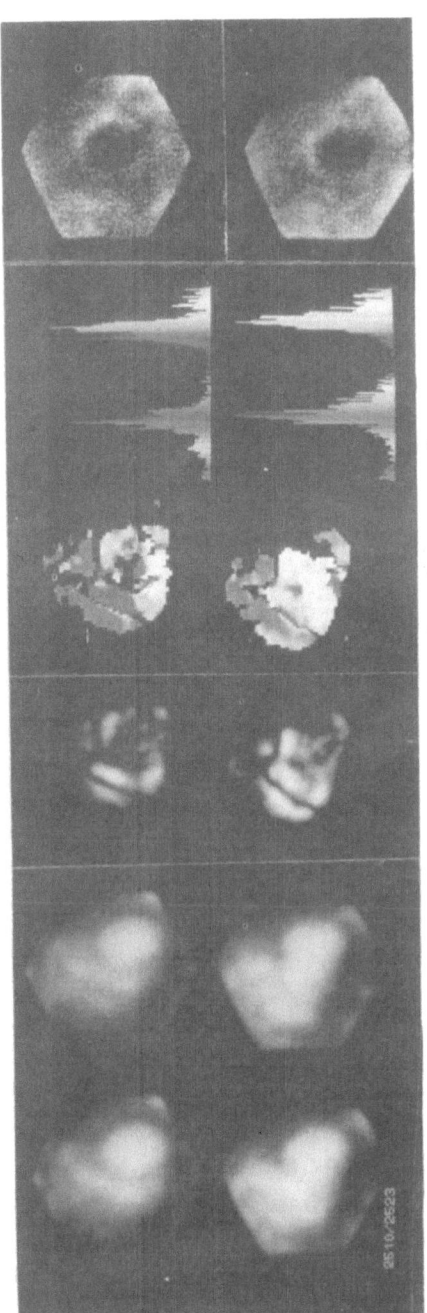

Fig. 12. Results from RNV (diastole, systole, amplitude, phase and phase histogram) and myocardial scintigraphy in a patient with extended transmural infarction. Above: LAO-40 view, below: anterior view.

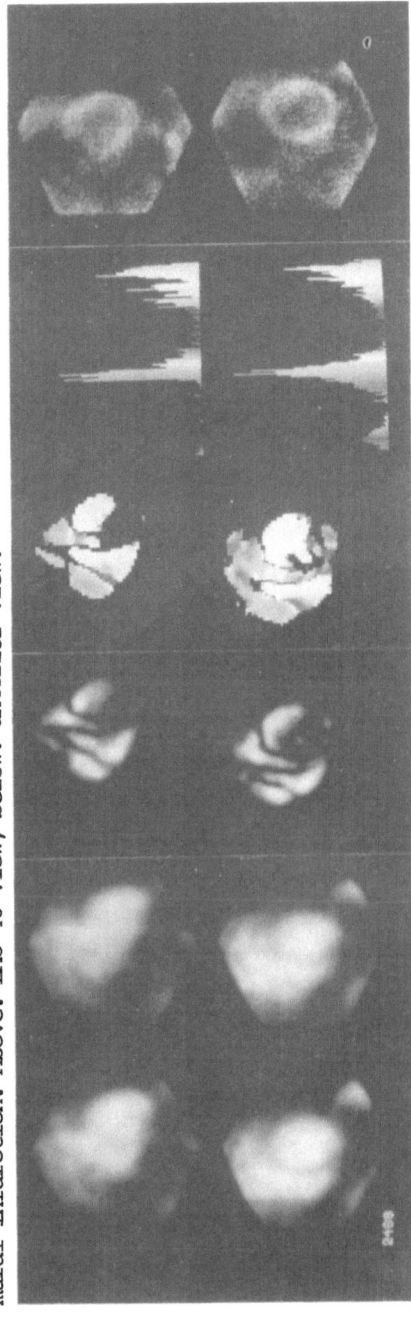

Fig. 13. Results of RNV and myocardial scintigraphy in anterior (above) and LAO-40 view (below) in a patient with primary cardiomyopathy.

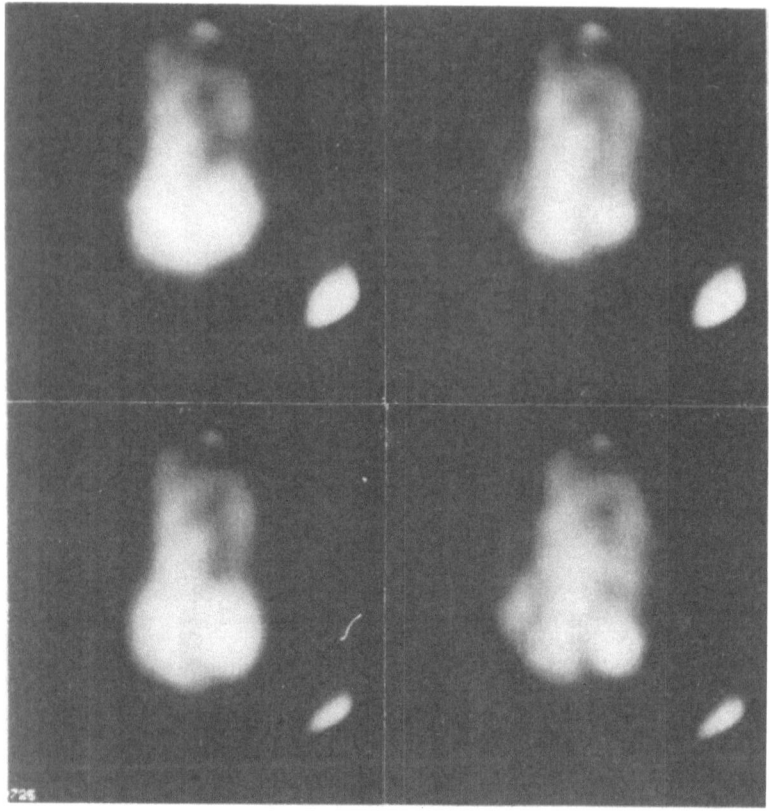

Fig. 14. Diastolic and systolic images at rest (above) and under exercise (below) in a patient with CAD and exercise induced akinesis of the apex and hypokinesis of the postero-lateral wall of the left ventricle.

On the other hand, fig 13 shows diastole, systole, amplitudes, phases and myocardial scintigrams of a patient with progressive primary cardiomyopathy. The left ventricle is also massively enlarged. The contraction of the ventricle in the basal region of the heart is relatively good, whereas the antero-lateral wall is shown to be hypo- to akinetic and the apex is quite distinctly dyskinetic. However, in contrast to the myocardial scintigram in fig 12, the ^{201}Tl scintigram of this patient shows a more or less homogeneous perfusion of the heart, even in the dyskinetic apical area. These findings are typical for a primary cardiomyopathy.

If, however, the case history of the patient is not

typical for CAD, then the assessment of motility disorders, which do not change significantly during exercise compared to the rest study, is not enough to justify the diagnosis of a CAD with previous myocardial infarction. If, for clinical reasons, it is only possible to perform a rest study, the case for diagnosing CAD will be strengthened if ^{201}Tl scintigraphy reveals perfusion abnormalities which are topographically concordant with the wall motion abnormalities. It is true that a hypoperfusion accompanied by a hypokinesis could also be due to a specific infiltration - e.g. in patients with sarcoidosis - but this diagnosis is unlikely, since this disease is not very prevalent. If it is only possible to perform a RNV, wall motion abnormalities induced merely through exercise become decisive in diagnosing CAD. In our patient population, specificity of RNV in diagnosing CAD was 100% in those cases in which only exercise-induced wall motion abnormalities were counted. Exercise-induced wall motion abnormalities are defined as those which arise as the result of exercise or those which, although present in the rest-state, are severely aggravated by exercise. An example is given in fig 14.

In most publications to date, the problem of a differential diagnosis between CAD and primary cardiomyopathy has not been very thoroughly discussed. Since COCM is not diagnosed very often in a normal patient population, this problem does not arise very often in practice and so the incorrect diagnosis of COCM as CAD would only minimally impair the specificity of RNV in the diagnosis of CAD. However, in the patient population examined in our hospital with RNV, around 15% were found to have a COCM, which lent a new importance to the differential diagnosis between CAD and COCM and often made a ^{201}Tl scintigraphy necessary.

Regional hypo- or akinesia of the apex of the left ventricle is often observed in patients with severe aortic-valve regurgitation (17). Naturally, this disease is diagnosed by auscultation and should figure in the case history of the patient prior to scintigraphical examination. Differential

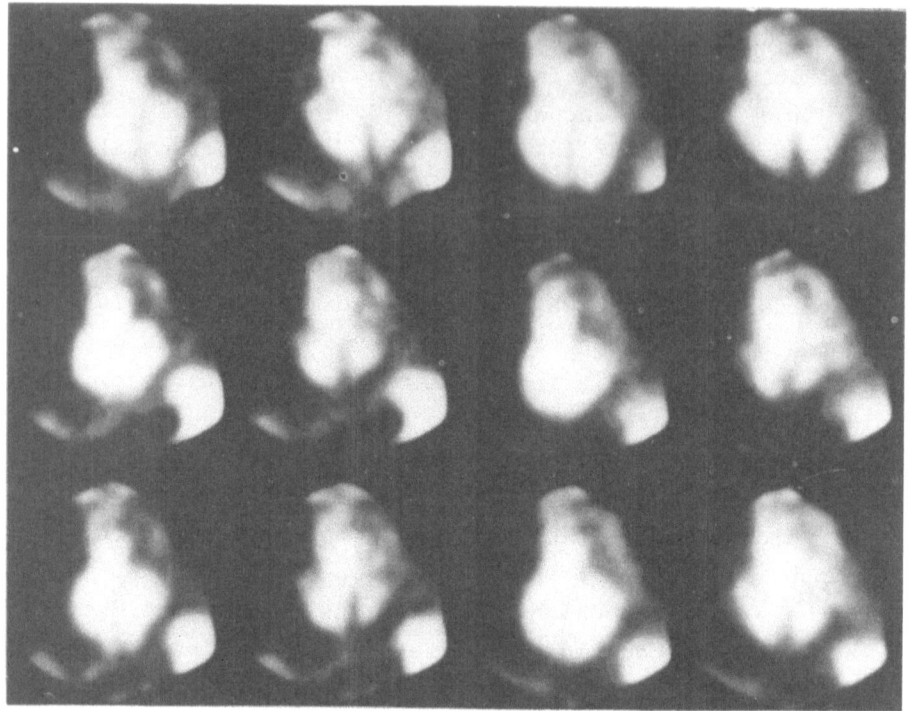

Fig. 15. Diastolic and systolic images at rest (left) and during exercise
(right) without a drug (upper line) and 2 and 5 hours after administration of Nifedipine ;(below): The Ca-antagonist prevents the myocardium
from an exercise induced coronary spasm (from 7).

diagnostic problems could arise, however, in the case of a
physician interpreting the scintigrams without first making a
short clinical examination and if the case history of the
patient is incomplete as well. However, the basal parts of
the left ventricle in these patients do usually reveal a
hyperkinesis. In addition, a hemodynamically significant
regurgitation could be demonstrated scintigraphically by
comparing right and left ventricular stroke counts. In
patients with competent valves and without an intracardial
shunt, the quotient from left to right ventricular stroke
counts varies between 0.8 and 1.4, whereas a value above 1.4
is only observed in patients with shunt or regurgitation.

If stress tests are performed in connexion with the
diagnosis of CAD, all drug treatments with beta-blocking
agents and Ca-antagonists must be discontinued for a

sufficient period of time. Beta-blockers limit the maximum
heart rate during exercise, which can mean that the myocardium
will be preserved from becoming ischemic. The effect of Ca-
antagonists is more complex.

Angina pectoris is caused by a (stress-induced) myocardial
ischemia. In some patients, the organically fixed stenoses
are sufficient to limit the perfusion under stress. In other
patients, however, especially those with low-grade stenoses,
exercise-induced spasms can increase the effect of the stenoses
and finally lead to angina. Ca-antagonists seem to have two
therapeutic uses, firstly to reduce the pre-load by widening
the periphery and on the other hand to prevent the onset of
spasms.

We studied a group of 21 patients at rest and under exercise without drugs and after administration of Nifedipin. All
these patients showed a significant global and/or regional
deterioration in left ventricular function without drugs.
After Nifedipin, 60% of the patients responded with either no
or a significantly diminished deterioration in heart function
under exercise (25). An example for the effect of Nifedipin is
given in fig 15, showing an exercise-induced akinesia of the
apex of the left ventricle at 50W work load prior to Nifedipin
whereas 2 hours later following drug administration, left
heart function was normal even at a work load of 100W. Whereas in the control study EF had decreased significantly and
the endsystolic volume had increased by about 100% under exercise, EF raised from 65% to 74% and the ESV decreased by 30%
2 hours after drug treatment. Even 5 hours later Nifedipine
was effective and the exercise induced increase in ESV was
limited to 20% as compared to 100% prior to drug treatment.

In patients with a bundle-branch block or with ST-segment
depression during digitalis, it is not possible to diagnose a
CAD with exercise EKG. However, digitalis doet not interfere with a radionuclide study, and the ascertainment of an
exercise-induced regional or global wall abnormality justifies
the diagnosis of CAD. In patients with a bundle-branch block,
regional wall motion can look pathologically due to the ab-

172

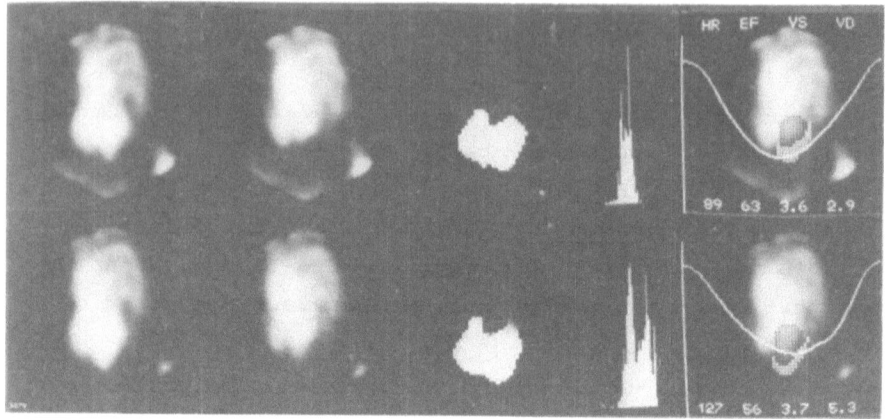

.Fig. 16. Diastolic, systolic and phase images with phase histograms and time-activity curves at rest (above) and under exercise (below) with an exercise induced left bundle-branch block (from 7).

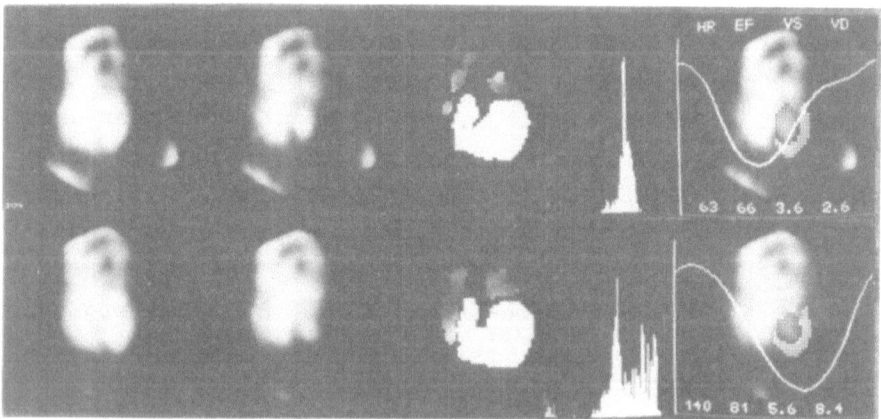

Fig. 17. Diastolic, systolic and phase images with phase histograms and time-activity curves at rest and under exercise in a patient with exercise induced left bundle-branch block due to CAD and deterioration of global and regional heart function under exercise.

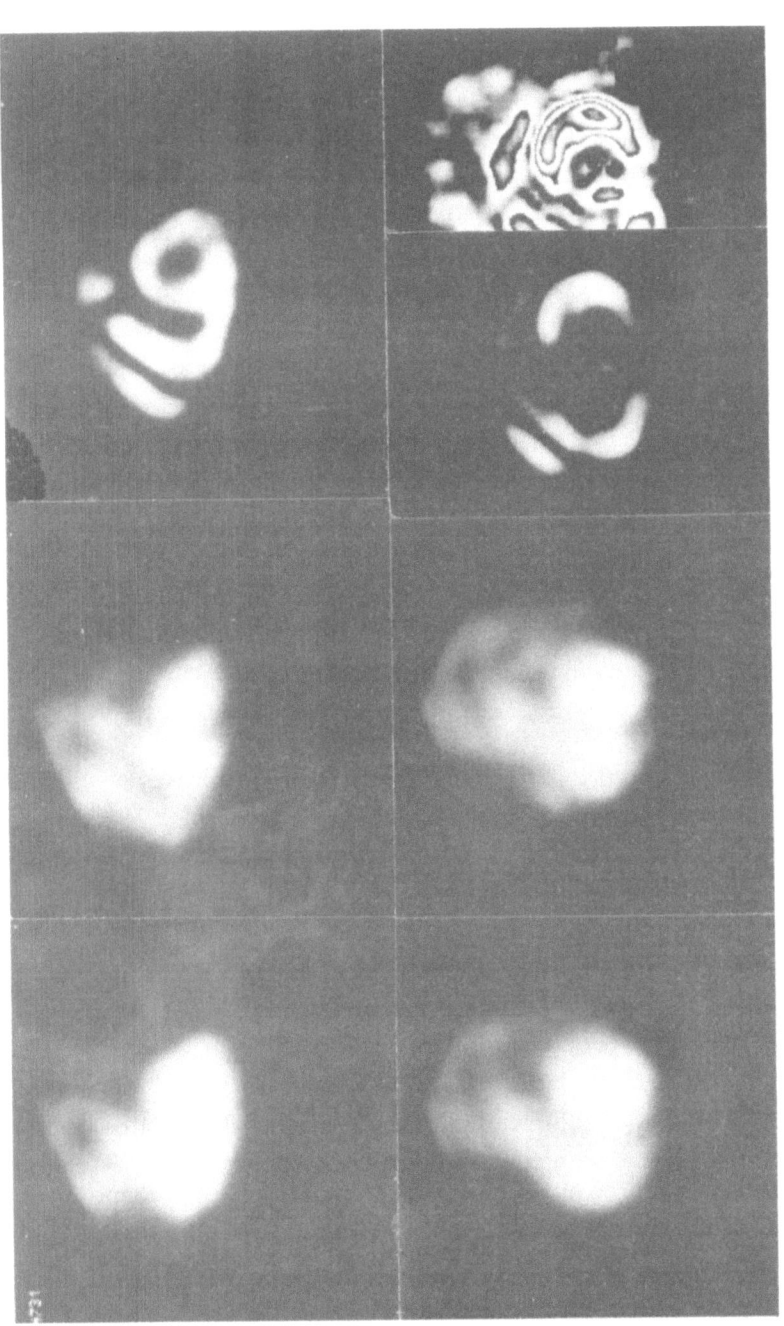

Fig. 18. Diastolic, systolic and amplitude images in anterior (above) and LAO-40 view (below). An aneurysm can only be detected in the parametric image of the amplitude in the LAO-40 view. For a better visualization, the very right image is contrast enhanced, showing the dyskinetic area as a small spot (arrow).

normal electric conduction. The regional wall disorders can
increase in concordance with the increase in disturbances of
the electric conduction, making a diagnosis of CAD impossible
from the interpretation of the regional wall motion alone. In
these patients, the global behaviour of the left ventricular
pump function can be decisive for the diagnosis of CAD. If
the EF of the left ventricle increases during exercise and
the endsystolic volume decreases, a CAD is very unlikely even
if the regional wall abnormalities seem to increase. On the
other hand, CAD is very likely if the global function deteriorates. Figs 16 and 17 show diastole, systole, phases, phase
histograms and time-curves of 2 patients, who both developed
a bundle-branch block during exercise. In the case of the
patient in fig 16, ESV decreased during exercise while EF
increased from 66 to 81%. Therefore, a CAD seems very unlikely,
despite the fact that the apex appears to be hypokinetic
during exercise. In contrast to this, the patient in fig 17
showed a marked increase in enddiastolic volume and EF fell
from 63 to 56%. In this case, the deterioration in the function of the left heart can not be explained by the disorders
in the electric conduction alone, and in fact the diagnosis
of a CAD was proved to be correct by contrast angiography.

In the case of patients with suspected ventricular
aneurysm, an exact diagnosis is essential on account of the
therapeutic implications. Whereas an aneurysm necessitates an
anticoagulative therapy, this is not indicated in the absence
of an aneurysm on account of the side effects. Using RNV, an
aneurysm can be diagnosed by a dyskinesia. The Fourier analysis
technique may be of especial help in this particular investigation, if the aneurysm can not be recorded at a lateral edge
in the usual views. If an aneurysm is found in the middle of
the ventricle near the septum, a paradoxical movement can be
shown by means of the amplitude and phase images, as seen in
fig 18. In this patient, only the amplitude image in connection with the phase image (which is not reproduced, because a
black and white representation is not adequate) revealed a

dyskinesia, whereas none of the views demonstrated a dyskinetic movement of a lateral wall.

The Fourier analysis technique is the most sensitive method of evaluation which one can use for the investigation of small regional wall motion disorders. However, regional phase retardation can not be taken as proof of the presence of CAD, since it can also result from essentially global disorders in the left ventricular function. A "phase retardation" of the lateral wall of the ventricle can be observed in many patients with incompetent valves, primary cardiomyopathies and especially in patients suffering from hypertension. However, most of these patients also have a global retardation in left ventricular filling, as is documented by the filling rate VD = $(-dV/dt)_{max}$/EDV. Therefore, when a retardation of phases is observed laterally, especially in the postero-lateral wall, this abnormality can only be accounted for as the first sign of regional wall motion abnormality due to CAD, if a global reduction of the compliance can be excluded. Otherwise, all the heart diseases cited above, and above all hypertension, must be taken into account in the differential diagnosis.

Conclusion

The RNV is a very important non-invasive method of diagnosis for cardiologists, since heart function can be assessed both globally and regionally at rest, under ergometric and pharmaceutical intervention for a period of some hours. In many cases, the assessment of regional wall motion is the only accurate method of producing an exact diagnosis and reliably controlling surgical and medical therapy. The experienced investigator can very often evaluate regional heart function using the cine mode representation by itself. But in doubtful cases, when the investigators have not a great deal of experience or as a means of standardization regional motility, quantifying, operator-independent methods such as the computation of the regional ejection fraction and the Fourier analysis method, with the demonstration of the dynamics of the bearing heart by means of 2 static images of the amplitudes and phases, are extremely helpful and important.

REFERENCES

1. Tennant R, Wiggers CJ, The effect of coronary occlusion on myocardial contraction. Amer. J. Physiol. 112:3651, 1935.

2. Burow RD, Strauss HW, Singleton R, Pond M, Rehn T, Bailey IK, Griffith LC, Nicoloff E, Pitt B, Analysis of left ventricular function from multiple gated acquisition cardiac blood pool imaging. Circulation 56:1024, 1977.

3. Green MV, Brody WR, Douglas MA, Borer JS, Ostrow HG, Line BR, Bacharach SL, Johnston GS, Ejection fraction by count rate from gated images. J. nucl. Med. 19:880, 1978.

4. Pitt B, Strauss HW, Myocardial perfusion imaging and gated cardiac blood pool scanning: Clinical application. Amer. J. Cardiol. 38:739, 1976.

5. Rigo P, Strauss HW, Taylor D, Murray M, Kelly DT, Weisfeldt M, Pitt B, Left ventricular function in acute myocardial infarction evaluated by gated scintigraphy. Circulation 50:678, 1974.

6. Zaret BL, Strauss HW, Hurley PJ, Natarajan TK, Pitt B, Noninvasive scintiphotographic method for detecting regional dysfunction in man. New Engl. J. Med. 284:1165, 1971.

7. Berger HJ, Reduto LA, Johnstone DE, Borkowsky H, Cohen LS, Langou RA, Gottschalk A, Zaret BL, Global and regional left ventricular response to bicycle exercise in coronary artery disease: Assessment by quantitative radionuclide angiocardiography. Amer. J. Med. 66:13, 1979.

8. Berman DS, Salel AF, DeNardo GL et al, Clinical assessment of left ventricular regional contraction patterns and ejection fraction by high resolution gated scintigraphy. J. nucl. Med. 16:865, 1975.

9. Borer JS, Bacharach SL, Green MV, Kent KU, Epstein SE, Johnston GS, Real-time radionuclide cineangiography in the noninvasive evaluation of global and regional left ventricular function at rest and during exercise in patients with coronary artery disease. New Engl. J. Med. 296:839, 1977.

10. Klein G, Sauer E, Bauer R, Wirtzfeld A, Sebening H, The comparison of the effects of AR-L 115 BS and Dobutamin in patients with severe cardiac failure. Arzneimittel-Forsch.. Drug Res. 31:257, 1981.

11. Sauer E, Dressler J, Sebening H, Hör G, Lutilsky L, Bofilias I, Weber N, Pabst HW, Blömer H, Nichtinvasive Erfassung der Dynamik des linken Ventrikels. Bestimmung der linksventrikulären Auswurffraktion der Ventrikelvolumina und der regionalen Wandbewegung durch die EKG-getriggerte Herzbinnenraumszintigraphie. Dtsch. med. Wschr. 103:1199, 1978.

12. Sauer E, Sebening H, Dressler J, Lutilsky L, Klein G, Ulm K, Hör G, Pabst HW, Blömer H, Linksventrikuläre Funktionsbeurteilung in Ruhe und unter Ergometerbelastung mit der Herzbinnenraumszintigraphie bei koronarer Herzkrankheit. Herz/Kreislauf 11:286, 1979.

13. Bauer R, Sauer E, Langhammer H, Pabst HW, Radionuklidventrikulographie bei Herzrhythmusstörungen. Nukl. Med. Suppl. 18:224, 1981.

14. Marshall RC, Berger HJ, Costin JC et al, Assessment of cardiac performance with quantitative radionuclide angiocardiography. Sequential left ventricular ejection fraction, normalized left ventricular

ejection rate and regional wall motion. Circulation 56:820, 1977.

15. Pabst HW, Bauer R, Sauer E, Optimale Datenaufnahme und -auswertung bei der Hernzbinnenraumszintigraphie. Vergleich von first pass und Aufnahmen im steady state. In: Systeme und Signalverarbeitung in der Nuklearmedizin. Pöppl SJ, Pretschner DP (eds), Springer Verlag Berlin-Heidelberg, pp 59-67.

16. Schad N, Nichtinvasive Darstellung der Wandbewegung und Schlag-volumenverteilung des linken Ventrikels nach Myokardinfarkt. Fort-schr. Röntgenstr. Nuklearmed. 124:201, 1976.

17. Sebening H, Sauer E, Bauer R, Kalhofer E, Lutilsky L, Änderung der linksventrikulären Funktion nach Aortenklappenersatz bei Aorten-insuffizienz. Z. Kardiol. 70:304, 1981.

18. Bauer R, Haluszczynski I, Pabst HW, Langhammer H, Bachmann W, In-vivo / in-vitro labeling of red blood cells with Tc-99m. Eur. J. Nucl. Med. 8:218, 1983.

19. Maddox DE, Wynne J, Uren R, Parker JA, Idoine J, Siegel LC, Neill JM, Cohn PF, Holman BL, Regional ejection fraction: A quantitative radionuclide index of regional left ventricular performance. Circulation 59:1001, 1979.

20. Standke R, Hör G, Maul FD, Fully automated sectorial equilibrium radionuclide ventriculography. Eur. J. Nucl. Med. 8:77, 1983.

21. Maddox DE, Holman BL, Wynne J, Idoine J, Parker JA, Uren R, Neill JM, Cohn PF, Ejection fraction image: A noninvasive index of regional left ventricular wall motion. Amer. J. Cardiol. 41:1230, 1978.

22. Adam WE, Sigel H, Geffers H, Kampmann F, Bitter F, Stauch M, Analyse der regionalen Wandbewegung des linken Ventrikels bei koronarer Herzerkrankung durch ein nichtinvasives Verfahren (Radionuklid-Kinematographie). Z. Kardiol. 66:545, 1977.

23. Bauer R, Sauer E, Langhammer H, Pabst HW, Parametric images of amplitudes and phases in analysing regional heart function. Nukl. Med. Suppl. 19:80, 1982.

24. Bauer R, Methodische Untersuchungen zur Herzbinnenraumszintigraphie und ihre Andwendung in der Diagnose und Differentialdiagnose der Koronarer Herzerkrankung. Habilitationsschrift Technische Universi-tät, München (1983).

25. Bauer R, Kiefl S, Sauer E, Sebening H, Pemsl M, Schön H, Langhammer H, Pabst HW, Wirkung von Nifedipin bei koronarer Herzkrankheit. Nukl. Med. Suppl. (in press).

EVALUATION OF REGURGITATION IN AORTIC AND MITRAL VALVE
INSUFFICIENCY

H. KLEPZIG Jr, G. HÖR

INTRODUCTION

The quantification of regurgitated blood-volume in patients
with aortic or mitral valve regurgitation is still difficult.
Usually, angiographic methods are used to evaluate valvular
incompetence. However, it is highly desirable to have a sensitive and specific non-invasive diagnostic procedure especially
for severely ill patients, in cases with dubious severity of
regurgitation and for follow-up studies. Radionuclide techniques proved to be a reliable tool.

Non-invasive radiological methods were tested for establishing a relation between heart size and left ventricular volume.
Lewis (1) found a close linear relationship between these investigations in patients with isolated aortic regurgitation. However, this procedure proved to be inadequate (2). Similarly,
the criteria originally established by Rackley and Hood (3)
(enlarged left ventricle, normal ejection fraction, left heart
failure) are inconclusive in diagnosing left ventricular volume
overload due to aortic or mitral regurgitation.

Angiographic techniques

Two angiographic methods are used in the clinical routine.
1. Semiquantitative method: The valvular regurgitation can be
   quantified in four or five grades of severity (4-14). The
   following criteria are used:
- The amount of contrast medium appearing in the left ventricle (or left atrium) after injection into the aortic
  root (or left ventricle,respectively).
- The number of cycles necessary for clearing the contrast
  material.

The reliability of this semiquantitative method can be influenced by the size of the ventricular or atrial cavity and accordingly by the distribution volume of the contrast material, by cardiac
arrhytmias and the position of the catheter during the injection.
In general, this method reveals clinically sufficient values (15).

Angiographic regurgitant fraction: The second more precise
technique is the method of Sandler and Dodge (16): The amount
of blood regurgitated into the left ventricle and left atrium
is calculated from the difference between the left ventricular
stroke volume, determined by the left ventricular cineangiography,
and effective stroke volume, determined by Fick's principle. This
difference as a fraction of left ventricular stroke volume is
considered to represent the angiographic regurgitant fraction.

Even this method has its limits. It is sometimes difficult
to assess the exact enddiastolic and endsystolic boundaries of
the left ventricle during cineangiography. Second, it is necessary
to determine the left and right ventricular stroke volume simultaneously. However, the reproducibility of cardiac output measurement during left ventricular cineangiography is poor, probably
due to the influence of deep inspiration and occuring arrhythmias
(17). Finally, arrhythmias induced by contrast material will limit
the value of this method, since the heart rate and ventricular
pressure at the time of angiography must be comparable to the
rate and pressure at the time of determination of cardiac output.
Nevertheless, this method represents the most reliable invasive
technique available.

Radionuclide techniques

Several radionuclide methods were developed earlier to determine the regurgitated blood volume in patients with left-sided
valvular incompetence (18,19). Attempts by Morch et al (19) to
quantitate mitral regurgitation using continuous infusion of
^{133}Xe were abandoned. Today, two basically different methods are
used in the daily routine.

Left-right ventricular (lv-rv) stroke volume ratio. The ratio
of left and right ventricular stroke volume is well established
to assess left-sided valvular incompetence (17,20-39). It

quantitates left ventricular volume overload without separating
mitral and aortic regurgitation. The ratio is calculated as the
ratio of enddiastolic-endsystolic count-rate differences of the
left and right ventricle.

$$a = \frac{counts \quad lv \quad (EDV \quad - \quad ESV)}{counts \quad rv \quad (EDV \quad - \quad ESV)}$$

Five different techniques are used to evaluate the lv-rv stroke
volume ratio:
- fixed single enddiastolic region of interest (20)
- separate enddiastolic and endsystolic region of interest
  (25)
- evaluation of ventricular stroke counts directly from the
  stroke volume image (30)
- evaluation of ventricular stroke counts from Fourier phase
  image (35)
- first-pass investigation (36).

Most authors determine the lv-rv stroke volume ratio during
equilibrium radionuclide ventriculography. For patients without
valvular incompetence, the normal range of this parameter,
using a single enddiastolic region of interest, in our laboratory
is 0.7 - 1.7 (28). Kress et al (17) investigated 33 patients
with aortic and/or mitral regurgitation. Their study revealed
a moderate correlation between the scintigraphically and hemodynamically determined lv-rv stroke volume ratio (r= 0.75).
Taylor et al (34) found the reliability of this parameter to
be even lower: the spread of the values of stroke volume ratio
for the different regurgitation groups was so high to ensure
that this technique can not be regarded as an accurate method
of assessing left-sided valvular heart disease. In general, the
sensitivity is about 80%, the specificity 100% (17,28,34,37).
The reduced sensitivity, even in patients with distinct aortic
or mitral regurgitation, is mainly due to two problems:
First, for geometric reasons (40) (i.e. an overlap of the two
ventricles, different distances of left and right ventricle to
the gamma camera) equilibrium radionuclide lv-rv stroke volume
is normal up to about 1.7, corresponding to a regurgitant

fraction of 41%. By using the first-pass technique (36), a slant hole collimator (26) or phase analysis (35), it was possible to approximate the lv-rv stroke volume ratio to the ideal value of 1.00 in healthy subjects. However, the reliability of these techniques is still under discussion.

Second, another even more important disadvantage of this parameter can not be overcome by these new techniques: in patients with left- and right-sided incompetence or shunt lesions the stroke volumes of both ventricles may be equivalent, leading to false-negative results.

Similarly to the values obtained by the method of Sandler and Dodge (16), the lv-rv stroke volume ratio is insufficient to differentiate aortic from mitral regurgitation: in patients with an incompetence of both left-sided valves, the total left ventricular regurgitation is determined, consisting of aortic and mitral regurgitation.

Radionuclide regurgitant fraction (Combined first-pass-/ equilibrium technique). This method goes a step further. It is based on the technique of Sandler and Dodge, and was initiated by Van Dyke (41) and Weber (42): the effective stroke volume is derived from the first-pass radionuclide ventriculography; the total left ventricular stroke volume is determined by equilibrium radionuclide ventriculography. The difference between these two volumes as a fraction of total left ventricular stroke volume is taken as the radionuclide regurgitant fraction (28). We studied the practical value of this technique in 24 patients with isolated aortic regurgitation. 16 men with normal valvular function served as control. All patients underwent ventricular and aortic cineangiography. The amount of aortic regurgitation was estimated semiquantitatively using the classification of Hunt (6):

- grade 0 corresponds to "no contrast material reflux into the left ventricle during aortography"
- grade 2 to 4 to increasing amounts of contrast material in the left ventricle
- and grade 5 to a reflux of contrast material clearly outlining the left ventricle with the density of ventricular contrast medium being equal to that of the aortic root within

three beats.

In addition, to determine the validity of the scintigraphic-ally derived enddiastolic volume, we calculated this volume in 16 patients with aortic regurgitation from the cineangiographic film. We used the biplane technique described elsewhere (43).

Within one day in patients with acute aortic regurgitation, and ten days in all others, prior or after cardiac catheterisa-tion, radionuclide ventriculography was performed.

First-pass technique: Cardiac output determination. In vivo-labelling of the red-blood cells was achieved by pre-injection of Sn pyrophosphate followed by a bolus injection of 15 mCi Tc^{99m} into a brachial vein (44). The first passage of the activ-ity through the heart was registered in LAO 45° position by a gamma camera-computer system (Picker small field of view camera 4/11, Informatek computer SIMIS 3). Two minutes later the "equilibrium activity" (c∞) was imaged in the same camera position. No background substraction was performed. The down-slope of the time-activity curve, generated from the list mode study using time intervals of one second, was extrapolated to baseline by a monoexponential fitting program (fig. 1). Accord-ing to the formula (below), the effective stroke volume (EffSV) was derived from the product of equilibrium count rate (c∞) and blood volume (BV) devided by the integral of the extra-polated time-activity curve of the first-pass study and the mean of the momentary heart rate (HR):

$$EffSV = \frac{c\infty \quad . \quad BV}{\int_{0}^{\infty} c(t) \quad . \quad dt \quad . \quad HR} \quad (41,42,45)$$

In favor of practical performance we predicted the blood-volume from the weight, height and sex of the patient (46).

Equilibrium technique: Total left ventricular stroke volume. Subsequently to the first-pass, equilibrium radionuclide ventric-ulography was performed in a one-step procedure: acquisition time 5 min, 64 frames, 32 . 32 pixels. The acquired data were processed

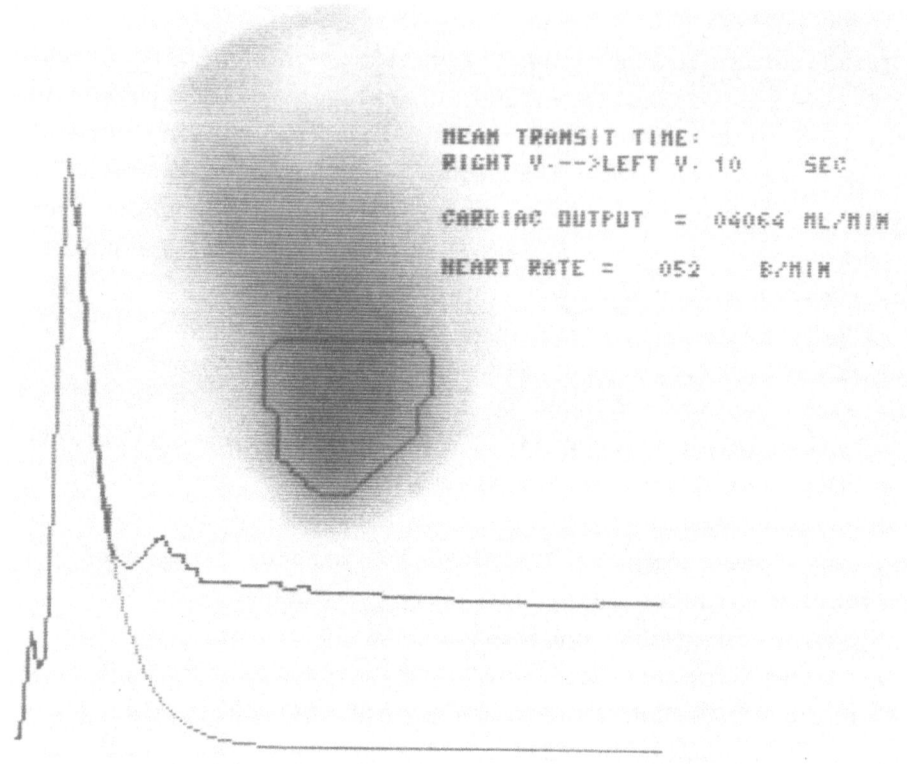

MEAN TRANSIT TIME:
RIGHT V.-->LEFT V. 10   SEC

CARDIAC OUTPUT = 04064 ML/MIN

HEART RATE =   052   B/MIN

Fig. 1. First passage of a bolus of 15 mCi Tc^{99m} through the heart, registered in LAO 45°. The downslope of the time-activity curve was extrapolated to baseline by a monoexponential fitting program (see text).

by a fully automated computer program (47-49). Left and right ventricular enddiastolic region of interest were set automatically, using functional and morphological criteria. Background activity, used for background correction, was taken sectorically in the endsystolic image outside the left ventricular region of interest, but only at the lateral wall.

The following parameters were calculated:
- radionuclide lv-rv stroke volume ratio
- global left ventricular ejection fraction (EF)
- left ventricular enddiastolic volume (EDV), using a geometric approach; the enddiastolic region of interest is assumed to consist of cylindrical slices, each of them with the height of one image element (fig 2). According

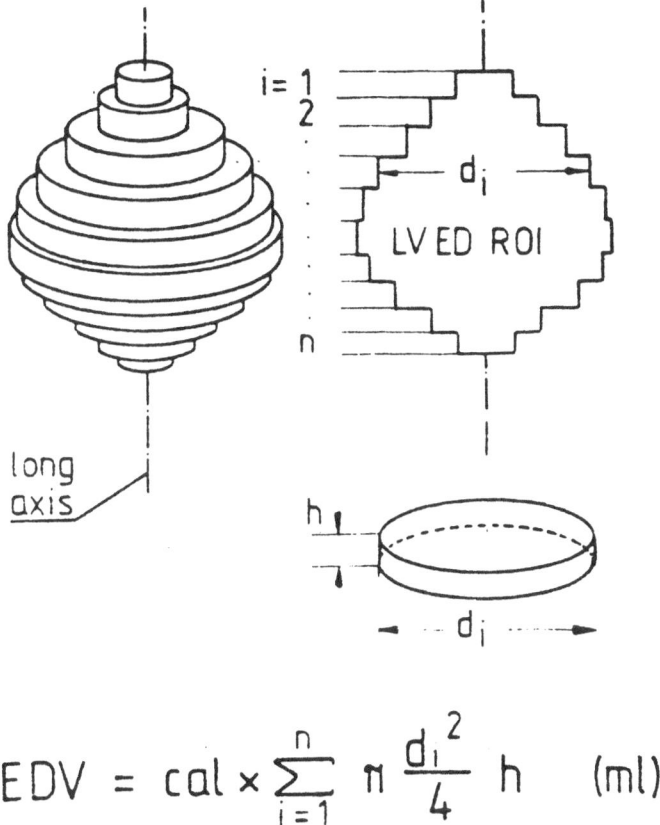

$$EDV = cal \times \sum_{i=1}^{n} \pi \frac{d_i^2}{4} h \quad (ml)$$

Fig. 2. Calculation of the radionuclide enddiastolic volume (see text).

to the formula in fig 2, the enddiastolic volume is calculated with a calibration factor (cal) in consideration of the spacial dimension of one image element
- total left ventricular stroke volume as a product of ejection fraction and enddiastolic volume

LVSV = EF . EDV.

The regurgitated blood-volume (RBV) was calculated from the difference of total and effective left ventricular stroke volume:

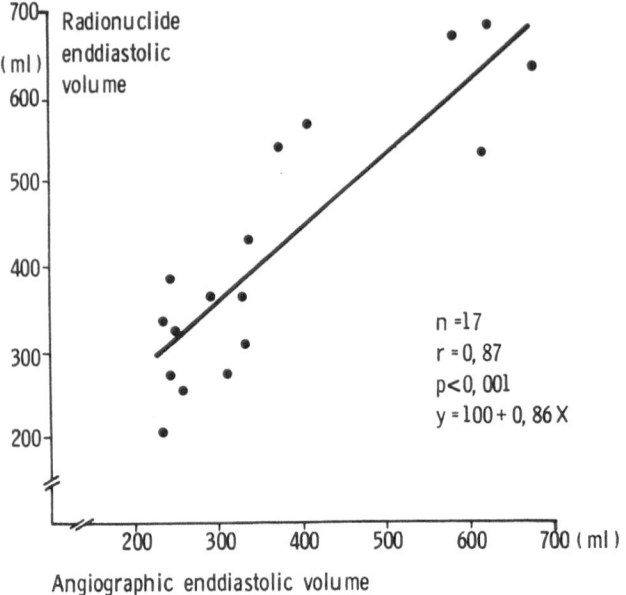

Fig. 3. The radionuclide and angiographic enddiastolic volume is compared in 17 patients with aortic regurgitation. The values correlate closely (r= 0.87).

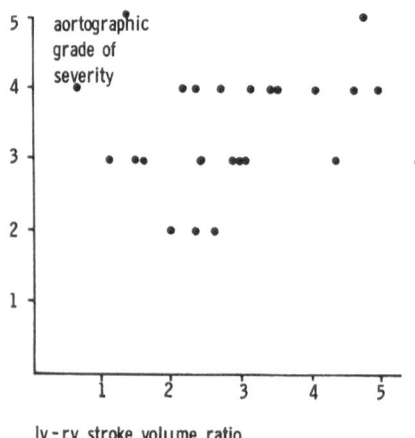

Fig. 4. Comparison of the radionuclide lv-rv stroke volume ratio and the aortographic grade of severity in 24 patients with aortic regurgitation.

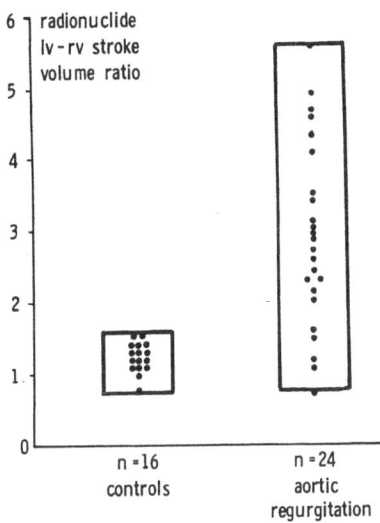

Fig. 5. Sensitivity and specificity of the radionuclide lv-rv stroke volume ratio in 24 patients with aortic regurgitation.

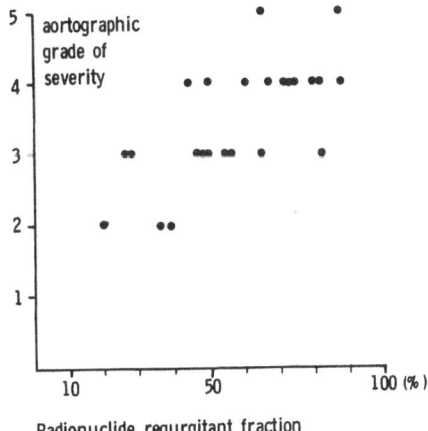

Fig. 6. Comparison of the radionuclide regurgitant fraction and the aortographic grade of severity in 24 patients with aortic regurgitation.

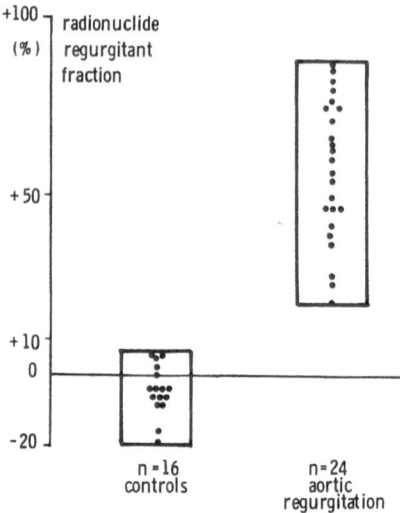

Fig. 7. Sensitivity and specificity of the radionuclide regurgitant fraction in 24 patients with aortic regurgitation.

$$RBV = EF \cdot EDV - EffSV$$

The radionuclide regurgitant fraction was taken as the ratio of the regurgitated blood-volume and the total left ventricular stroke volume.

Radionuclide vs angiographic results: The results of our study are shown in figs 3-7.

The individual paired data for radionuclide and angiographic enddiastolic volume are demonstrated in fig 3. The values correlate closely (r= 0.87).

The radionuclide lv-rv stroke volume ratio and aortographic grade of severity of aortic regurgitation are compared in fig 4. Fig 5 shows that 5 of 24 patients with aortic regurgitation had lv-rv stroke volume ratios within the normal range, corresponding to a sensitivity of 79%. Specificity was 100%.

The sensitivity of lv-rv stroke volume ratio for detecting mild to severe valvular regurgitation using other previously mentioned methods ranges between 37,8 and 62,2% (30).

The sensitivity is said to increase when left the ventricular ejection fraction is greater than 35% (30). When excluding 5 patients with an ejection fraction lower than 35%, sensitivity in our study increases to 94%. The reduced sensitivity of this parameter in patients with an ejection fraction lower than 35% is probably due to a -clinically silent- additional pulmonic or tricuspid regurgitation, which lead to an increase of the right ventricular stroke volume.

The radionuclide regurgitant fraction and aortographic grade of severity of aortic regurgitation are compared in fig 6. Fig 7 demonstrates that in the control group the regurgitant fraction never exeeded +10%, whilst patients with aortic regurgitation never had values lower than +20%.

Sensitivity and specificity of the combined first-pass-/ equilibrium technique therefore were 100%.

Advantages of radionuclide regurgitant fraction. Consequently, the combined first-pass-/equilibrium radionuclide ventriculography shows many advantages. The overlap of the heart chambers plays only a minor role. The effective stroke volume, derived from the first-pass study, is not influenced by any valvular incompetence or shunt lesion within the left and right heart. The radionuclide regurgitant fraction can easily be determined during the daily routine. The time needed for the whole procedure is 15 min including 3 min for data processing. Patients with hemodynamically insignificant reflux were not represented in our study because they were not subjected to cardiac catheterisation. For these cases the accuracy of our technique can not be derived from this study.

Limitations of radionuclide regurgitant fraction. Several factors can influence the reliability of our technique. Similarly to the method of Sandler and Dodge and the lv-rv stroke volume ratio, an additional mitral regurgitation will contribute to the "total regurgitant fraction" consisting of mitral and aortic regurgitation. Gated cardiac blood-pool studies share the disadvantage not to be applicable to patients with atrial fibrillation or multifocal tachycardia (22).

We decided to predict the blood-volume from sex, weight and hight of the patient; the enddiastolic volume is calculated using a geometric approach. The potential disadvantages of both methods can probably be avoided when substituted by a counts-based method (50-52). However, in our opinion this distinctly invalidates the practicability of our method during the daily routine. Furthermore, counts-based methods are less reliable in patients with enddiastolic volumes larger than 300 ml (53), as observed in patients with aortic regurgitation. Fig 3 demonstrates, that our geometric model permits a reliable evaluation of the enddiastolic volume in patients with aortic regurgitation when compared with the enddiastolic volume, determined from the left ventricular cineangiography.

Until now, we have only limited experience regarding the reliability of the first-pass-/equilibrium technique in patients with mitral regurgitation. However, on theoretical grounds, we expect no significant differences.

Conclusions and outlook. Radionuclide techniques provide important information on cardiac performance in patients with left-sided valvular regurgitation. The radionuclide lv-rv stroke volume ratio represents a simple technique for non-invasive evaluation of aortic and mitral regurgitation. Disadvantage is the reduced sensitivity in a considerable number of patients. Radionuclide regurgitant fraction estimated by the combined first-pass-/equilibrium technique in all cases enables a reliable quantitative evaluation of the aortic regurgitation. Further efforts are necessary to develop new methods which can distinguish between aortic and mitral regurgitation, and which permit the separate determination of the amounts of aortic and mitral regurgitation in patients suffering from valvular incompetence of both left-sided valves. The detection of tricuspid valve insufficiency using Fourier phase and amplitude analysis was shown in a pilot study by Pavel et al (54).

ADDENDUM (received in proof).

Until December 1984 many advances concerning the combined first-pass-/equilibrium radionuclide ventriculography have been made:

-   the method has been validated for patients with mitral regurgitation;
-   for patients with combined aortic and mitral regurgitation;
-   and for patients with mild valvular incompetence regurgitant fraction between 20 and 40%).

Radionuclide regurgitant fraction correlated closely with angiographic regurgitant fraction. Reproducibility was high.

REFERENCES

1. Lewis RP, Bristow JD, Griswold HE, Radiographic heart size and left ventricular volume in aortic valve disease. Amer. J. Cardiol. 27:250, 1971.

2. Miller GAH, Kirklin JW, Swan HJC, Myocardial function and ventricular volumes in acquired valvular insufficiency. Circulation 31:374, 1965.

3. Rackley CE, Hood WP Jr, Quantitative angiographic evaluation and pathophysiologic mechanisms in valvular heart disease. Progr. cardiovasc. Dis. 15:427, 1973.

4. Calderón J, Cineangiographic diagnosis of aortic insufficiency. Angiology 18:723, 1967.

5. Cohn LH, Mason DT, Ross J Jr, Morrow AG, Braunwald E, Preoperative assessment of aortic regurgitation in patients with mitral valve disease. Amer. J. Cardiol. 19:177, 1967.

6. Hunt D, Baxley WA, Kennedy JW, Judge TP, Williams JE, Dodge HT, Quantitative evaluation of cineaortography in the assessment of aortic regurgitation. Amer. J. Cardiol. 31:696, 1973.

7. Mennel RG, Joyner CR Jr, Thompson PD, Pyle RR, Macvaugh H, The preoperative and operative assessment of aortic regurgitation. Amer. J. Cardiol. 29:360, 1972.

8. Runco V, Molnar W, Meckstroth CV, Ryan JM, The Graham Steel murmur versus aortic regurgitation in rheumatic heart disease. Amer. J. Med. 31:71, 1961.

9. Sellers RD, Levy MJ, Amplatz K, Lillehei CW, Left retrograde cineangiography in acquired cardiac disease. Technic, indications and interpretations in 700 cases. Amer. J. Cardiol. 14:437, 1964.

10. Amplatz K, Lester RG, Ernst R, Lillehei CW, Left retrograde cardioangiography: Its diagnostic value in acquired and congenital heart disease. Radiology 76:393, 1961.

11. Lyngborg K, Mitral regurgitation. Acta Med. Scand. p 594 (suppl) 1974.

12. Björk VO, Lodin H, Malers E, The evaluation of the degree of mitral insufficiency by selective left ventricular angiocardiography. Amer. Heart J. 60:691, 1960.

13. Gray IR, Joshipura CS, Mackinnon J, Retrograde left ventricular cardioangiography in the diagnosis of mitral regurgitation. Brit. Heart J. 25:145, 1963.

14. Honey M, Gough JH, Katsaros S, Miller GAH, Thuraisingham V, Left ventricular cine-angiocardiography in the assessment of mitral regurgitation. Brit. Heart J. 31:596, 1969.

15. Frank MJ, Casanegra P, Nadimi M, Migliori AJ, Levinson G, Measurement of aortic regurgitation by upstream sampling with continuous infusion of indicator. Circulation 33:545, 1966.

16. Sandler H, Dodge HT, Hay RE, Rackley CE, Quantitation of valvular insufficiency in man by angiocardiography. Amer. Heart J. 65:501, 1963.

17. Kress P, Geffers H, Stauch M, Nechwatal W, Sigel H, Bitter F, Adam WE, Evaluation of aortic and mitral valve regurgitation by radionuclide ventriculography: Comparison with the method of Sandler and Dodge. Clin. Cardiol. 4:5, 1981.

18. Hildner FJ, Pierson WR, Barold SS, Linhart JW, Samet P, Isotope quantitation of aortic insufficiency compared to cineangiography in man. Ann. Thorac. Surg. 8:84, 1969.

19. Morch JE, Klein SW, Richardson P, Froggatt G, Schwartz L, McLoughlin M, Mitral regurgitation measured by continuous infusion of 133-Xenon. Amer. J. Cardiol. 29:812, 1972.

20. Rigo P, Alderson PO, Robertson RM, Becker LC, Wagner HN Jr, Measurement of aortic and mitral regurgitation by gated cardiac blood pool scans. Circulation 60:306, 1979.

21. Boucher AC, Okada RD, Pohost GM, Current status of radionuclide imaging in valvular heart disease. Amer. J. Cardiol. 46:1153, 1980.

22. Bough EW, Gandsman EJ, North DL, Shulman RS, Gated radionuclide angiographic evaluation of valve regurgitation. Amer. J. Cardiol. 46:423, 1980.

23. Henze E, Schelbert HR, Wisenberg G, Ratib O, Schön H, Assessment of regurgitant fraction and right and left ventricular function at rest and during exercise: A new technique for determination of right ventricular stroke counts from gated equilibrium blood pool studies. Amer. Heart J. 104:953, 1982.

24. Mendelson S, Carlson CJ, Rapaport E, A new method for quantification of aortic regurgitation during cardiac catheterization. Amer. J. Physiol. Heart Cir. Physiol. 8:121, 1980.

25. Sorensen SG, O'Rourke RA, Chaudhuri TK, Noninvasive quantitation of valvular regurgitation by gated equilibrium radionuclide angiography. Circulation 62:1089, 1980.

26. Gandsman EJ, North DL, Shulman RS, Bough EW, Measurement of the ventricular stroke volume ratio by gated radionuclide angiography. Radiology 138:161, 1981.

27. Chevigné M, Rigo P, Quantification of isolated regurgitation by gated cardiac blood pool scan. Eur. J. Nucl. Med. 7:39, 1982.

28. Klepzig H Jr, Standke R, Kunkel B, Maul FD, Hör G, Kaltenbach M, Kombinierte First-pass- / Äquilibrium-Radionuklid- Ventrikulographie zur nicht-invasiven Beurteilung der Schwere einer Aorteninsuffizienz (Combined first-pass-/equilibrium radionuclide ventriculography for non-invasive evaluation of aortic valve incompetence). Z. Kardiol. 71:661, 1982.

29. Konstam MA, Wynne J, Holman BL, Brown EJ, Neill JM, Kozlowski J, Use of equilibrium (gated) radionuclide ventriculography to quantitate left ventricular output in patients with and without left-sided valvular regurgitation. Circulation 64:578, 1981.

30. Nicod P, Corbett JR, Firth BG, Dehmer GJ, Izquierdo C, Markham RV Jr, Hillis LD, Willerson JT, Lewis SE, Radionuclide techniques for valvular regurgitant index: Comparison in patients with normal and depressed ventricular function. J. nucl. Med. 23:763, 1982.

31. Manyari DE, Nolewajka AJ, Kostuk WJ, Quantitative assessment of aortic valvular insufficiency by radionuclide angiography. Chest 81-170, 1982.

32. Alderson PO, Radionuclide quantification of valvular regurgitation. J. nucl. Med. 23:851, 1982.

33. Bezossi M, Clare J, Santinga J, Thrall J, Pitt B, Exercise lv/rv stroke index ratios measured by gated blood pool scans in aortic regurgitation pre and post valve replacement. J. nucl. Med. 21:49, 1980.

34. Taylor DN, Harris DNF, Condon B, Ogilvie B, Ackery DM, Fleming J, Goddard BA, Radionuclide evaluation of valvular regurgitation. Brit. J. Radiol. 55:204, 1982.

35. Makler PT, McCarthy DM, Velchik MG, Goldstein HA, Alavi A, Fourier amplitude ratio: A new way to assess valvular regurgitation. J. nucl. Med. 24:204, 1983.

36. Janowitz WR, Fester A, Quantitation of left ventricular regurgitant fraction by first pass radionuclide angiocardiography. Amer. J. Cardiol. 49:85, 1982.

37. Lam W, Pavel D, Byrom E, Sheikh A, Best D, Rosen K, Radionuclide regurgitant index: Value and limitations. Amer. J. Cardiol. 47:292, 1981.

38. Thompson R, Ross I, Elmes R, Quantification of valvar regurgitation by cardiac gated pool imaging. Brit. Heart J. 46:629, 1981.

39. Urquhart J, Patterson RE, Packer M, Goldsmith SJ, Horowitz SF, Litwak R, Gorlin R, Quantification of valve regurgitation by radionuclide angiography before and after valve replacement surgery. Amer. J. Cardiol. 47:287, 1981.

40. Strauss HW, McKusik KA, Boucher CA, Bingham JB, Pohost GM, Of linens and laces: The eight anniversary of the gated blood pool scan. Sem. Nucl. Med. 9:296, 1979.

41. Van Dyke D, Anger HO, Sullivan RW, Vetter WR, Yano Y, Parker HG, Cardiac evaluation from radioisotope dynamics. J. nucl. Med. 13:585, 1972.

42. Weber PM, Dos Remedios LV, Jasko IA, Quantitative radioisotopic angiocardiography. J. nucl. Med. 13:815, 1972.

43. Schulz W, Kaltenbach M, Neues Verfahren zur Bestimmung der Röntgenvergrösserung bei angiographischen Ventrikelvolumenbestimmungen. (New method of estimating X-ray magnification on angiographic volume determinations). Z. Kardiol. 67:554, 1978.

44. Pavel DG, Zimmer AM, Patterson VN, In vivo labeling of red blood cells with 99m-Tc: A new approach to blood pool visualization. J. nucl. Med. 18:305, 1977.

45. Parker H, Weber PM, Van Dyke DC, Davies H, Steele P, Sullivan R, Evaluation of central circulatory dynamics with the radionuclide angiogram. In: Cardiovascular nuclear medicine. Strauss W, Pitt B, James A Jr (eds), The CV Mosby Comp, St. Louis, p 67, 1974.

46. Ciba-Geigy AG, Wissenschaftliche Tabellen. 8th ed. Basel, p 66, 1981.

47. Hör G, Standke R, Maul FD, Munz D, Äquilibrium-Radionuklid-Ventrikulographie bei koronarer Herzkrankheit. Diagnostik 15:116, 1982

48. Standke R, Hör G, Fully automatic sectorial radionuclide ventriculography. Informatek Newsl. 4:63, 1981

49. Standke R, Hör G, Maul FD, Fully automated sectorial equilibrium radionuclide ventriculography: Proposal of a method for routine use

(exercise and follow-up). Eur. J. Nucl. Med. 8:77, 1983.

50. Massie BM, Kramer BL, Gertz EW, Henderson SG, Radionuclide measurement of left ventricular volume: comparison of geometric and counts-based methods. Circulation 65:725, 1982.

51. Slutsky R, Karliner J, Ricci D, Kaiser R, Pfisterer M, Gordon D, Peterson K, Ashburn W, Left ventricular volumes by gated equilibrium radionuclide angiography: A new method. Circulation 60:556, 1979.

52. Dehmer GJ, Lewis SE, Hillis LD, Twieg D, Falkhoff M, Parkey RW, Willerson JT, Nongeometric determination of left ventricular·volumes from equilibrium blood pool scans. Amer. J. Cardiol. 45:293, 1980.

53. Strauss HW, McKusick KA, Bingham JB, Cardiac nuclear imaging: Principles, instrumentation and pitfalls. Amer. J. Cardiol. 46:1109, 1980.

54. Pavel DG, Handler B, Lam W, Meyer-Pavel C, Byrom E, Pietras R, A new method for the detection of tricuspid insufficiency. J. nucl. Med. 22:4, 1981.

^{195m}GOLD FOR ASSESSMENT OF CARDIAC FUNCTION

F.J.Th. WACKERS, H.J. BERGER, P.B. HOFFER, R.C. LANGE,
B.L. ZARET

INTRODUCTION

Tc^{99m} is currently the radionuclide of choice for assessing cardiac function by either the first-pass or multigated equilibrium radionuclide angiocardiography. However, its relative long half-life of 6 hours pose some practical limitations to the clinical use of the radiotracer. For example, using Tc^{99m} labelled pharmaceuticals that are cleared primarily by the kidneys or reticulo-endothelial system, the total number of first-pass studies that can be performed in sequence and the dose per study are limited (3 studies and 10 mCi, respectively). In addition the minimal time interval between sequential first-pass studies using these radiopharmaceuticals is longer than desirable, especially during exercise, and should be at least 10 min. Employing Tc^{99m} labelled red cells for gated cardiac blood-pool imaging, serial assessment of cardiac function can be performed. However, the half-life of Tc^{99m} necessitates delay of imaging with other radionuclides, such as ^{201}Tl, for at aleast 24 hours. In the present chapter, we will discuss our initial clinical experience with ^{195m}Gold, a new short-lived (30.6 sec) radiotracer, which permits a number of interesting clinical applications (1,2).

The generator

The results reported in this chapter were obtained with generators manufactured by Byk-Mallinckrodt, Petten, The Netherlands (3). Other ^{195m}Mercury/^{195m}Gold-generators have been developed and are used for clinical studies (4,5). ^{195m}Gold is the daughter of the long-lived parent ^{195m}Mercury (half-life of 41.6 hours). Table 1 shows the decay scheme of ^{195m}Mercury.

Table 1. Decay scheme of [195m]Mercury

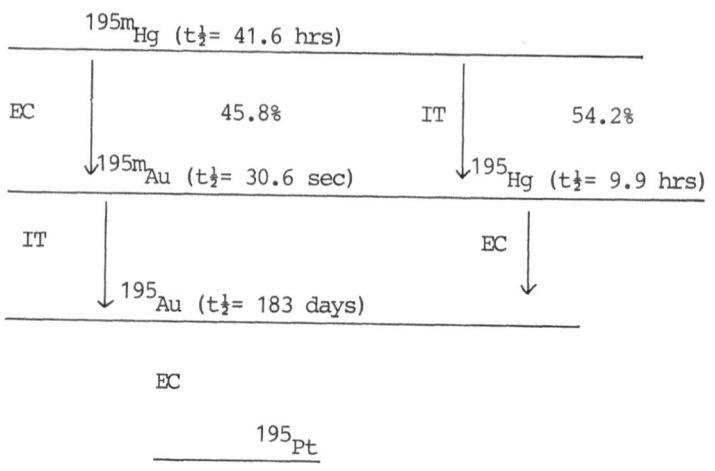

Hg = mercury;   Au = gold;   Pt= platinum

The principal gamma emissions of [195m]Gold are at 262 keV (68%), and of [195m]Mercury at 262 keV (32%), 388 keV (3%) and 560 keV (8%). Short-lived [195m]Gold can be obtained from a table top generator. The prototype [195m]Mercury/[195m]Gold generator (Byk-Mallinckrodt, Petten, The Netherlands) consists of a 9x12 lead housing, containing a 5x1 cm glass column with an inlet at one end and an outlet at the other (figs 1,2).[195m]Mercury is adsorbed on inorganic material in this column. The column can be flushed with an aqueous sodium-thiosulfate/sodium-nitrate eluent. The daughter, [195m]Gold, is eluted from the column. Only small amounts of [195m]Mercury and [195]Gold are present in the eluate, in equilibrium with [195m]Gold.

Quality control
    Careful quality control and analysis of performance of each individual generator is crucial and should be performed before administration of eluate to patients (1). First, the generator has to be flushed with at least 40 ml of eluent to wash off [195m]Mercury and [195]Mercury, freed from the column by radioautolysis (fig 3). Subsequently, the total volume of

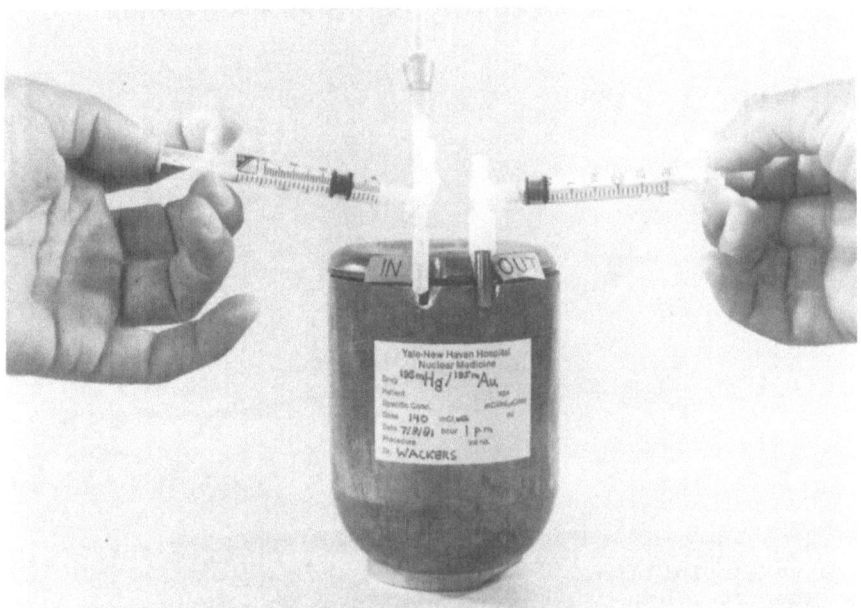

Fig. 1. The [195m]Mercury/[195m]Gold generator. Because of medium-energy 262 keV photon emissions, heavier lead shielding than shown in this figure required for clinical use. (Reproduced with permission from Ref. 1).

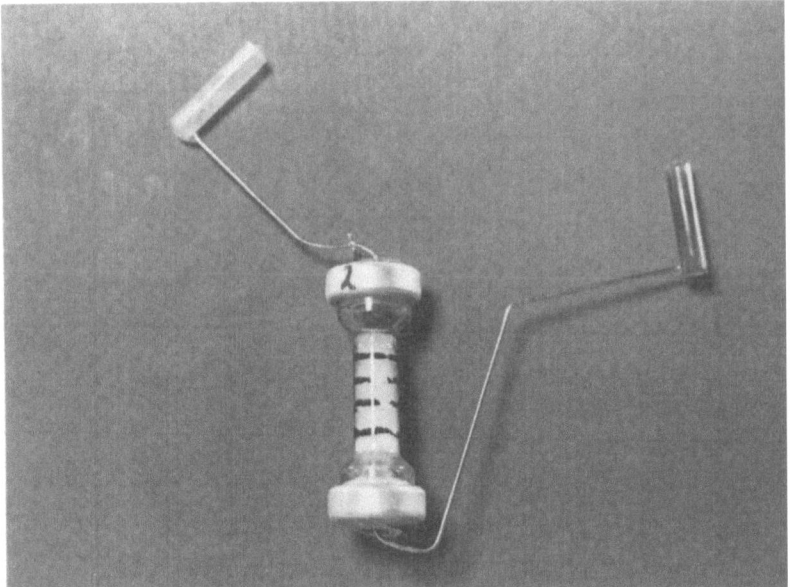

Fig. 2. The glass column (5x1 cm), in which the parent [195m]Mercury is adsorbed on inorganic material. The inlet (white) and outlet (dark) by which the column is flushed with eluent are shown.

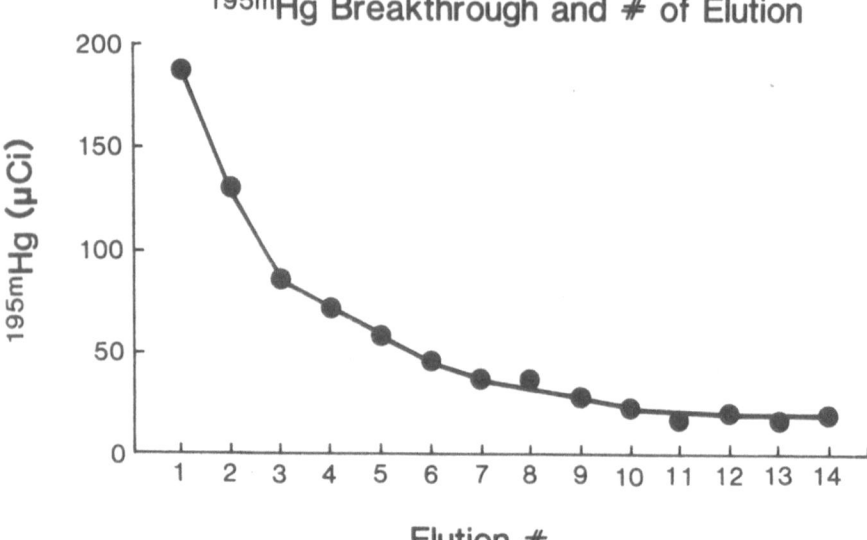

Fig. 3. After a period of rest, ^{195m}Mercury and ^{195}Mercury are freed from the generator column by radioautolysis. These long-lived radio-nuclides have to be washed off before clinical use of the generator. Initially, the eluate will contain a high amount of ^{195m}Mercury, which decreases rapidly after repeat elutions. The breakthrough of ^{195m} Mercury in the eluate usually is stable after approximately 10 elutions (20 ml of eluent). With frequent use of the generator, this amount will further decrease.

Table 2. Estimated comparative radiation dose to human organs for ^{195m}Gold and Tc^{99m}

Organ	^{195}Au(^{195m}Hg) rads/20 mCi (20 μCi)*	Tc^{99m}DTPA rads/20 mCi
Kidney	0.34	1.8
Liver	0.07	
Spleen	0.09	
Ovaries	0.003	0.31
Testes	0.001	0.21
Whole body	0.007	0.12

* Radiation dose is determined mainly by 20 μCi of ^{195m}Hg in the eluate

eluate is to be measured in a standard dose calibrator (model CRC-17, Capintec) to determine the amount of [195m]Gold (calibrator setting: 106) obtained, and breakthrough of [195m]Mercury (calibrator setting: 521). Prior to use of a generator for clinical study, the activity of [195m]Gold in the eluate is to be measured 15 sec after elution because this represents the approximate time at which the radioactive bolus is injected in a patient. Furthermore, the amount of [195m]Mercury breakthrough in the eluate is measured 15 min after elution. A typical prototype generator contained approximately 170 mCi of [195m]Mercury on the column. At 15 sec after elution, the amount of [195m]Gold ranged from 37 to 60 mCi (mean 23 ± 8), depending on the day after calibration. The yield of [195m]Gold at the time of elution, therefore, was 39 ± 6% (expressed as percent of [195m]Gold activity on the generator). The [195m]Mercury breakthrough per 2 ml of eluate ranged from 5 to 50 µCi (mean 32 ± 12 µCi). The yield of [195m]Gold and the breakthrough of [195m]Mercury was stable for the prototype generators over a period of 7 days. The human radiation dose was estimated on the basis of biodistribution studies of [195m]Mercury and its descendents [195m]Gold, [195]Mercury and [195]Gold in animals at 48 hours after injection (1,6,7). The target organ for [195m]Mercury and its products are the kidneys which receive 0.017 rads per µCi of [195m]Mercury (1). Comparative dosimetric values for [195m]Gold and Tc[99m] are shown in table 2. To limit radiation dose to the kidneys to 5 rad, as recommended by U.S. Food and Drug Administration guidelines, the maximum amount of [195m]Mercury than can be injected in a patient should not exceed 295 µCi. Therefore, the total number of sequential injections permitted per patient ranged from 6 to 95 (mean 10 ± 4).

[195m]Gold first-pass angiocardiography

The most promising and most logical application of this new ultra-short-lived radioisotope is first-pass angiocardiography. The first preliminary experimental and clinical results have been reported by our group and also by others (1,2,8-11). Compared to studies with Tc[99m], considerable reduction in

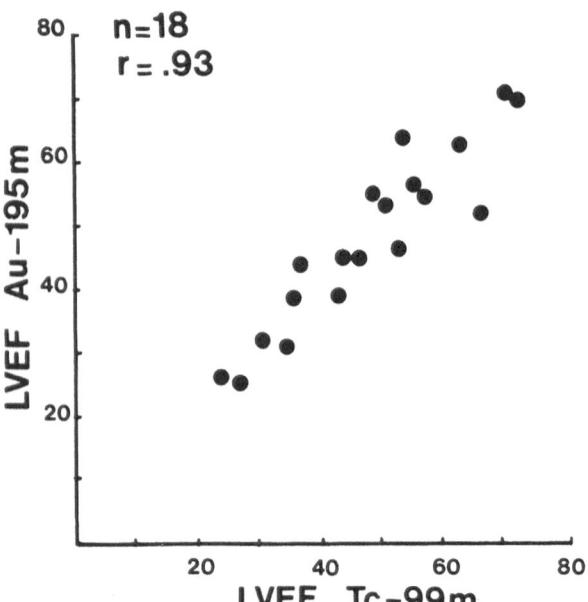

Fig. 4. Correlation of left ventricular ejection fraction (LVEF) determined by first-pass angiocardiography with Tc99m and 195mGold (195mAu)
in 18 patients.

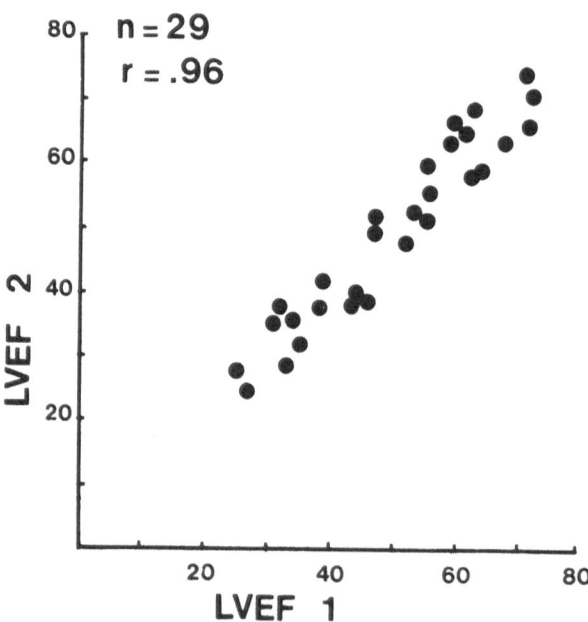

Fig. 5. Reproducibility of left ventricular ejection fraction (LVEF)
determined twice with 195mGold (195mAu) by first-pass angiocardiography.

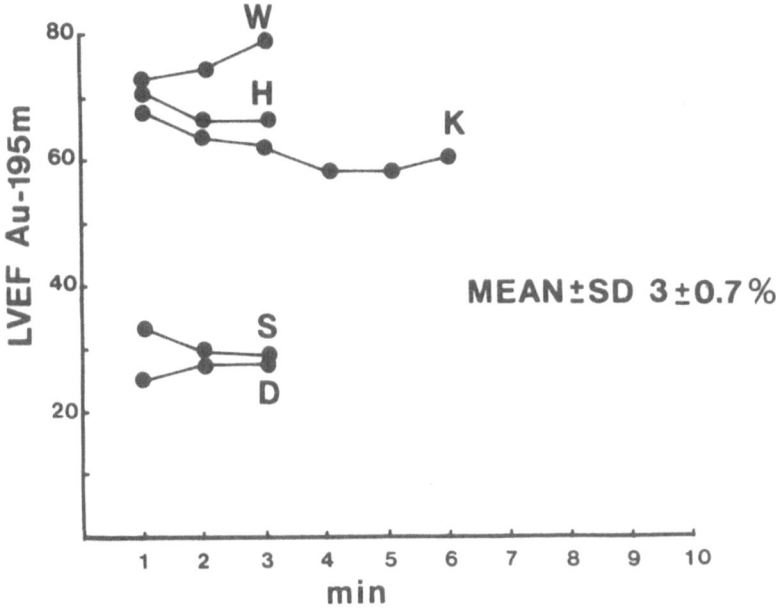

Fig. 6. Reproducibility of rapid sequential determinations (1-min intervals of left ventricular ejection fraction (LVEF) with 195mGold (195mAu) in 5 patients. The mean interstudy difference was 3 ± 0.7%.

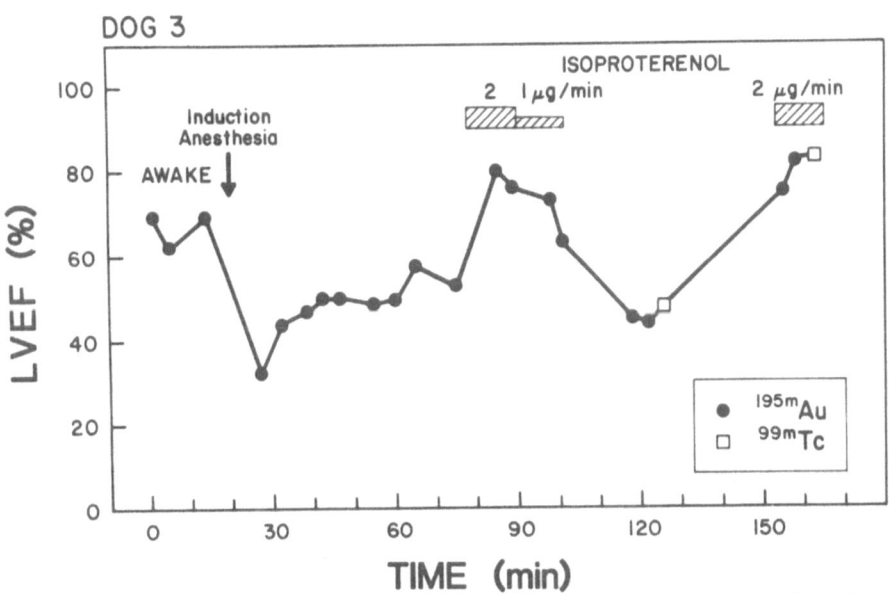

Fig. 7. Rapid serial assessments of left ventricular ejection fraction (LVEF) using 195mGold (195mAu) in an experimental animal. Rapid changes in LVEF by induction of anesthesia with chlorose-urethane and isoproterenol unfusion can be demonstrated. Note the good reproducibility during stable phases and the excellent agreement with LVEF determinations using Tc99m. (Reproduced with permission from Ref. 1).

patient radiation dose per study can be achieved (1). Of practical importance is that the short half-life of the radioisotope
allows for rapid serial assessment of left ventricular ejection
fraction. The background build-up of radioactivity between
serial studies is minimal. This background activity is mainly
from accumulation of ^{195m}Mercury in subdiaphragmatic organs.
Employing a multicrystal gamma camera, first-pass studies with
^{195m}Gold were of excellent quality, indistinguishable from
those with Tc^{99m}. There was good temporal separation of the
right and left heart phases during the first transit of radioactive bolus through the central circulation. The mean (±
standard deviation) count rate acquired in the whole field of
view, uncorrected for decay, during the left ventricular phase
of the bolus was 211,128 ± 13,271 counts per sec (166 studies).
The mean count rate in the end-diastolic region of interest
over the left ventricle, decay and background corrected, was
9,326 ± 1,056 counts. These count rates are equal to, or
slightly greater than those obtained with 15 mCi of Tc^{99m}:
182,462 ± 12,260 counts per second in the whole field of view
during the left ventricular phase and 4,260 ± 728 counts in
the end-diastolic region of interest over the left ventricle.
As mentioned above, the background build-up during sequential
studies using ^{195m}Gold was negligible, ranging from 3-12 percent of counts in the end-diastolic region of interest.

Left ventricular ejection fraction at rest assessed with
Tc^{99m}-DTPA and ^{195m}Gold correlated well (r = 0.93) in 18
patients who had both studies (fig 4). The absolute mean interstudy difference was 4 ± 4%. Mean left ventricular ejection
fraction with Tc^{99m} was 47 ± 14% and with ^{195m}Gold 47 ± 14%.
Repeat left ventricular ejection fraction determined by consecutive ^{195m}Gold studies also corresponded closely (r = 0.96)
in 29 patients (fig 5). The absolute mean interstudy difference
was 4 ± 2%. Mean left ventricular fraction was 50 ± 14%, respectively. In 5 patients, who had multiple determinations of
left ventricular ejection fraction at rest with ^{195m}Gold at
one-minute intervals, the mean absolute interstudy difference
between concecutive studies was 3 ± 0.7% (fig 6).

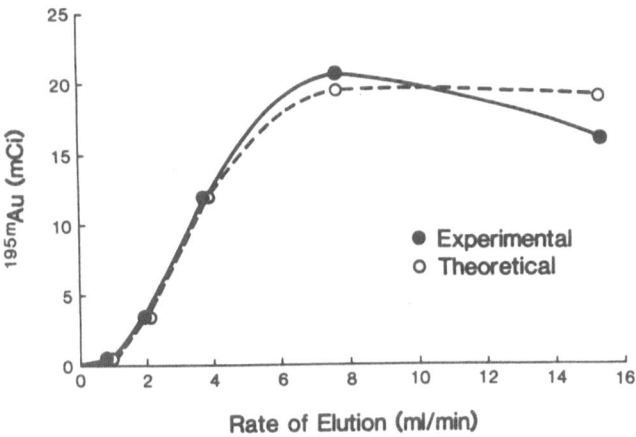

Fig. 8. The yield of ^{195m}Gold (^{195m}Au) by continuous elution of the generator is a function of the rate of elution. At any rate of elution, a steady state of ^{195m}Gold activity is achieved after 1-2 min. The highest possible yield is obtained at an elution rate of 7.6 ml/min.

In experimental animals, we demonstrated the feasibility of obtaining multiple determinations of left ventricular ejection fraction with ^{195m}Gold first-pass studies at rest and during a variety of physiologic and pharmacologic interventions (fig 7) (1). This approach will be particularly relevant clinically in evaluating patients whose hemodynamic status is changing rapidly, such as those experiencing cardiac reflex events. This new radionuclide also makes it possible to monitor cardiac performance frequently over a prolonged period of time, a feature that may be desirable in the acute phase of myocardial infarction.

Continuous elution of the ^{195m}Mercury/^{195m}Gold generator

Since conventional single crystal gamma camera's are limited in count rate capability, this equipment is not ideally suited for performing first-pass studies. For example, typical count rates obtained in the left ventricular enddiastolic region of interest employing a single-crystal gamma camera range from 500-1000 counts, whereas using a multicrystal count density is considerably higher, ranging from 4000 to 8000 counts.

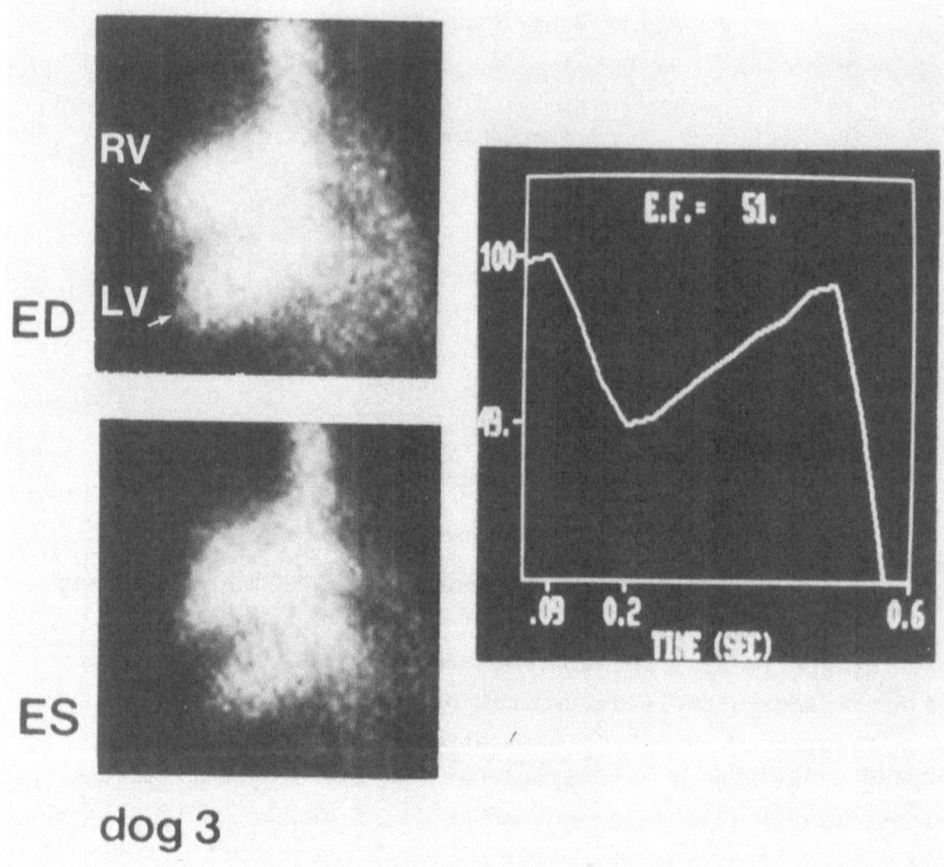

dog 3

Fig. 9. Gated cardiac blood-pool imaging with 195mGold by continuous elution of the generator. The study is performed in a closed-chest dog. End-diastole (ED) and end-systole (ES) of right (R) and left (L) ventricle (V) are shown at the left. At the right, the time-activity curve is shown from which left ventricular ejection fraction (EF) was calculated (51%).

Since the statistical error in calculation of ejection fraction is inversely related to count density obtained, we explored the feasibility of obtaining higher count rates by continuous elution of the generator for imaging with a single crystal gamma camera. The yield of ^{195m}Gold activity by continuous elution of the generator is a function of the rate of elution. The highest yield and steady state is achieved at an elution rate of approximately 7.5 ml per min (fig 8). In contrast, the ^{195m}Mercury breakthrough per volume unit of eluate is constant

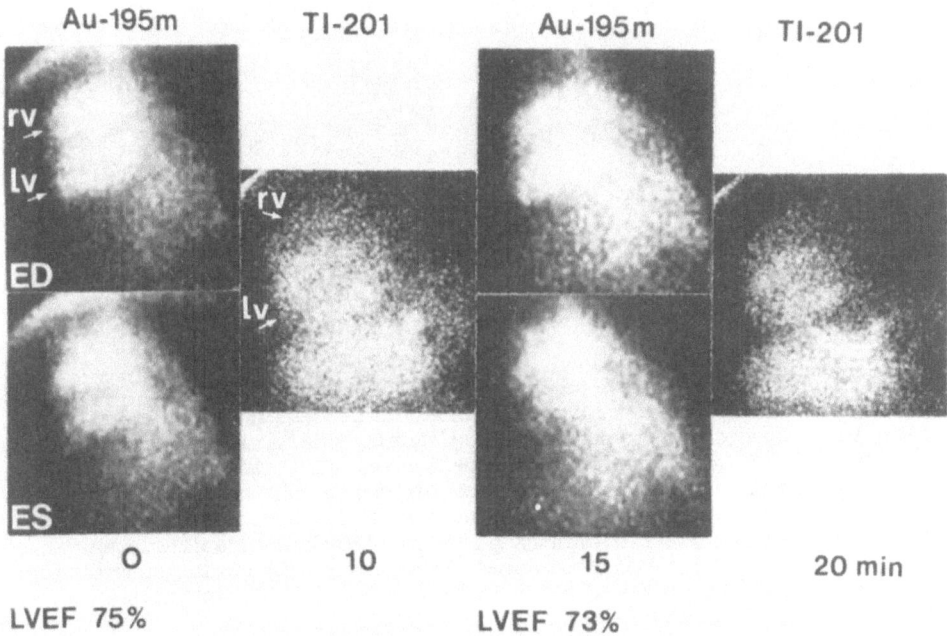

Fig. 10. Alternating 5 min ^{195m}Gold (^{195m}Au) gated cardiac blood-pool imaging and 10 min ^{201}Tl myocardial imaging in an experimental closed-chest dog. Left ventricular ejection fraction (LVEF) is reproducibly calculated. ^{201}Tl myocardial images are unaffected by continuous infusion of ^{195m}Au. ED= end-diastole; ES= end-systole; RV= right ventricular; LV= left ventricular.

and independent of the rate of elution. Therefore, performing continuous elution of the generator in patients, the breakthrough of ^{195m}Mercury per ml of eluate should be measured. The maximal volume of eluate (containing 295 µCi of ^{195m} Mercury) that can be administered to a patient can then be calculated. For individual generators, this varied in our experience from a total volume of 12 ml to 120 ml and, accordingly, the maximum infusion time from 2 to 7 min.

208

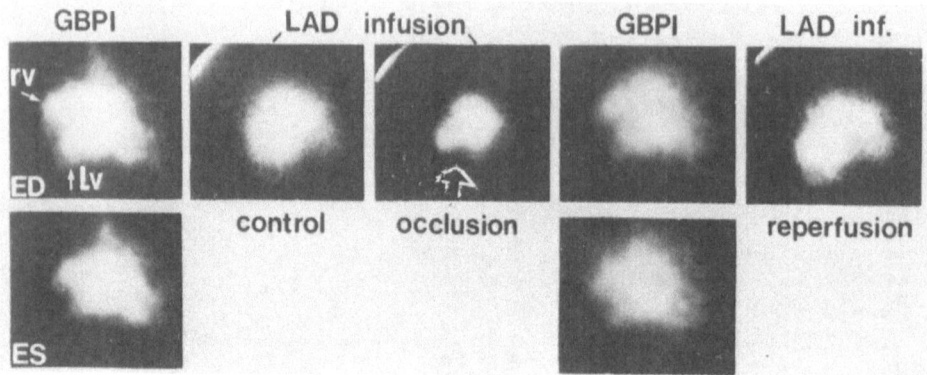

Fig. 11. Gated cardiac blood-pool imaging (GBPI) with 195mGold, alternated
with infusion of 195mGold in the left anterior descending (LAD) coronary
artery in an open-chest experimental dog. During GBPI, right (R) and left
(L) ventricle (V) are visualized in end-diastole (ED) and end-systole (ES).
During LAD infusion, the distribution of blood-flow of the LAD is shown
(control). After occlusion of the LAD with a snare, a wedge-shaped defect
(open arrow) in the distribution of LAD blood-flow can be appreciated.
Subsequent GBPI shows a moderate anterior regional wall motion abnormality.
After release of the snare, the full territory of the LAD again is
visualized by 195mAu LAD infusion.

Intravenous and intracoronary infusion of ^{195m}Gold

Employing continuous elution of the ^{195m}Mercury/^{195m}Gold
generator, two modes of administration were investigated
initially in experimental animals (12,13). Continuous elution
and administration by intravenous route resulted in steady-
state equilibrium blood-pool activity, whereas continuous
elution by intracoronary route resulted in visualization of
the myocardial vascular bed, distal to the perfused coronary
artery (12-14). The short half-life of ^{195m}Gold allows rapid
alternation of these two modes of administration. In addition,
it allows for alternating imaging with radiopharmaceuticals
with a different predominant energy spectrum, e.g., ^{201}Tl. In
experimental animals, we demonstrated the feasibility of
performing multigated ^{195m}Gold steady-state cardiac blood-pool
imaging, alternated with ^{201}Tl myocardial imaging (figs 9,10)
(13). We also performed alternating ^{195m}Gold cardiac blood-

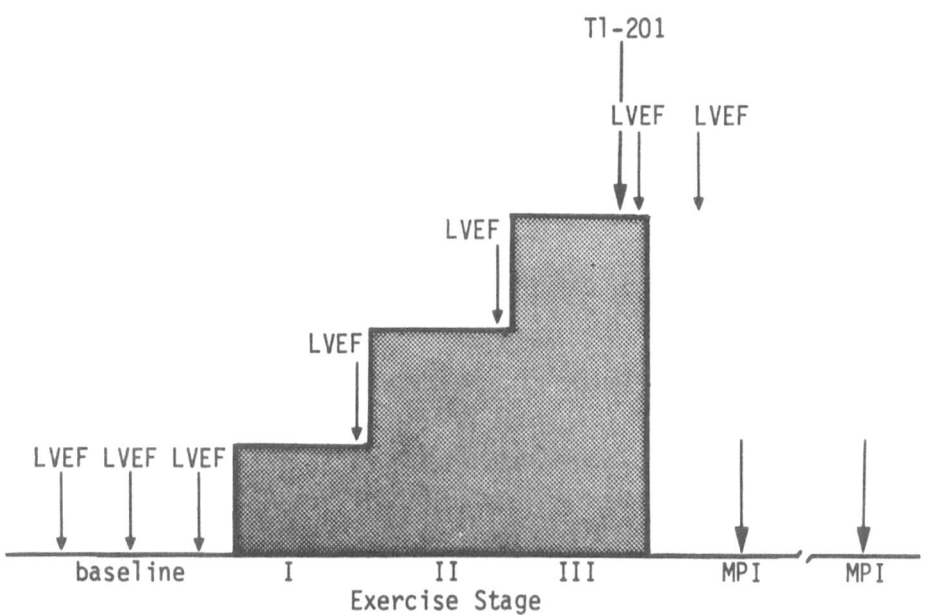

Fig. 12. Protocol of combined ^{195m}Gold and ^{201}Tl stress imaging. Serial baseline left ventricular ejection fraction (LVEF) is determined by ^{195m}Gold first-pass studies on a multicrystal gamma camera. At the end of each 3 min stage of exercise, LVEF is determined. When the patient appears to approach the end point of exercise, ^{201}Tl is injected. The patient is then encouraged to exercise for at least one more minute. At the very peak of exercise, LVEF is determined again, after which the patient stops exercising. Within 1 min of discontinuation of the stress test, LVEF determination is repeated. Subsequently, post-exercise and delayed ^{201}Tl myocardial perfusion imaging (MPI) is performed using a single crystal gamma camera.

pool imaging and ^{195m}Gold selective blood-flow imaging (12). Temporary occlusion of the infused coronary artery resulted in a defect on the intracoronary infusion images and changes in regional wall motion of the equilibrium cardiac blood-pool images (fig 11). In addition, we explored the feasibility of visualizing myocardial perfusion by continuous infusion in the aortic root as was described using ^{81m}Kr by Selwyn et al (15). It appears, however, that the 30.6 sec half-life of ^{195m}Gold is too long for this purpose. After 1 to 2 min of aortic root infusion, we obtained equilibrium cardiac blood-pool images, rather than visualization of myocardial perfusion.

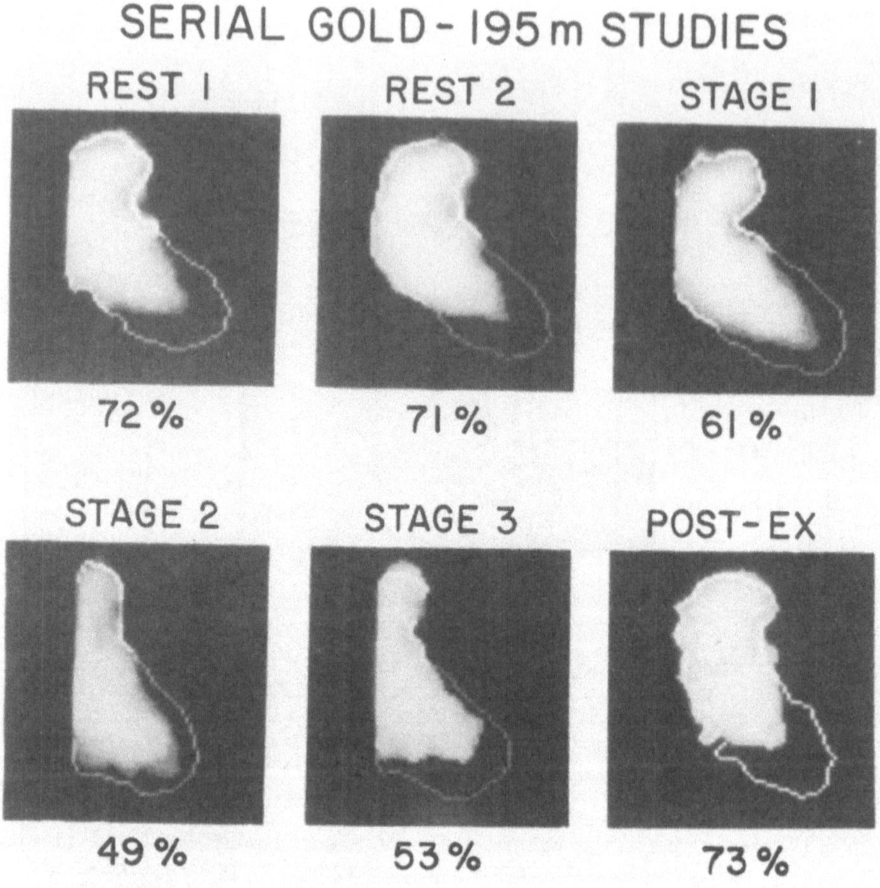

210

SERIAL GOLD-195m STUDIES

Fig. 13. Serial first-pass radionuclide angiocardiography with 195mGold in a patient. The end-systolic images are superimposed over the end-diastolic outlines. At rest, left ventricular ejection fraction (LVEF) is stable: 72%, 71%. During exercise, LVEF decreases gradually and is 53% at peak (stage 3) of exercise. Within 1 min after termination of exercise (Post-Ex), LVEF has returned to baseline value. (Reproduced with permission from Ref. 2).

Clinical studies with 195mGold

Serial first-pass radionuclide angiocardiography. The short half-life of 195mGold permits the performance of sequential first-pass radionuclide angiocardiography. In 25 patients with known or suspected coronary artery disease, 195mGold first-pass studies were obtained with a computerized multi-crystal gamma camera at rest, at the end of each 3 min stage

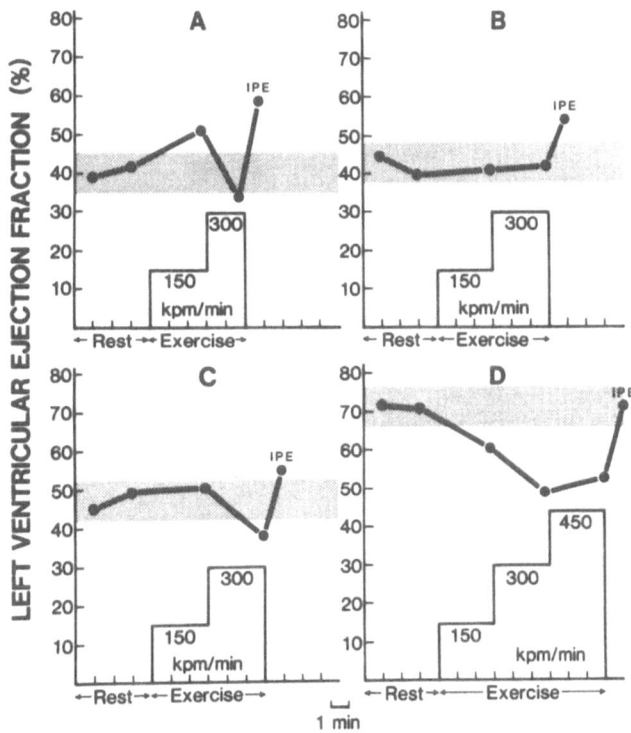

Fig. 14. Examples of patterns (A,B,C,D) of abnormal left ventricular reserve observed in patients with coronary artery disease. The shaded zone indicated the anticipated variability of 5% absolute in either direction of left ventricular ejection fraction at rest. Changes beyond this zone are significant changes. Left ventricular ejection fraction (LVEF) at rest, at the end of each stage of exercise, and immediately post-exercise (IPE) is shown. The exercise level is indicated as kpm/min. Pattern A: Initial increase of LVEF followed by a decrease of LVEF, compared to maximal value. Pattern B: No change in LVEF during exercise. Pattern C: No change in LVEF during initial submaximal phases of exercise followed by a decrease. Pattern D: Progressive decrease of LVEF during exercise. (Reproduced with permission from Ref. 2).

EXERCISE

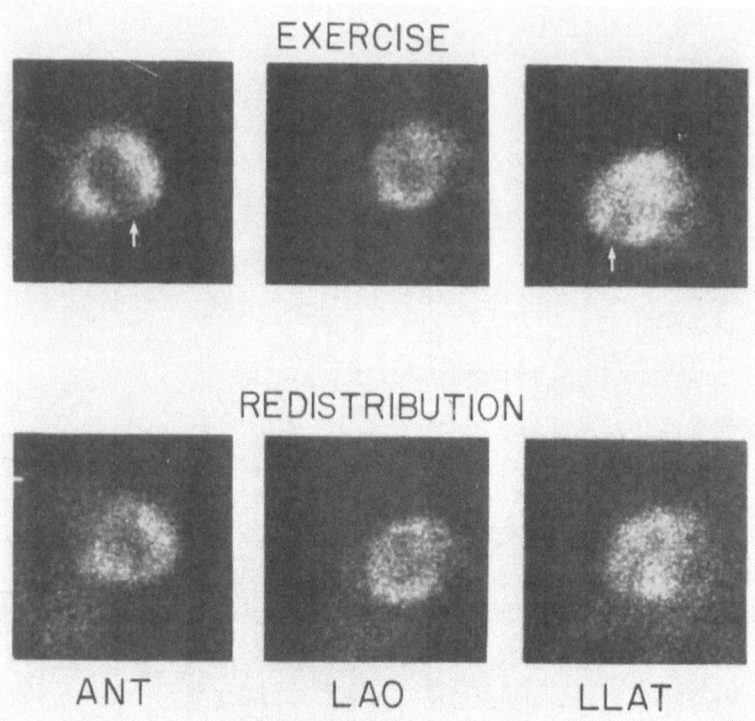

REDISTRIBUTION

ANT   LAO   LLAT

Fig. 15. ^{201}Tl myocardial stress scintigraphy in a patient who received 7 injections of ^{195m}Gold during the stress test. The ^{201}Tl images are of good quality showing an inferoapical perfusion defect (arrows) immediately after exercise, which fills in at delayed (redistribution) imaging. ANT= anterior. LAO= left-anterior-oblique. LLAT= left-lateral. (Reproduced with permission from Ref. 2).

of exercise, and immediately after exercise (2). In 13 patients, assessment of left ventricular function during exercise with ^{195m}Gold was combined with ^{201}Tl stress scintigraphy (fig 12). In this group of patients, 21 exercised to symptom-limited fatique. 4 patients discontinued exercise because of angina pectoris; 8 patients (including 3 with angina) had ischemic electrocardiographic response (>1 mm) horizontal ST-segment depression). Fig 13 shows a representative example of sequential first-pass studies with ^{195m}Gold in a patient.

Comparing mean resting left ventricular ejection fraction with ejection fraction at peak exercise, abnormal exercise left ventricular reserve was demonstrated in 20 of 25 patients.

THALLIUM-201
Routine   After Au-195m

LAO

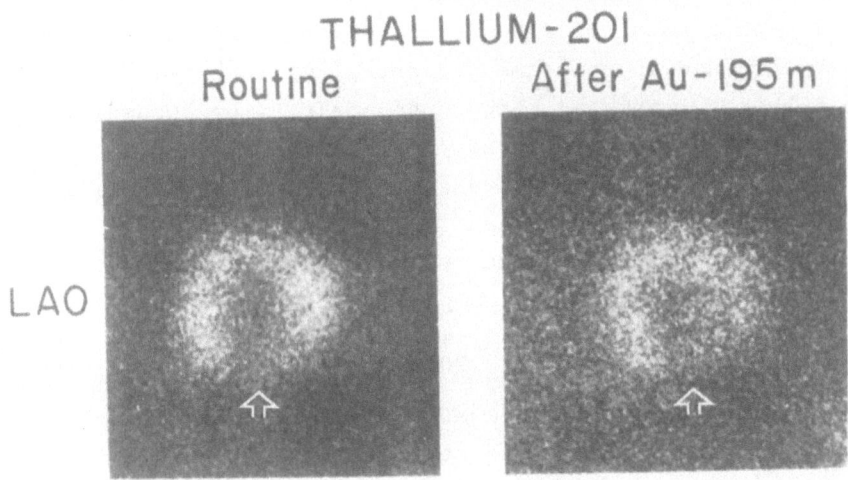

Fig. 16. ^{201}Tl stress scintigraphy in a patient who received a total of 12 injections of ^{195m}Gold (^{195m}Au) containing a total of 250 µCi of ^{195m}Mercury, prior to ^{201}Tl imaging (right). A stress-induced infero-apical defect is present. At the left for comparison, a ^{201}Tl stress image in the same patient (same workload and heart rate) without pre-ceding injections of ^{195m}Gold. Although there is increased background activity from accumulated ^{195m}Mercury, both images are of diagnostic quality. (Reproduced with permission from Ref. 2).

In this relatively small number of patients, various abnormal patterns were observed, illustrating the diagnostic potential of serial studies during exercise (fig 14). Interestingly, in 12 of the patients with an abnormal functional response and 4 of those with normal response, left ventricular ejection fraction immediately after exercise was significantly (<0.01) greater than at rest. The multiple ^{195m}Gold first-pass studies prior to myocardial imaging with ^{201}Tl, did not affect the diagnostic quality of analog ^{201}Tl images. Nevertheless, after administration of eluate, there was measureable background activity in the 80 keV ^{201}Tl window, originating from ^{195m} Mercury breakthrough accumulated in the kidneys and liver.

In the whole field of view 380 cpm/μCi of ^{195m}Mercury injected
was measured. Fig 15 shows excellent quality ^{201}Tl images
in a patient who received 7 injections of ^{195m}Gold. Fig 16
compares a ^{201}Tl image after a total of 12 injections of
^{195m}Gold and a total of 250 μCi of ^{195m}Mercury administered,
to that obtained in the same patient after routine ^{201}Tl stress
test. Although increased background activity by accumulated
^{195m}Mercury can be appreciated, the ^{201}Tl image is of adequate
diagnostic quality. This extraneous source of radioactivity
should be considered, but quantitative analysis of ^{201}Tl
kinetics should be unaffected, since background activity is
stable over a 2-4 hours period post-exercise. The ^{201}Tl images
were of good technical quality in all 13 patients. In 3 patients
with atypical chest pain, the ^{201}Tl images were entirely normal.
The regional wall motion on exercise ventriculograms in these
patients was also normal. The remaining 10 patients had
abnormal ^{201}Tl images showing evidence of either myocardial
infarction or exercise-induced myocardial ischemia or both. In
all 10 patients, regional left ventricular wall motion was
abnormal during exercise at the anatomic site of ^{201}Tl perfusion
defects.

The results of combined ^{195m}Gold exercise studies and ^{201}Tl
stress scintigraphy illustrate the diagnostic potential of this
method. It is of clinical significance that combined imaging
with ^{195m}Gold and ^{201}Tl allows assessment of both functional
response to exercise and the presence of exercise-induced myocardial hypoperfusion, as well as ^{201}Tl kinetics during a single
exercise session. Once the conventional tracer Tc^{99m} is administered to a patient, ^{201}Tl myocardial imaging generally cannot
be performed for at least 24 hours so that technically acceptable images can be obtained. Several studies have shown the
complimentary value of performing exercise myocardial perfusion
imaging and left ventricular function studies in patients with
coronary artery disease (16-20). By obtaining these studies
simultaneously, they may provide a more reliable assessment
of functional significance of coronary artery stenosis. This
combined technique also has obvious advantages in relation to

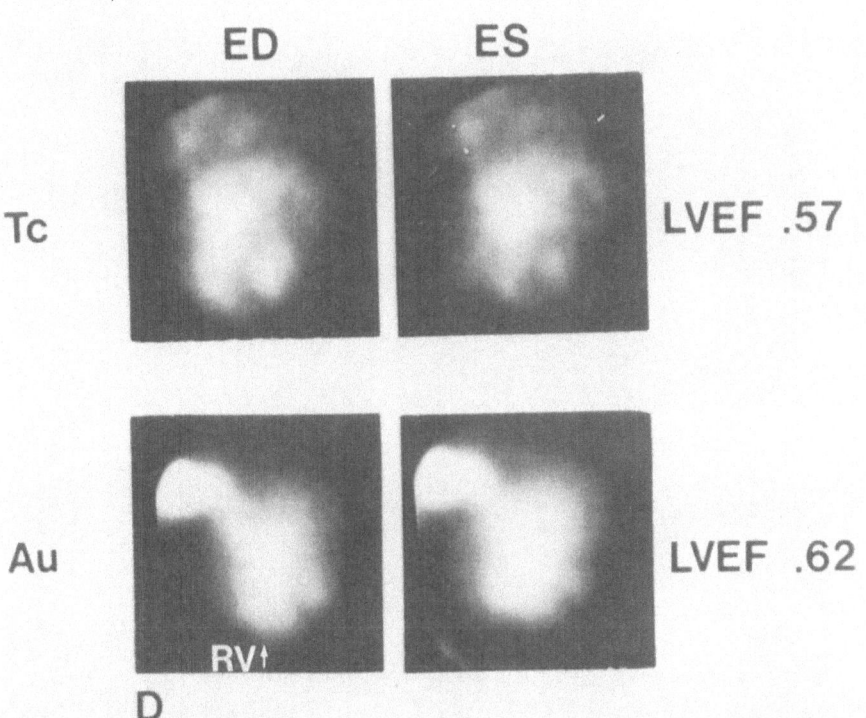

Fig. 17. Multigated cardiac blood-pool imaging (left-anterior-oblique view) with Tc99m-labelled red cells (Tc) and 195mGold continuous infusion (Au) in a patient. The end-diastolic (ED) and the end-systolic (ES) images are shown. Due to the short half-life of 195mGold, the right heart is "hotter" than the left heart. The infusion of 195mGold was performed via the right arm. The entering of 195mGold in the thoracic cavity via the subclavian vein is noted on the Au images as the "hot spot" in the left upper corner. Compared to the Tc image, the Au image shows relatively greater activity in the right ventricle (RV) than the left ventricle. The septum is less well defined in the Au study. Left ventricular ejection fraction (LVEF), employing standard processing techniques, shows good agreement in this patient with normal cardiac function.

cost-effectiveness of patient evaluation because only one exercise test is needed to obtain this information. Even with the development of new Tc99m-labelled myocardial perfusion imaging agents, this combined approach will be feasible because of the difference in primary photopeak of the radionuclide.

195mGold multigated cardiac blood-pool imaging

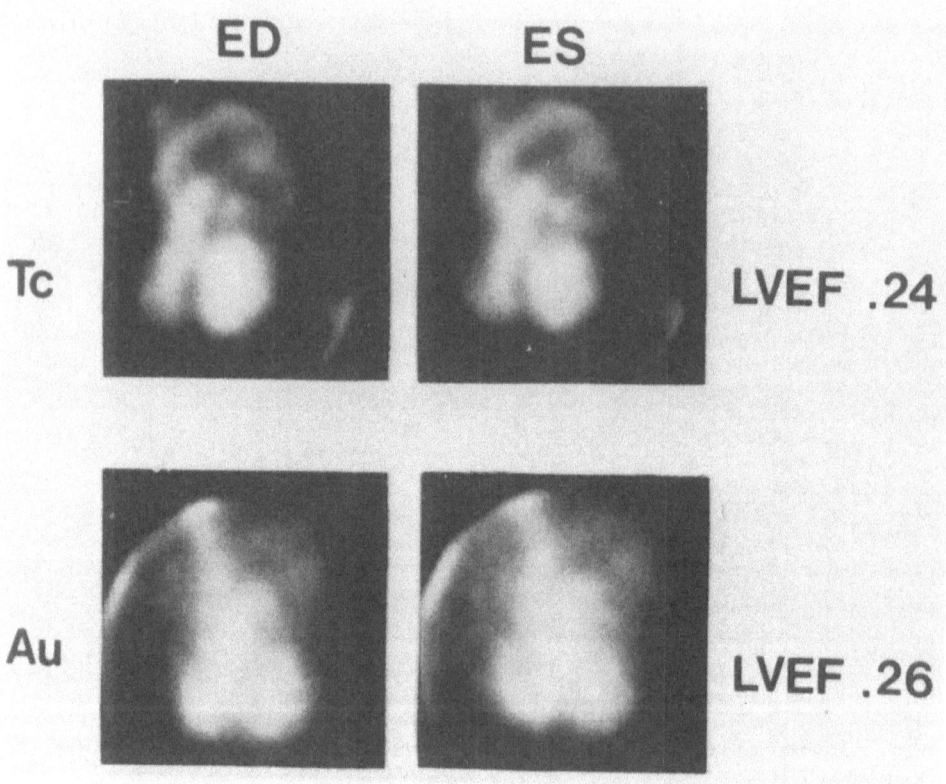

ED   ES

Tc   LVEF .24

Au   LVEF .26

Fig. 18. Multigated cardiac blood-pool imaging in the left anterior position with Tc99m (Tc) and 195mGold (Au). The format is the same as in fig 17. In this patient with poor left ventricular function, calculation of LVEF with either radionuclide agrees closely.

Employing continous i.v. infusion of 195mGold at 7.5 ml/ min, we performed multigated cardiac blood-pool imaging in 15 patients (14). Excellent count rates were obtained in end-diastole (11,122 ± 4,837 counts), using 5 min acquisitions with a single crystal camera equipped with medium energy collimator. The images were of good quality and showed typically more radioactivity in the right ventricle than in the left ventricle with minimal subdiaphragmatic activity (fig 17,18). Left ventricular ejection fraction calculated in the usual manner from 195mGold studies correlated well (r= 0.80)

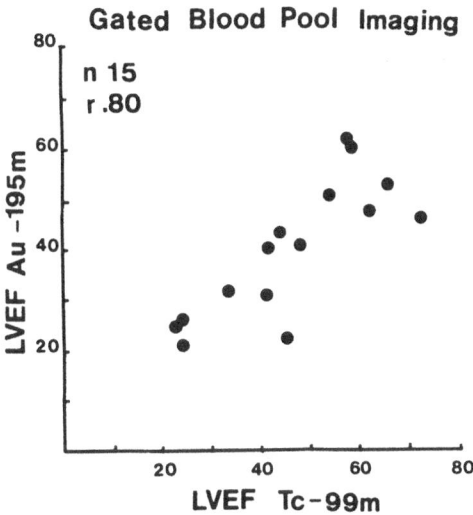

Fig. 19. Left ventricular ejection fraction (LVEF) determined by gated cardiac blood-pool imaging using Tc99m-labelled red cells (Tc-99m) and 195mGold continuous infusion (Au-195m).

with multigated Tc99m cardiac blood-pool imaging (fig 19). Also, regional wall motion analysis of the 195mGold equilibrium studies agreed closely with that of Tc99m studies. In 5 patients, rapidly alternating 195mGold gated cardiac blood-pool studies and 201Tl myocardial perfusion imaging was performed (fig 20). Thus, gated cardiac blood-pool imaging with 195mGold is feasible in patients using continuous generator elution and a conventional single crystal gamma camera. Intermittent discontinuation of infusion allows concomitment serial 201Tl myocardial imaging. Thus, also employing this alternative mode of administration, the physical properties of 195mGold make alternating assessment of both left ventricular function and myocardial perfusion possible.

Future for 195mGold angiocardiography
Our excellent results with both 195mGold first-pass radio-nuclide angiocardiography and 195mGold equilibrium cardiac blood-pool imaging have been reproduced and confirmed by other investigators (8-11). Presently (July, 1983)., approximately

218

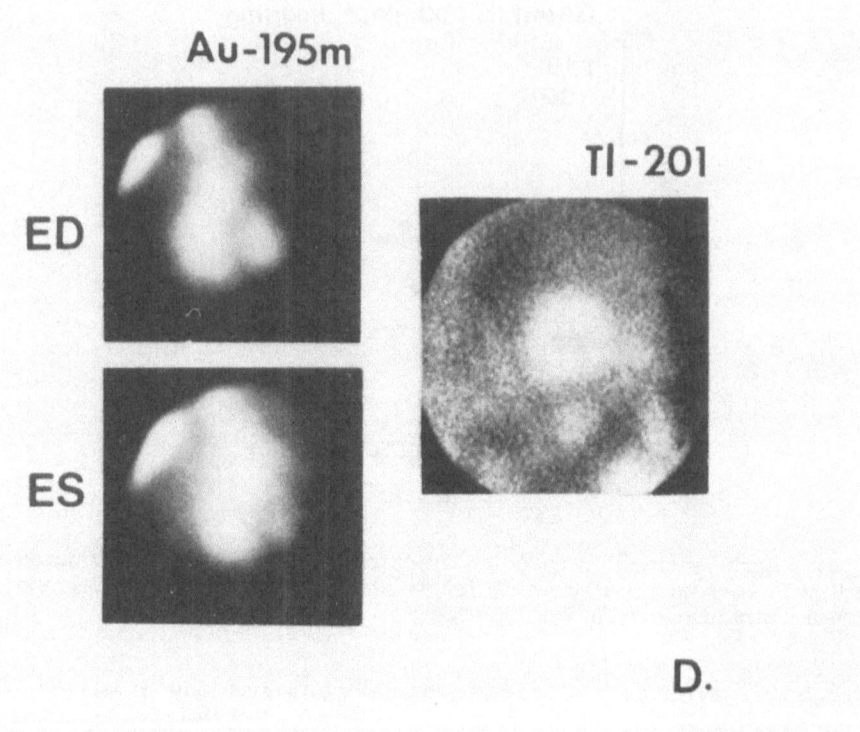

Au-195m

ED

ES

Tl-201

D.

Fig. 20. Alternating ^{195m}Gold (Au-195m) gated cardiac blood-pool imaging and ^{201}Tl myocardial imaging at rest in a patient with normal left ventricular function. Good quality images are obtained with both radioisotopes. The ^{201}Tl image is of good quality, and apparently unaffected by the infusion of ^{195m}Gold for 5 min shortly before myocardial imaging.

500-600 patients have been studied at various centers. It is beyond question that the most promising application is that of first-pass studies combined with myocardial perfusion imaging in patients suspected of coronary artery disease. In addition, when rapid changes in left ventricular function are anticipated, such as during exercise, cold pressor test, or pharmacologic interventions, ^{195}Gold is an ideal imaging agent for rapid sequential assessment of cardiac performance. Schad et al (21) recently have demonstrated in patients that coronary blood-flow can be visualized by intracoronary injection of ^{195m}Gold. functional images, displaying appearance and disappearance time of the radionuclide, potentially provide similar information as has been reported using digital contrast radiography. The obvious advantage of a radionuclide method is that, contrary to X-ray contrast material, no pharmacologic effect on the coronary vasculature precludes reliable serial assessments.

For exercise studies, the first-pass technique offers distinct technological advantages over multigated equilibrium cardiac blood-pool imaging. The first-pass data are acquired over a short period of time and left ventricular ejection fraction is derived from 3 to 5 cardiac cycles. Therefore, first-pass left ventricular ejection fraction reflects more accurately left ventricular function at a distinct point in time during exercise, than multigated equilibrium ejection fraction which is acquired over several hundred heartbeats and represents a "average" value. With the expected technical improvement of gamma camera's permitting acquisition of higher count rates, the first-pass technique may well become the method of choice for performing cardiac studies during exercise. Medium-energy collimation, detector shielding, and adequate crystal thickness to maintain both intrinsic resolution and sensitivity will be additional requirements to use the new generation camera's for ^{195m}Gold studies.

220

REFERENCES

1. Wackers FJTh, Giles RW, Hoffer PB, Lange RC, Berger HJ, Zaret BL, Gold-195m, a new generator-produced short-lived radionuclide for sequential assessment of ventricular performance by first-pass radionuclide angiocardiography. Amer. J. Cardiol. 50:89, 1982.

2. Wackers FJTH, Stein R, Pytlik L, Plankey MW, Lange R, Hoffer PB, Sands MJ, Zaret BL, Berger HJ, Gold-195m for serial first pass radionuclide angiocardicgraphy during upright exercise in patients with coronary artery disease. JACC 1, September 1983.

3. Panek KL, Lindeyer J, Van der Vlugt HC, A new generator system for production of short-living Au-195m radioisotope. J. nucl. Med. 23:108, 1982.

4. Brihaye C, Guillaume M, Lavi W, Cogneau M, Development of a reliable Hg-195m/Au-195m generator for the production of Au-195m, a short-lived nuclide for vascular imaging. J. nucl. Med. 23:1114, 1982.

5. Bett R, Cuninghame JG, Sims HE, Willis HH, Dymond DS, Flatman W, Stone DL, Elliott AJ, Development and use of the Hg 195m-Au 195m generator for first pass radionuclide angiography of the heart. J. Lab. Comp. Radiopharm. 19:1444, 1983.

6. Lange RC, Wackers FJ, Giles RW, Hoffer PB, Berger HJ, Zaret BL, Dosimetry for Hg-195m and its descendants. J. nucl. Med. 23:87, 1982.

7. Ackers JG, De Jong RBJ, Arnhem TNO, Dosimetry consequences of eluates from Hg-195m/Au-195m. J. nucl. Med. 23:68, 1982.

8. Fazio F, Gerundini P, Maseri A, Giardi M, Margonato A, Aiazzi L, Fregoso A, Milanesi L, Bencivelli W, Clinical assessment of left ventricular ejection fraction with short-lived 195m-Au. J. nucl. Med. Allied Sci. 26:105, 1982.

9. Schon HR, Schad N, Nickel O, Breit A, Blomer H, Au-195: A promising new agent for first-pass radionuclide angiography (FPRNA) in man. Circulation 66:351, 1982.

10. Mena I, Narahara KA, De Jong R, Maublant J, Gold-195m, an ultra-short-lived generator-produced radionuclide: Clinical application in sequential first pass ventriculography. J. nucl. Med. 24:139, 1983.

11. Dymond DS, Elliot AT, Flatnan W, Stone D, Bett R, Cuninghame G, Sims H, The clinical validation of Gold-195m: A new short half-life radio-pharmaceutical for rapid, sequential, first-pass angiocardiography in patients. JACC 1:85, 1983.

12. Wackers FJTh, Various modes of administration of Gold-195m. Potential clinical applications. Proceedings of International Symposium on Short-lived Radionuclides. ACNP, Washington DC, 1983, (in press).

13. Giles R, Hoffer P, Lange R, Zaret B, Wachers F, Serial alternating assessment of ventricular performance and myocardial perfusion using Gold-195m and Thallium-201. J. nucl. Med. 23:80, 1982.

14. Wackers FJ, Giles R, Hoffer P, Lange R, Plankey M, Berger HJ, Zaret BL, Rapidly alternating gated cardiac blood-pool and myocardial perfusion imaging using Gold-195m and Thallium-201. J. nucl. Med. 24:76, 1983.

15. Selwyn AP, Fox U, Shillingford JP, Myocardial imaging with extractable cations and inert tracers: The effects of flow and metabolism. Clin. Cardiol. 1:60, 1978.

16. Caldwell JH, Hamilton GW, Sorensen SG, Ritchie JL, Williams DL, Kennedy JW, The detection of coronary artery disease with radio-nuclide techniques: A comparison of rest-exercise thallium imaging and ejection fraction response. Circulation 61:610, 1980.

17. Johnstone DE, Sands MJ, Berger HJ, Reduto LA, Lachman AS, Wackers FJTh, Cohen LS, Gottschalk A, Zaret BL, Comparison of exercise radionuclide angiocardiography and thallium-201 myocardial perfusion imaging in coronary artery disease. Amer. J. Cardiol. 45:1113, 1980.

18. Elkayam U, Weinstein M, Berman D, Maddahi J, Staniloff H, Freeman M, Waxman A, Swan HJC, Forrester J, Stress thallium-201 myocardial scintigraphy and exercise technetium ventriculography in the detection and location of chronic coronary artery disease: Comparison of sensitivity and specificity of these noninvasive tests alone and in combination. Amer. Heart J. 101:657, 1981.

19. Kirschenbaum HD, Okada RD, Boucher CA, Kushner FG, Strauss HW, Pohost GM, Relationship of thallium-201 myocardial perfusion pattern to regional and global left ventricular function with exercise. Amer. Heart J. 101:734, 1981.

20. Tubau J, Witztum K, Froelicher V, Jensen D, Atwood E, McKirnan D, Reynolds J, Asburn W, Noninvasive assessment of changes in myo-cardial perfusion and ventricular performance following exercise training. Amer. Heart J. 104:238, 1982.

21. Shad N, Schon HR, Nichel O, Breit A, Blomer H, Gold-195m for first-pass radioangiocardiography and intracoronary administration. Proceedings of the International Symposium on short-lived Radio-nuclides. ACNP, Washington DC, 1983, (in press).

III. MYOCARDIAL PERFUSION

DIAGNOSTIC UTILITY OF Tl^{201} IMAGING

R. SCHMOLINER, R. DUDCZAK

INTRODUCTION

Since its introduction into medical diagnosis, Tl^{201} scintigraphy has provided important information concerning the non-invasive assessment of myocardial perfusion. The technique has been demonstrated to be of major importance in patients with suspected and documented coronary artery disease and provided also useful information in a variety of other cardiac disorders like cardiomyopathy, valve disease, right ventricular hypertrophy, and cardiac involvement in systemic diseases like sarcoidosis (1-19). The major clinical application of Tl^{201} imaging was reported in the field of coronary artery disease. In comparison to older noninvasive diagnostic tests considering ECG changes during exercise, Tl^{201} scintigraphy in combination with stress procedures has yielded high values of sensitivity and specificity in the detection of patients with coronary artery disease. Apart from the usual form of physical stress applying bicycle or treadmill exercise, the potential value of Tl^{201} imaging has been considerably increased by the possibility to provoke stress conditions using high doses of intravenously given dipyridamole. This special type of stress is regarded as an important alternative in many patients unable to exercise adequately (20-28). As our group has gained great experience with Tl^{201} imaging following dipyridamole, the following paper will primarily focus on the description of our findings with this technique in patients with suspected or known coronary artery disease (27,28).

Method

Background. Tl^{201} which was first introduced into medical diagnosis in 1973 by Lebowitz is a potassium analog with a physical half life of 74 hours (29). After intravenous injection the isotope distributes over the body as a function of distribution of cardiac output (4). Since the myocardium receives approximately 5% of the cardiac output and myocardial extraction fraction for Thallium is around 87% in the initial distribution phase, approximately 4% of the injected Tl^{201} goes to the heart, with more than 90% in the other body organs which serve as a large reservoir of Thallium outside the heart. The blood acts as the transport vehicle between these 2 compartments. At basic conditions the uptake of Tl^{201} in the heart correlates well with blood-flow, however, at exceedingly high flow levels that are in excess of the myocardial needs, myocardial uptake of Tl^{201} is no longer linearly related to blood-flow implying a progressive decrease in extraction fraction (4,23,24). This characteristic feature must be taken into account in Tl^{201} imaging following coronary vasodilation by dipyridamole.

When injected at rest conditions Tl^{201} reflects myocardial perfusion and viability at rest, injection of the tracer at stress conditions provides information about perfusion and viability under stress. Hypoperfused regions do not take up Tl^{201} adequately which is visualized by a scintigraphic defect. During the following hours of the redistribution phase Tl^{201} enters the myocardium from the systemic pool and it also washes out of the myocardium. Based on these findings, Tl^{201} defects in the initial scintigrams may be categorized as reversible and irreversible. The irreversible process is usually associated with the presence of myocardial scars, reversible defects are related with the presence of viable, but under stress conditions hypoperfused myocardium. Thus single-dose Tl^{201} imaging following stress with redistribution imaging some, preferably 4 - hours later provides diagnostic information about myocardial perfusion and viability during both stress and rest conditions.

Tl^{201} decays by electron capture to Hg^{201} emitting X-rays of 69-83 KeV and gamma rays of 167 KeV and 135 KeV. For clinical Tl^{201} imaging the energy window is a 20% window centered on the Hg^{201} X-ray photopeak (4). A low energy, parallel hole, all purpose collimator ensures satisfactory imaging results, a conventional gamma camera system (either large field of view or mobile) with the dedicated computer systems was used in our studies reported below.

Some authors have described the use of special collimators, like 7 pin hole, additionally single photon emission computed tomography (SPECT) has been regarded to be of potential value (19,22). However, at present time it appears that SPECT offers little additional benefit compared with planar Thallium imaging as the increased cost of a SPECT system should be taken into account as discussed recently (19).

Stress protocols in Tl^{201} imaging

Dipyridamole as a potent coronary vasodilating agent has been known to provoke ischemic pain and electrocardiographic changes in patients with severe coronary artery stenoses (30-36). This agent can cause a coronary steal phenomenon which has contributed to the change of the indication for intravenous dipyridamole from a therapeutic to an exclusively diagnostic one. The possibility to use aminophylline i.v. as a specific and immediate antagonist to dipyridamole increases the safety of the test in clinical practice (37-39). The following protocol has been used by us in a great number of patients:

After an overnight fast the patients are given 0.50 mg dipyridamole per kg bodyweight intravenously within 5-10 min under continuous ECG monitoring in supine position. Immediately thereafter 2 mCi of Tl^{201} is injected. In the cases with severe anginal pain and/or ischemic ST-segment changes 240 mg aminophylline is given 3 min or later after Tl^{201} injection, in few cases nitroglyzerin is necessary in addition to aminophylline to reverse the side effects of dipyridamole. Imaging is started 5 min after Tl^{201} injection with the 45° LAO view

followed by the anterior and left lateral views. A preset
count rate of 500 k or a preset time of 8 min should be chosen
for each projection. 4 hours later redistribution images are
obtained in the same views as before.

Instead of dipyridamole i.v. physical exercise may be
performed. The patients are stressed in supine or sitting
position using either bicycle exercise or treadmill stress
testing according to a standard graded exercise protocol. In
most laboratories a symptom limited protocol is applied exercising the patients until shortness of breath, leg fatigue,
chest pain, or positive ECG response (at least 0.2 mV down-
sloping ST-change) occur. 30-90 sec before the anticipated
end of exercise 2 mCi of Tl^{201} is injected i.v. The imaging
procedure starting 5 min after Tl^{201} injection conforms to the
protocol described above in dipyridamole-Tl^{201} imaging.

Image interpretation

a) Qualitative analysis. Fig 1 demonstrates the 3 conventional views and the division into the typical myocardial segments.
The unprocessed and processed scintigrams are interpreted
visually by at least 2 observers without knowledge of the
clinical and angiographic data of the patients. Each of the
segments is interpreted subjectively and scored according to
a grading system (0 = no activity, 1 = grossly diminished
activity, 2 = slightly diminished activity, 3 = normal activity).

Isolated defects in the apical region are considered a
normal variant. A reversible defect is defined as an increase
in activity from grade 0 or 1 in the initial image to grade
2 or 3 in the delayed image for any ventricular segment except
the apical regions. An irreversible defect is defined as a
stress and delayed grade 0 or 1 defect. Both reversible and
irreversible defects are considered positive for coronary
artery disease, irreversible defects representing a scar and
reversible defects representing transient ischemia. Cases with
disagreement of the observers are conventionally resolved by
consensus or, if still equivocal, by an additional quantitat-

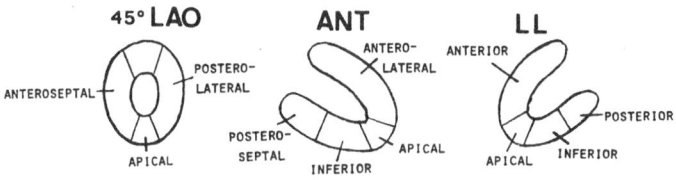

Fig. 1. Schematic representation of myocardial segments in the 3 conventional views (45° LAO, anterior, left lateral).

ive analysis. The anterior, anteroseptal, and anterolateral regions are considered to be supplied by the left anterior descending artery (LAD), the posteroseptal and inferior regions by the right coronary artery, the posterolateral wall is assumed to represent the distribution of the left circumflex artery (12,13,16,40,41).

b) Computer analysis. Computers are playing an increasingly important role in Tl^{201} acquisition, processing, and display (2-4,6,42). Computer processing of the images is directed toward image enhancement and quantitation. The primary method of background subtraction has now become the method first described by Goris as bilinear interpolative background subtraction (43). This technique has been used to correct for the nonuniformity of the background, both spatially and as a function of time. After background subtraction the images are smoothed using a standard algorithm for nine-point weighted averaging. From the smoothed images circumferential maximum count profiles of the myocardial Tl^{201} activity are generated, quantitating the segmental activity as an angular function referenced from the center of the left ventricular cavity 2-4,6,22,44) (fig 2).

The profiles are obtained for the stress and redistribution images and are compared to the statistical limits of normal. In addition to circumferential profiles, regional wash-out rates may be calculated as a percent wash-out from stress to the approximately 4 hour redistribution time (3,4, 44,45). In normal cases regional wash-out rates should be

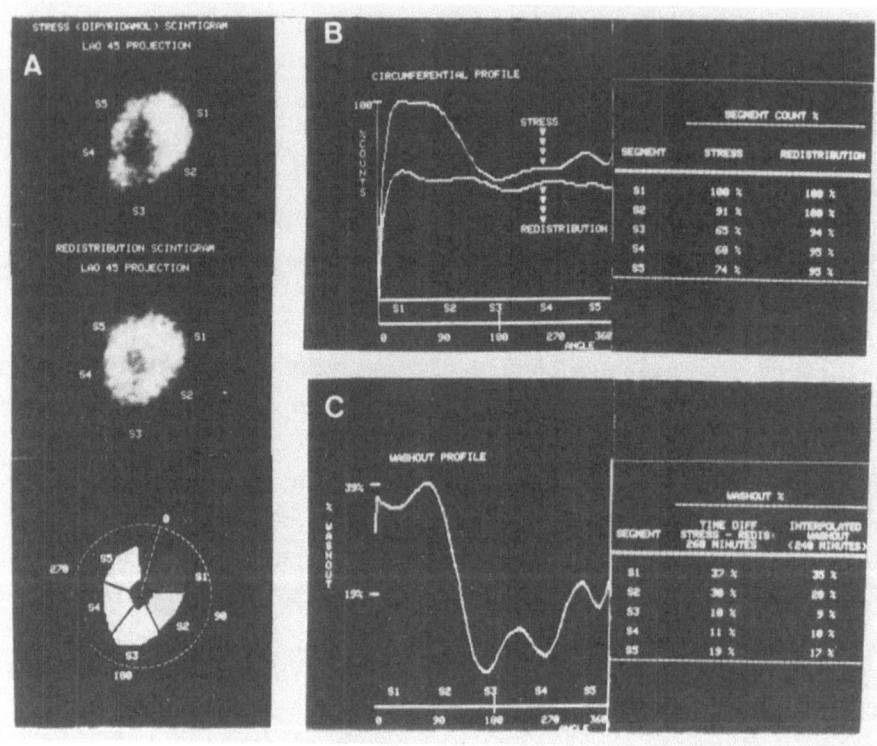

Fig. 2. Example of quantitative Tl201 analysis in a patient with coronary artery disease (100% LAD, 90% LCx, 50% RCA stenoses, normal left ventricle). Data acquisition time 8 min.

A (left panel): Dipyridamole and redistribution images, 45° LAO view, after bilinear interpolative background subtraction. Reversible perfusion defects in the anteroseptal, apicoinferior and lower posterolateral regions. For further analysis the myocardium is subdivided into 5 segments.

B (upper right panel): Circumferential profiles quantitating the segmental activity as an angular function, in addition the relative count rates for each segment compared with the maximum segment are depicted showing markedly reduced count rates in the segments with reversible hypoperfusion.

C (lower right panel): Wash-out profile and segmental wash-out rates. Reduced wash-out in the hypoperfused segments as expected. As the time between stress and redistribution imaging may vary in different patients, the wash-out rates are interpolated to exactly 4 hours assuming a monoexponential decline. Since early redistribution of Tl201 into transiently ischemic regions may occur, imaging should generally start as soon as possible. For wash-out calculations, however, a second LAO view (15-20 min post Tl^{201} injection) should be obtained.

uniform from all myocardial regions. In ischemic regions Tl^{201} wash-out should be reduced which means that myocardial clearance rates are delayed compared with normal regions. Although this approach of Tl^{201} wash-out analysis seems very attractive from theoretical reasons, this technique has to be regarded very cautiously at present because of some major limitations to be discussed.

It has been demonstrated that the reproducibility of Tl^{201} wash-out parameters following dipyridamole studied in the same patient twice at intervals of at least 1 week is within a wide range. The absolute figures of wash-out vary greatly from one study to the repeat study which seems to be a major limitation of this approach (45). Furthermore, the influence of other factors on myocardial Tl^{201} wash-out has been clearly demonstrated. Glucose-insulin-potassium infusion and the ingestion of a high-carbohydrate meal exhibited considerable influence on Tl^{201} wash-out kinetics (46,47). Massie and co-workers have shown that in normal patients myocardial Tl^{201} wash-out is slower when the tracer is injected during submaximal exercise compared to maximum exercise (40). So a number of various factors have been defined which possibly affect Tl^{201} myocardial clearance rates. A comprehensive basic examination in this respect is still lacking which seems, however, necessary before such criteria can be applied to the interpretation of clinical Tl^{201} study results (47).

The major advantage to be expected from quantitative analysis is to minimize some of the problems associated with subjectivity of visual analysis of Tl^{201} scintigrams. It could be demonstrated that quantitation enhances significantly the capability of predicting multivessel disease (4,44). On the other hand, sole reliance on a computer-derived quantitative scan interpretation of Tl^{201} uptake and wash-out parameters may be hazardous, or as it was summarized by Beller in a recent review: Quantitation of images alone does not insure

improved sensitivity and specificity (2). It must be emphasized
that qualitative or visual scrutiny of myocardial images is
necessary for identification of artifacts and normal variations. A basic problem of Tl^{201} imaging is a poor signal-to-
noise ratio and statistical count deficiencies that preclude
reliable identification of diseased arteries (42). In contrast
to positron emission computed tomography, Tl^{201} scintigraphy
is inherently not a quantitative technique so that according
to Gould the method of quantitative Tl^{201} analysis should be
more correctly termed "computer mapping" of conventional
planar data (42).

c) Qualitative versus quantitative analysis of Tl^{201} scintigrams following dipyridamole. In order to study the potential
value of a quantitative analysis including bilinear interpolative background subtraction and circumferential profile
analysis in contrast to a visual, more or less qualitative
analysis, we compared our results in 61 patients refered for
Tl^{201} imaging following dipyridamole i.v. Wash-out analysis
was not included in this comparison because of the limitations
cited above.

48 patients had angiographically proven coronary artery
disease (1-vessel-disease n=16, 2-vessel-disease n=16, 3-
vessel-disease n=16). Positive scintigraphic results (reversible or irreversible perfusion defects) were found in 38
patients (79%) by qualitative analysis and in 41 (85%) by the
quantitative approach, however, in 1 patient a defect was
defined by the latter method in a region supplied by a non-
stenotic coronary artery. Thus 40 out of 48 patients with
coronary artery disease (83%) were diagnosed as having CAD in
the correct localization. So although the quantitative analysis
was somewhat more sensitive, the difference did not reach
statistical significance.

Qualitative and quantitative analysis were in complete
agreement in 43 out of 48 patients with coronary artery
disease (90%). In 5 patients quantitative analysis could
detect one additional stenosis. Subtracting one case with a
false positive regional defect finding, the regional sensitiv-

ity was 70% for the quantitative and 66% for the qualitative
method (no significant difference).

12 patients out of 13 (92%) with normal coronary arteries
were correctly diagnosed as normal by the qualitative method,
whereas true negative results by quantitative analysis were
found in 10 out of 13 cases, for a specificity of 77%. So the
application of a quantitative method could not provide an
essential improvement of diagnostic accuracy.

This result agrees with an editorial by Gould published
in "Circulation" who concluded that for routine clinical diagnosis and management visual interpretation of standard Thallium
images obtained by planar gamma camera scintigraphy is most
appropriate for analysing myocardial perfusion (42). Computer
imaging may add impartiality and ease of interpretation, but
has not been shown to improve diagnostic accuracy (42). Considering our own results and in accordance with the referenced
opinion the following clinical data presented for Tl201 imaging
following dipyridamole i.v. were achieved primarily by the
quantitative analysis described above.

Patients

Our findings in 258 unselected patients (220 male, 38
female) are presented who were refered for coronary angiography because of typical or atypical chest pain. Tl201
following dipyridamole i.v. was performed in close temporal
connection with angiography (in the majority interval between
1 day and 1 week). Patients with recent myocardial infarctions
(within 2 months), unstable angina, after coronary artery
surgery, and patients with clinical, echocardiographic and/or
angiographic signs for cardiomyopathy or valve disease were
excluded from this study. All coronary stenoses of at least
70% reduction of luminal diameter were accepted as hemodynamically significant. The left ventricular contraction was assessed in the 30° RAO angiogram.

52 patients had normal coronary arteries, 206 patients
demonstrated coronary stenoses, 1-vessel-disease was present
in 75 patients (normokinetic left ventricular contraction

n=34, asynergic contraction n=41), 2-vessel disease in 73
patients (normokinetic n=32, asynergic n=41) and 3-vessel
disease in 58 patients (normokinetic n=31), asynergic n=27).

Results

1) Overall specificity and sensitivity of Tl^{201} imaging
following dipyridamole. True negative results were obtained in
49 out of 52 cases for a specificity of 94%. True positive
results (reversible or irreversible perfusion defects) could
be found in 173 out of 206 cases with coronary artery disease,
for a sensitivity of 84%.

Fig 3. The global sensitivity values showed a progressive
increase according to the number of narrowed vessels (1-VD
77%, 2-VD 84%, 3-VD 93%).

Fig 4. A positive Tl^{201} scintigram with a reversible
perfusion defect in a patient with coronary artery disease is
demonstrated in fig 4.

Fig 5. When subdividing the patients with CAD into 2
groups with either normokinetic or asynergic left ventricular
function, a significant difference in overall sensitivity
could be calculated. In patients with normokinetic left
ventricles the number of false negative Tl^{201} results was
comparably higher yielding a lower sensitivity of 71% as
contrasted to the 95% sensitivity in patients with asynergies
(p <0.001).

Fig 6. In the patients with asynergies the global sensitivity was equally high in 1-vessel disease (95%), 2-vessel
disease (93%) and 3-vessel disease (100%).

Fig 7. In the patients with normal left ventricular
contraction sensitivity was lowest in 1-vessel disease (56%),
somewhat higher in 2-vessel disease (72%) and satisfactorily
high only in 3-vessel disease (87%).

Fig 8. The typical example of a false negative result in
a patient with 2-vessel disease is demonstrated in fig 8.

2) Probability analysis in noninvasive scintigraphic diagnosis of coronary artery disease. The interpretation of a
test result in a given patient requires more than only

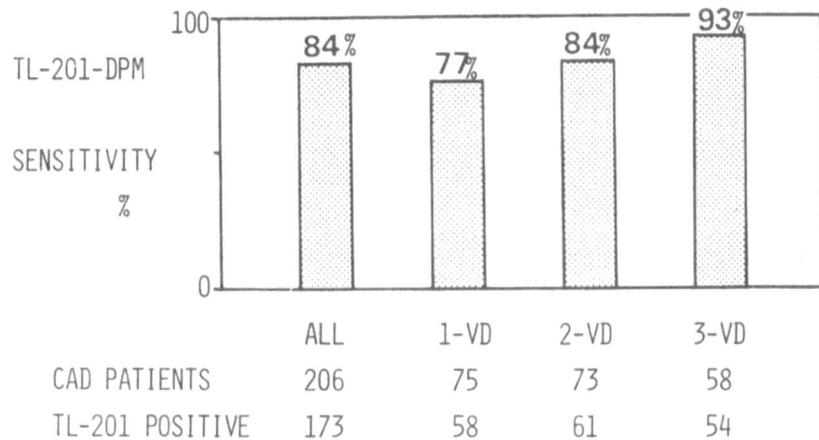

Fig. 3. Sensitivity of Tl^{201} imaging following dipyridamole, values for all patients with CAD and for the subgroups according to the number of narrowed vessels.

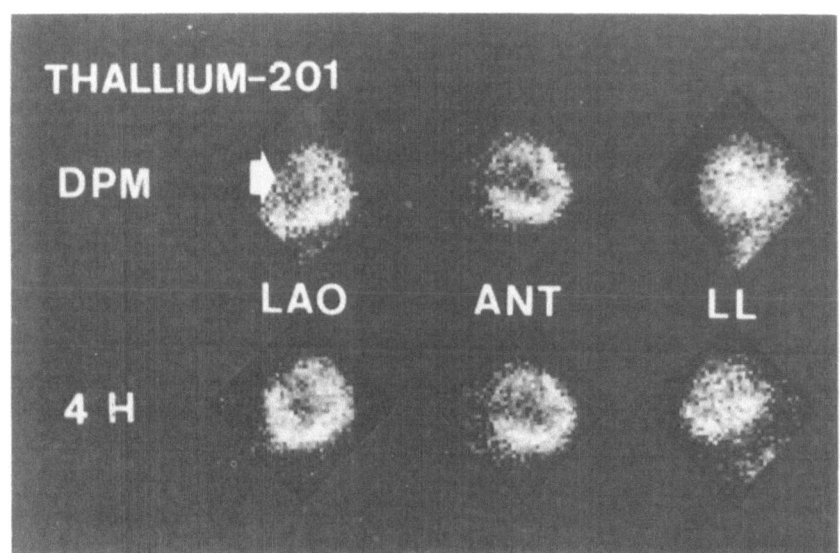

Fig. 4. Tl^{201} images following dipyridamole (DPM, upper panel) and 4 h later (4 H, lower panel) of a patient with 3-vessel disease (95% proximal LAD, 90% LCx, 100% RCA stenoses) and normokinetic left ventricle. Reversible anteroseptal perfusion defect (arrow).

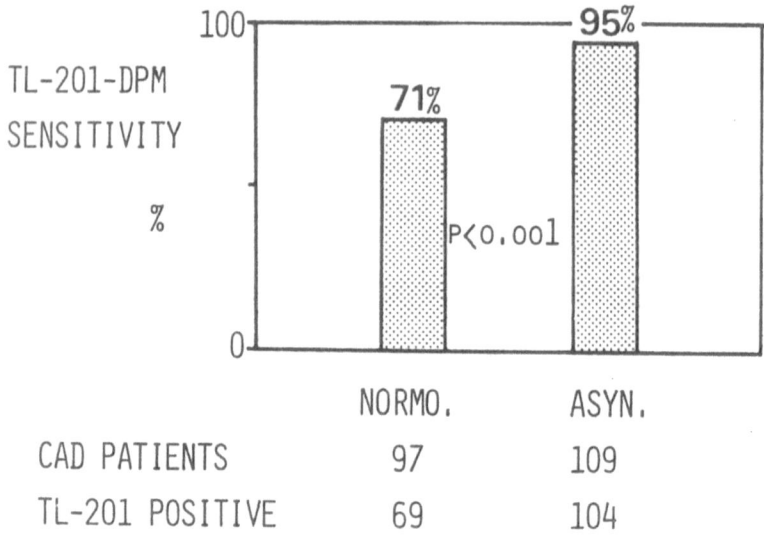

Fig. 5. Different sensitivity of Tl^{201} imaging following dipyridamole in patients with normokinetic (NORMO) and asynergic (ASYN) left ventricles.

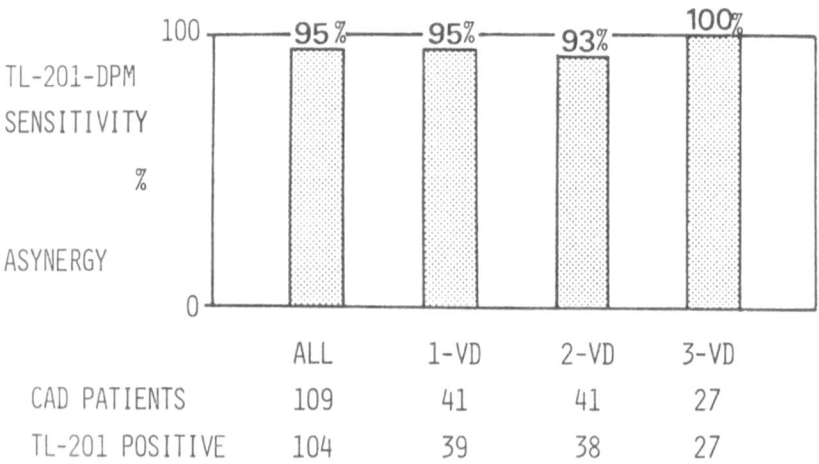

Fig. 6. Sensitivity values of Tl^{201} imaging following dipyridamole in patients with asynergic left ventricles.

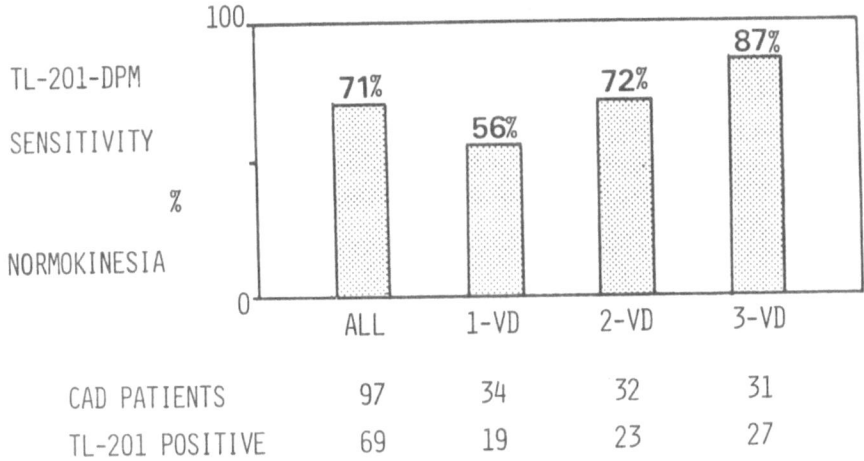

Fig. 7. Sensitivity values of Tl201 imaging following dipyridamole in patients with normokinetic left ventricles.

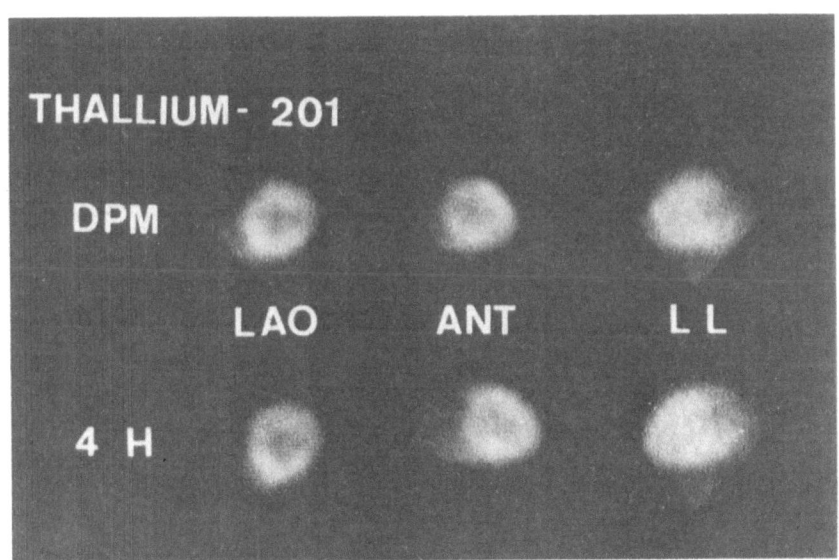

Fig. 8. False negative Tl201 images following dipyridamole in a patient with 2-vessel disease (80% distal LAD, 75% RCA stenoses) and normal left ventricle.

consideration of sensitivity and specificity of the applied method. According to Bayes' Theorem, the posttest probability of disease depends greatly on the pretest probability of the patients studied which is at least as important as the sensitivity and specificity of the method (4,14,49,50,51). This concept implies that in most instances of medical diagnosis a test result causes primarily a change in the probability for the presence of disease and not a dichotomic yes or no decision. A positive test result increases the probability, this increase is strictly depending on the pretest probability of the individual patient. In patients with negative test results the posttest probability is lower than the pretest probability, again this decrease depends on the probability of each single patient before the test.

As we have shown above, Tl^{201} imaging following dipyridamole has a significantly different sensitivity in patients with asynergic or normokinetic ventricles. The application of our reported values for sensitivity and specificity and the calculation of posttest probability according to Bayes' Theorem leads to the diagrams in fig 9 and fig 10.

The curves in fig 9 depict the posttest probability for a positive (upper curve) and negative (lower curve) Tl^{201} result in patients with asynergies and normal controls, whereas the curves in fig 10 pertain to CAD-patients with normokinetic ventricles opposed to normal cases. The different sensitivity values for the 2 groups of patients explain the different shape of the lower curves for negative Tl^{201} findings. For all ranges of pretest probability the 2 curves depicted show a greater distance in the patients with asynergy than with normokinesia. A negative finding excludes more or less the presence of coronary artery disease with asynergy, a positive finding increases greatly the probability of disease. In clinical practice the curves of fig 10 seem more important as they must be applied in patients with suspected coronary artery disease and normokinesia. As it can be derived from the literature, the major diagnostic benefit by the Tl^{201} scintigram can be expected in patients with low to inter-

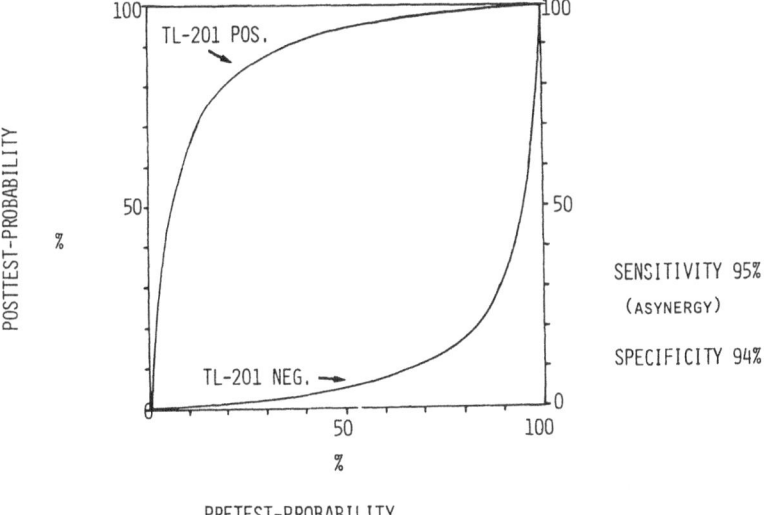

Fig. 9. Relation of pretest and posttest probability for positive and negative Tl201 scintigraphy following dipyridamole in patients with asynergic left ventricles and normal controls.

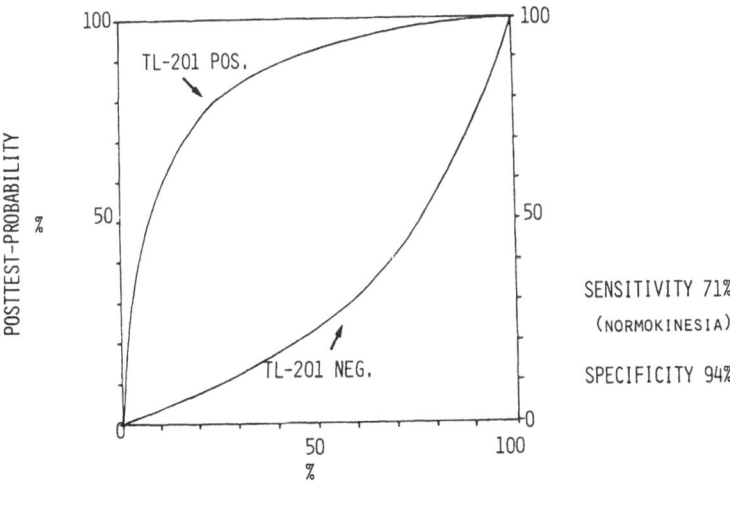

Fig. 10. Relation of pretest and posttest probability for positive and negative Tl201 scintigraphy following dipyridamole in patients with normokinesia.

mediate pretest probability (20-60% range) irrespective of the test result. A positive test will greatly increase, a negative decrease the probability for coronary artery disease. In both extremes of probability (either very low or very high) the diagnostic yield of scintigraphy is comparatively lower than in the 20-60% range. The consideration of this concept of probability analysis enables a better indication for the performance of the scintigraphic test. The comparatively low diagnostic value in the very low pretest probability range confirms that this test can not be advised as a screening technique in an asymptomatic population. The relative small gain in diagnostic information in all patients with very high probability must be considered in so far that a negative result can never exclude the presence of disease with reliability, although the positive test will prove the presence of disease in such a patient. Each single test result in a given patient must be discussed in this very important context of probability analysis which requires the pretest probability classification of the patient according to age, sex, symptoms, and risk factors (4,14,15,17,18,48,49,50,51).

3) Results of Tl^{201} imaging following dipyridamole in regard to the 3 major coronary vessels.

a) Regional sensitivity.

Fig 11. True positive regional scintigraphic defects following dipyridamole were found in 67% (108/162) of LAD stenoses, 60% (80/133) of right coronary artery stenoses, and in 38% (38/100) of left circumflex stenoses. So a significantly smaller number of left circumflex than LAD and RCA stenoses could be detected scintigraphically (p <0.001).

In similarity to global sensitivity, also regional sensitivity values must be differentiated according to the regional wallmotion of the myocardial segment related with the specific vessel.

Fig 12. For all vessels with relation to asynergies the regional sensitivity was high, 98% for the LAD, 88% for the RCA, and 94% for the LCx. In the great majority of these cases the scintigraphic defects were irreversible represent-

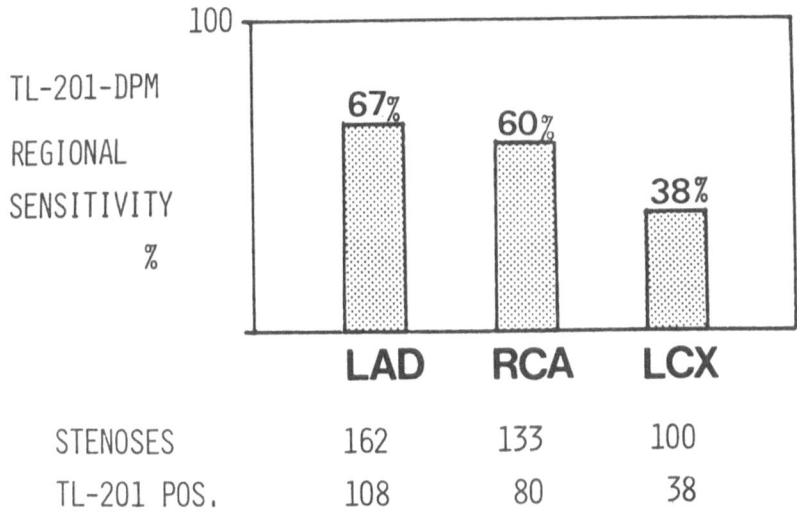

Fig. 11. Regional sensitivity of Tl^{201} imaging following dipyridamole for LAD, right coronary artery (RCA) and left circumflex artery (LCx).

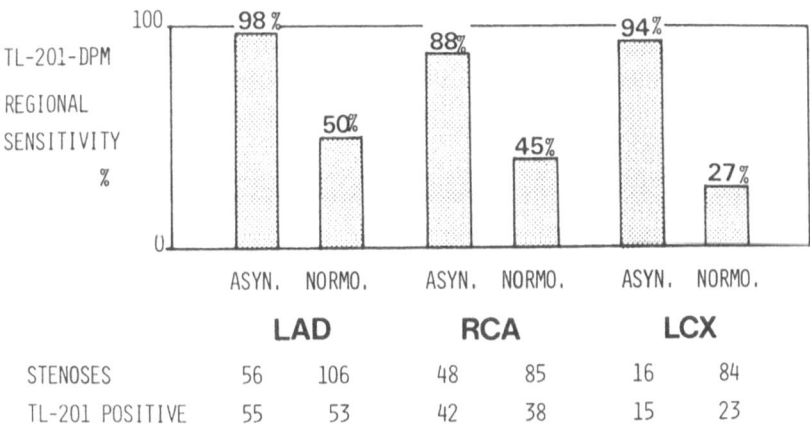

Fig. 12. Subdivision of regional sensitivity of Tl^{201} imaging following dipyridamole according to the contraction of the corresponding wall segment (asynergic or normokinetic).

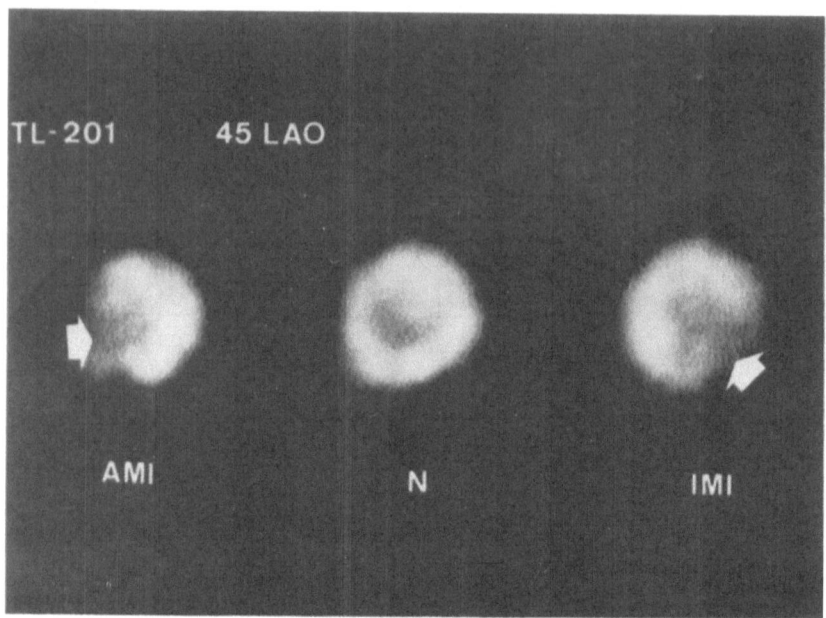

Fig. 13. 4 hour redistribution Tl^{201} images in patients with old anterior myocardial infarction (AMI, left panel) and inferior myocardial infarction (IMI, right panel) in comparison to a normal control case (N), 45° LAO views.

ing myocardial scars. Such irreversible defects were found in 89% of LAD, 81% of LCx, and 73% of RCA stenoses with relation to asynergy, so in the distribution of 82% of all asynergy-related vessels persistent scintigraphic defects could be noted. Narrowed vessels supplying normokinetic segments were detected less frequently yielding regional sensitivity values of 50% for the LAD, 45% for the RCA, and 27% for the LCx. Although most defects in the vascular bed of these noninfarct stenoses were reversible, there were also 15% (15/97) irreversible defects in the 4 hour images.

Fig 13. Typical findings in the redistribution images in patients with anterior and inferior myocardial infarctions are demonstrated in fig 13.

Because of the outstanding role of the LAD for the myocardial blood-supply, we performed a special consideration of Tl^{201} findings following dipyridamole in LAD stenoses located either proximal or distal in comparison to the first septal perforator artery.

While scintigraphy correctly detected 79% (66/84) of proximal LAD stenoses, only 54% (42/78) of the distal LAD stenoses were recognized which was a significant difference (p <0.001). The major difference between the 2 locations could be demonstrated in stenoses with relation to normo-kinetic left ventricular wall segments. Only 36% (20/56) of distal LAD stenoses with normokinesia had scintigraphic defects in at least one typical LAD region while 66% (33/50) of proximal LAD stenoses with relation to normokinetic wall segments were detected (p <0.002). There was no difference between the 2 locations of LAD stenoses with relation to asynergic wall segments (proximal 97% detected, distal 100% detected).

As the blood-supply to the interventricular septum is derived primarily from the LAD, stenoses in this vessel might be expected to cause abnormalities in septal perfusion. There-fore we attempted to examine the extent of jeopardized septal myocardium assessed by Tl^{201} perfusion imaging.

An abnormal antero septal myocardial perfusion (visualized in the 45° LAO view) was found in 61% (51/84) of proximal LAD stenoses and 37% (29/78) of the cases with distal LAD disease (p <0.01). Thus a normal septal stress perfusion could not exclude proximal LAD disease, in addition septal perfusion abnormalities could not be regarded as specific findings for patients with proximal LAD disease.

An abnormal antero septal stress perfusion was induced by dipyridamole with approximately the same frequency in proximal stenoses related either to asynergy or normokinesia and in distal LAD stenoses related to asynergy. In noninfarct related distal LAD disease abnormalities in the septum were detected significantly less frequently.

b) Regional specificity. We could find only 3 false positive scintigrams in 52 patients with normal coronary arteries which corresponded to LAD segments in 2 cases and to the LCx region in 1 case. Thus the regional specificity was equally high for the LAD (96%), LCx (98%), and RCA (100%).

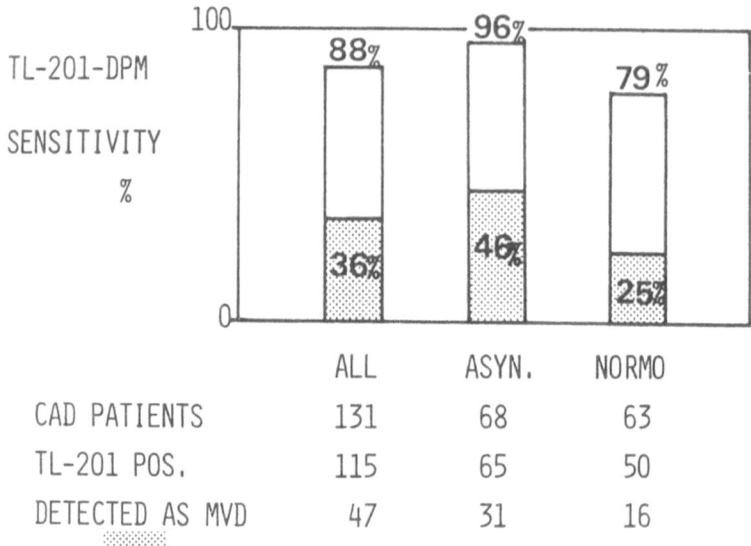

Fig. 14. Sensitivity of Tl^{201} imaging following dipyridamole in the assessment of 1) CAD and 2) multivessel disease in all patients with multivessel disease.

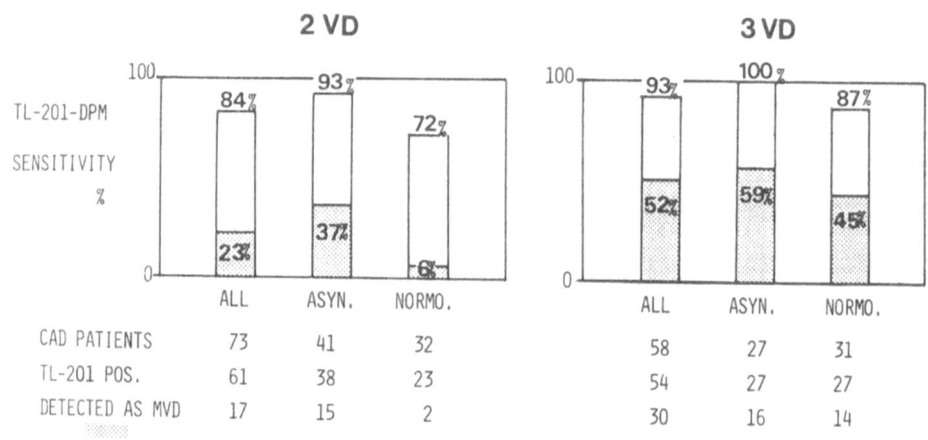

Fig. 15. Sensitivity values according to fig 14 in the subgroups of 2 vessel disease and 3 vessel disease.

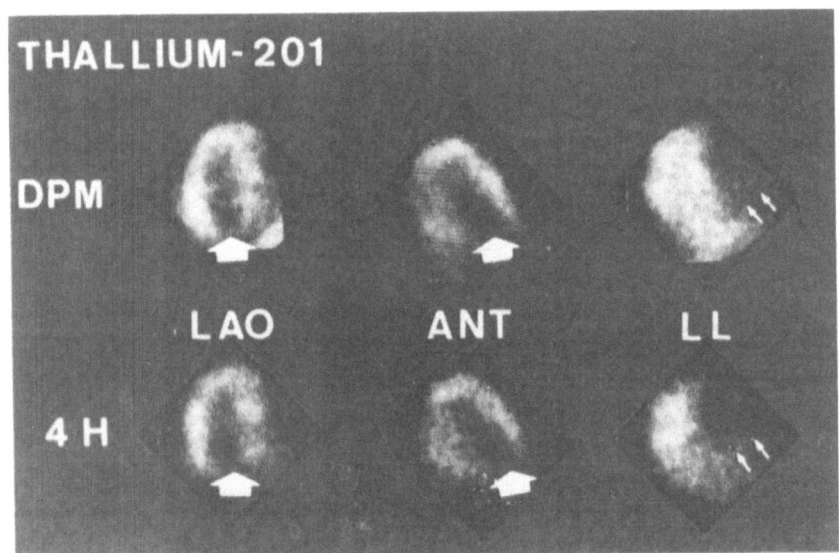

Fig. 16. Tl^{201} images after dipyridamole and 4 hours later in a patient with 3 vessel disease (80% LAD, 100% RCA, 100% LCx stenoses) and inferior as well as apical akinesis. Irreversible perfusion defects in the inferior and apical regions (arrows), no perfusion abnormality in the postero lateral region "supplied" by the LCx.

Infrequently there were some problems in the detection of hypoperfused inferior wall segments. In 5 patients with CAD and compromised blood-supply to the inferior wall, the scintigraphic defects - although correct in location - were attributed to the false coronary vessel according to the diagram in fig 1. So it might be suggested to diagnose preferably only inferior wall hypoperfusion and not to address specifically one vessel as being narrowed and responsible for the hypoperfusion.

4) <u>Problems of the method in coronary multivessel disease</u>.

Fig 14. Out of 131 patients with multivessel disease (2-VD and 3-VD) 88% were correctly diagnosed by scintigraphy

246

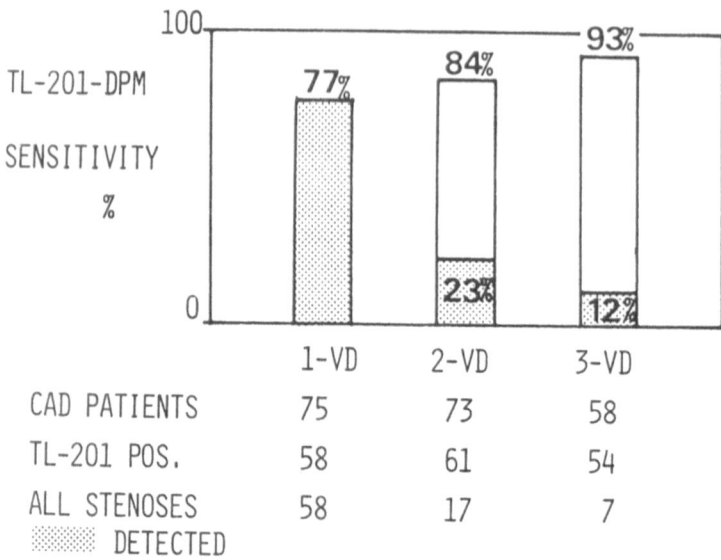

	1-VD	2-VD	3-VD
CAD PATIENTS	75	73	58
TL-201 POS.	58	61	54
ALL STENOSES DETECTED	58	17	7

Fig. 17. Sensitivity of Tl^{201} imaging following dipyridamole in 1) the assessment of CAD and 2) detection of all stenotic vessels in 1-VD , 2-VD and 3-VD resp.

as having CAD, however, the presence of defects in at least 2 different vascular regions allowed the correct diagnosis of multivessel disease in only 36% of these patients. The subdivision of the patients into cases with normokinesia and asynergy demonstrated a better diagnostic accuracy for the detection of multivessel disease in patients with asynergy than with normokinesia (46% vs 25% correct MVD diagnoses).

In order to study possible influences of the extent of CAD on the scintigraphic quantification of vessel involvement, we separated the patients with multivessel disease into cases with 2 vessel disease and 3 vessel disease.

Fig 15. Among the 73 cases with 2 vessel disease only 23% were correctly diagnosed as having 2-VD. The rate of detected multivessel involvement was higher in the 2-VD cases with than without asynergies (37% vs 6%).

Out of 58 patients with 3-VD 52% were correctly classified by scintigraphy as multivessel disease. This does not imply

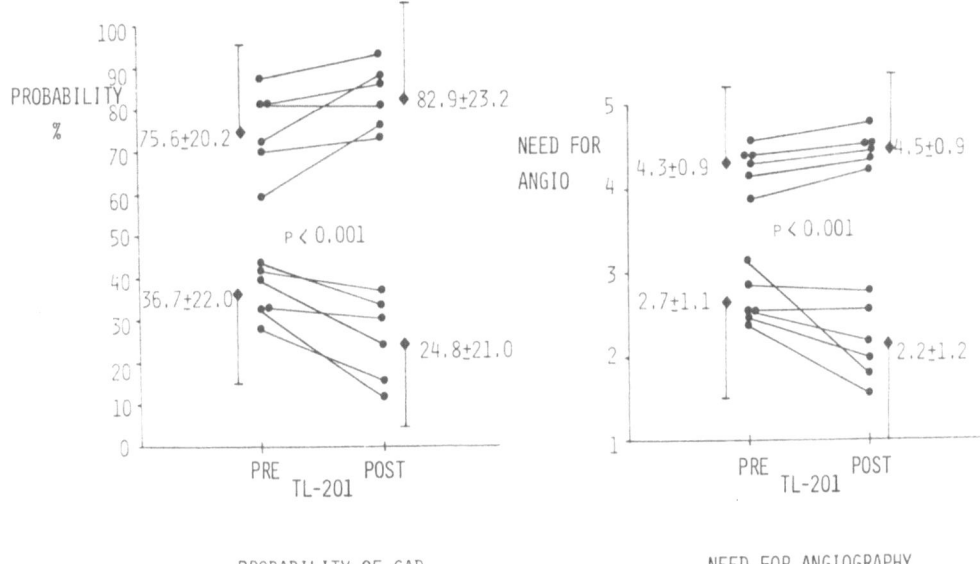

PROBABILITY OF CAD   NEED FOR ANGIOGRAPHY

Fig. 18. Influence of Tl^{201} imaging following dipyridamole on the estimated probability for CAD and need for coronary angiography in patients with CAD (upper panel) and without CAD (lower panel). Mean values ±SD and individual values for all 6 physicians participating in the study.

that all of these cases were correctly diagnosed as 3-VD. The rate of correctly diagnosed multivessel involvement was some-what higher in the patients with than without asynergies (59% vs 45%).

Fig 16 shows the typical example of a patient with 3-VD and underestimation of the extent of coronary artery disease in the scintigraphic study.

Fig 17. In order to illustrate the ability of Tl^{201} imaging following dipyridamole to quantitate the number of diseased vessels, fig 17 presents our findings in the sub-groups with 1-VD, 2-VD and 3-VD.

All angiographically narrowed vessels were detected by scintigraphic abnormalities in the corresponding segments in

77% of the patients with 1-VD, 23% of 2-VD, and only 12% of 3-VD. These values were significantly lower than the overall sensitivity values in these subgroups for the qualitative detection of CAD as demonstrated in fig 17.

In not a single patient scintigraphy caused an overestimation of the number of angiographically diseased vessels.

5) Impact of Tl^{201} imaging following dipyridamole on clinical assessment and management of patients with chest pain. While studies of sensitivity and specificity of a new diagnostic test are the essential first step in its evaluation, a comprehensive appreciation of its role in clinical practice requires further information (52,53). Therefore we studied the influence of Tl^{201} imaging following dipyridamole on the clinical assessment of patients with chest pain in regard to the presence of coronary artery disease and the impact of the method on the estimated need for coronary angiography. This retrospective study comprised 60 patients without infarction who had been refered for both coronary angiography and Tl^{201} scintigraphy following dipyridamole i.v. Summaries of the 60 case histories were presented to 6 physicians of our cardiology department giving the following information:

age and sex; chest pain characteristics including location, duration, radiation, quality, precipitating and relieving factors; other cardiac symptoms; coronary risk factors; rest ECG; exercise ECG results including maximal stage, heart rate, symptoms, ST-segment changes, arrhythmias.

After reviewing the clinical summary the physicians were asked to estimate the probability for the presence of coronary artery disease in % (ranging from 0 - 100%, 0% = definitely no CAD, 100% = definitely CAD). In addition the need for coronary angiography was estimated on a 5-point-scale (1 = definitely not indicated, 5 = definitely indicated). After these baseline estimations the physicians were given the results of Tl^{201} imaging after i.v. dipyridamole and asked to revise their estimations of probability and need for angiography. The physicians did not know the rate of patients with and without CAD nor the sensitivity (74%) and specificity

(100%) of Tl^{201} scintigraphy in this certain group of patients.

Fig 18. In the 43 patients with CAD the mean baseline probability for all 6 physicians (258 estimations) was 75.6% ± 20.2. This judgement was increased highly significantly to 82.9% ± 23.2 (p <0.001) after receiving the Tl^{201} results. Thus the relative change of probability was 10% of the pre-Tl^{201} probability. In the cases with CAD the need for coronary angiography was 4.3 ± 0.9 without Tl^{201} and 4.5 ± 0.9 with Tl^{201},this 5% relative change was statistically significant (p <0.001).

In the 17 patients without coronary vessel disease (102 individual estimations) a significantly lower probability than in the patients with CAD was found (p <0.001). The pre-Tl^{201} value of 36.7% ± 22.0 was decreased to 24.8% ± 21.0 with the information of Tl^{201} which was a highly significant -32% relative change (p <0.001). In these patients without coronary stenoses the baseline need for angiography was judged 2.7 ± 1.1, with the information of the scintigraphic results the need decreased to 2.2 ± 1.2 (-19% relative change p <0.001).

Discussion

Tl^{201} imaging following physical exercise of the patients has provided important information about presence or absence of coronary artery stenoses. Several studies have examined the sensitivity and specificity of the exercise Thallium test in the diagnosis of coronary artery disease and compared these values with exercise stress testing (1,3,10,11,12,13,15,16, 17,18). In all of the studies Tl^{201} imaging has provided a better diagnostic information than the exercise ECG. According-ing to reports in the literature the mean sensitivity of exercise Tl^{201} is 83% and the mean specificity 90% (10).

The rate of true positive Tl^{201} findings is strictly depending on the performance of adequate physical exercise. Many patients however can not achieve intense and sufficient levels of exercise. This includes patients with symptomatic claudication, pulmonary disease, skeletal abnormalities, lack of physical training, and lack of motivation. In all of these cases an alternative stress test would be highly desirable.

It has been demonstrated that the intravenous administration of high-dose dipyridamole can cause anginal pain, ST-depression, and increase of diastolic pulmonary artery pressure, changes that also occur during exercise in patients with CAD (33,34,54). Using intracoronary Xe^{133} injection a coronary steal phenomenon following dipyridamole infusion could be clearly demonstrated by our group (33). The comparable diagnostic utility of exercise stress testing and of the so-called dipyridamole-test could be shown in several studies including our own (30,31,32,35,36).

Since the availability of Tl^{201} it seemed reasonable to combine the dipyridamole-test with myocardial Tl^{201} perfusion studies (20-28). The potential value of the dipyridamole-Tl^{201} method is still increased by the possibility to antagonize dipyridamole effects within a few minutes by the intravenous injection of aminophylline (38). As also methylxanthines can counteract the effects of dipyridamole, it should be pointed out that these studies must always be performed in fasted patients because also the intake of tea or coffee could block the vasodilation in response to dipyridamole (37, 38,55).

The mechanism of vasodilation following dipyridamole is considered to involve adenosine,inhibiting its degradation to inosine by blocking the enzym adenosine-deaminase (37,38,39, 55,56).

Using the described technique of Tl^{201} imaging following dipyridamole we could find in our patients a sensitivity of 84% and a specificity of 94% in the diagnosis of coronary artery disease. The high specificity value might partly be explained by the exclusion of patients from the study who might possibly have false positive scintigrams, like cardiomyopathies or valve disease (4). The sensitivity value described by us is in good agreement with reports in the literature about Tl^{201} imaging following physical exercise. Some extreme values are mainly due to different patient selection and different methods of data analysis.

As we could demonstrate there is a significant difference in sensitivity between patients with normokinetic and asynergic left ventricles (71% vs 95%,p <0.001). So one of the major determinants for a positive Tl^{201} finding is the presence of asynergy generally due to an infarction. Therefore the overall sensitivity must be the higher, the more patients with infarctions are included in a study. As older studies for Tl^{201} imaging following exercise comprised up to 75% of patients with infarction, the sensitivity values were disproportionately high (1,11,13). This fact is explained by the preselection of patients for such studies which are always performed in patients who have undergone coronary angiography. The majority of patients refered for angiography have suffered infarctions which in turn accounts for the predominance of these patients in scintigraphic studies.

In most patients with infarctions there is no doubt however about the presence of coronary artery disease as history and ECG can frequently confirm this diagnosis. In all cases with inconclusive history and inconclusive or negative ECG a major diagnostic information about the presence of an infarction scar can be expected by Tl^{201} imaging which helps to clarify the diagnosis with a similar reliability as 2-dimensional echocardiography as reported by us previously (57).

The comparatively low sensitivity in the patients with normokinetic left ventricles implies that a negative finding can not exclude coronary artery disease, although the presence of 3 vessel disease is very much unlikely with a negative Tl^{201} study (50,58).

The decision whether coronary artery disease is present or absent, does not only require the consideration of sensitivity and specificity, but also and at least as important the consideration of the pretest probability of the individual patient. As described above, the greatest diagnostic information by Tl^{201} imaging can be expected in the 20-60% range of pretest probability. In agreement with interpretations following Bayes' Theorem similar discussions have appeared in the literature about Tl^{201} imaging after exercise (10,14,15,18,49, 51). The curves depicted in fig 9 and fig 10 should always be kept in mind by the physician who orders a Tl^{201} study. The different shape of the curves for negative Tl^{201} results in fig 9 and fig 10 reflects the different sensitivity values found for patients with normokinesia and asynergy, respectively. The application of Bayes' Theorem leads to the main field of indication for Tl^{201} imaging following dipyridamole which can generally be recommended for patients with low to intermediate pretest probability of disease.

The calculation of regional sensitivity of the method in dependence on diseased vessels could clearly show that stenoses of the LAD and right coronary artery can be detected more frequently than left circumflex artery stenoses (67% vs 60% vs 38%). This fact is again in good agreement with results obtained by exercise Tl^{201} scintigraphy (10,12,16). The lower sensitivity for the left circumflex might be caused by the smaller mass of myocardium supplied by this vessel and the fact that the left circumflex artery can be evaluated in only one scintigraphic view (45° LAO).

There was a striking difference of scintigraphy to recognize stenoses supplying viable (normokinetic) or scarred (asynergic) myocardium. The rates of detected stenoses with relation to asynergy (ranging from 88% to 98%) verifies that the method is very reliable in detecting asynergies and corresponding narrowed vessels. In the majority of these asynergies the scintigraphic defects were irreversible and therefore also clearly visualized in the 4-hours scintigrams which allowed the reliable identification of myocardial scars caused by infarctions. In many of these patients however the presence of infarction scars can also be diagnosed by ECG or echocardiography which are considerably cheaper methods than Tl^{201} imaging. For the diagnosis of infarction scars the scintigraphic method should be restricted to cases with questionable findings in the other methods (57). The infrequent finding of irreversible defects in normokinetic segments indicates that in some of these segments the time neccesary for complete redistribution might be more than 4 hours as it was discussed previously for exercise Tl^{201} imaging (4,8).

There is some evidence that obstructions of the LAD have different prognostic, therapeutic, and surgical implications depending on the proximity of the lesions (7,9,16,59,60,61). Therefore we tried to define the usefulness of Tl^{201} imaging following dipyridamole in the assessment of LAD stenoses located either proximal or distal in regard to the first septal perforator branch (61). The method proved to be extremely useful in the prediction of LAD stenoses related to asynergies irrespective of the location. The test was less reliable in the diagnosis of proximal LAD stenoses supplying normokinetic segments and nearly useless in predicting noninfarct LAD stenoses distal to the first septal perforator. Therefore the value of the method is limited in estimating the extent of jeopardized myocardium supplied by the LAD although overall a significantly greater number of proximal than of distal LAD stenoses could be detected (79% vs 54%, p <0.001).

Antero septal stress perfusion defects could be induced more frequently in patients with proximal LAD disease, however, these defects were not specific for proximal LAD disease which is in agreement with previous data (9,16). Abnormalities in the antero septal area do not correlate with the location of LAD disease in relation to the first septal perforator. So it could be assumed that the first septal perforator might not be important as septal perfusion may depend on the total number of septal perforators or on the contribution of the right coronary artery to septal perfusion via the posterior septal perforator branches. Therefore the presence or absence of septal perfusion abnormalities may be regarded as relatively inaccurate in distinguishing between proximal and distal LAD disease which is in contrast to an older study that however seems questionable because of the rather small number of patients included (59).

In confirming our previous findings, the present study shows that in 88% of the patients with multivessel disease the presence of CAD could be documented scintigraphically (16,58).

The ability of Tl^{201} scintigraphy following dipyridamole to
predict the number of angiographically narrowed vessels was
considerably poorer than the overall sensitivity for diagnosing CAD. The presence of defects in at least 2 vascular
regions allowed the diagnosis of multivessel disease in only
36% of these patients. In only 23% of the patients with 2
vessel disease and 12% of the patients with 3 vessel disease
scintigraphy predicted correctly all narrowed vessels.

The explanation for this limitation of the method could be
that only the most severely involved areas of myocardium may
in fact become ischemic during coronary vasodilation with
dipyridamole. So the most severe lesion in a heart is usually
identified. Another explanation might be that seemingly normal
areas are in fact mildly ischemic, but this ischemia can not
be detected by the Thallium scintigram because this method is
only able to evaluate relative and not absolute perfusion. In
the important group of patients with asynergy caused by infarction, scintigraphy did not prove very useful in excluding
multivessel disease, however, a positive finding provided
reliable evidence for multivessel disease.

It could be argued that patients with multivessel disease,
but without evidence of severe ischemia in different vascular
regions, might have a relatively benign prognosis. However,
according to our experience the lack of perfusion defects in
several regions can not be regarded as evidence of hemodynamically irrelevant stenoses because even severe narrowings
gave frequently negative findings (58). This limitation might
partly be attributed to the nonquantitative nature of Thallium
scintigraphy and the fact that the presence of regional mal-
perfusion is determined only with reference to "normal"
regions which themselves might be underperfused.

Several approaches have been proposed to improve data
analysis by the application of quantitative procedures including profile analysis and wash-out determinations in Tl^{201}
exercise studies (2,3,4,44). As discussed above, such techniques can reasonably improve overall and regional sensitivity values also in Tl^{201} imaging following dipyridamole which

is however associated with a small loss in specificity. These problems seem even much greater for the analysis of Tl^{201} wash-out determinations following dipyridamole yielding obviously high regional sensitivity, but also unsatisfactorily low regional specificity which makes its application in clinical practice questionable. In addition other until now unresolved problems cited above, like lack of reproducibility of wash-out parameters and the possible influence of intake of food or drugs, seem major limitations which at present make the value of these parameters open to discussion for clinical nuclear cardiology (45-47).

In addition to determination of sensitivity and specificity of a diagnostic test, a comprehensive appraisal of the clinical value of a certain method requires further information (52). In our study concerning the clinical impact of Tl^{201} imaging we could demonstrate that the results of scintigraphy can improve significantly the clinical assessment of non-infarct patients with chest pain (53). The estimated probability of coronary artery disease was increased in patients with hemodynamically significant narrowings and decreased in patients with normal coronary arteries. Thus the knowledge of the results of Tl^{201} perfusion studies improved the diagnostic differentiation of patients with and without CAD in a highly significant extent. The relative change of probability for CAD was greater in the patients with normal coronary arteries than with narrowed vessels (-32% vs 10%). This fact is in good agreement with interpretations of Bayes' Theorem which have shown the greatest diagnostic yield of Tl^{201} in patients with low to intermediate pretest probability of disease (10,14,18,49,50,51).

Another important aspect of our study was the assessment of the clinical management of patients in regard to coronary angiography with the information of Tl^{201} scintigraphy. For all 6 participating physicians taken together, an improvement in the estimated need for angiography was documented. This influence was comparably greater in the patients without CAD. So it can be concluded that these patients benefit still

more from Tl^{201} studies than patients with CAD. It could be
speculated that the use of Tl^{201} scintigraphy could reduce the
number of such patients refered for coronary angiography.

Data presented in the literature and our own results prove
the outstanding importance of Tl^{201} imaging following exercise
or vasodilation using dipyridamole in the noninvasive diagnosis of patients with suspected or known CAD. The potential
clinical value of the method seems even to be higher because
it provides also important functional and pathophysiological
information in patients with known CAD to supplement the
anatomic abnormalities determined by coronary angiography. In
a comparative study performed in patients with CAD applying
Tl^{201} imaging following dipyridamole and radionuclide ventriculography at rest and during physical exercise we could find
a typical relation between stress perfusion and global left
ventricular ejection fraction response (28). Reversible Tl^{201}
defects usually predicted functional impairment of the left
ventricle with exercise, irreversible defects suggested impaired rest function with only minor further dysfunction
during exercise. Patients with false negative Tl^{201} scintigrams demonstrated normal rest ejection fraction which did
not change with exercise. This close connection between perfusion and function points to a possible role of radionuclide
studies for a better risk stratification of the patients. Thus
the noninvasive nuclear cardiology methods do not only provide
important diagnostic information, but also valuable functional
and even prognostic data that may be used in therapeutic
strategies in patients with coronary artery disease.

LITERATURE

1. Bailey IK, Griffith LSC, Rouleau J, Strauss HW, Pitt B, Thallium-201 myocardial perfusion imaging at rest and during exercise. Comparative sensitivity to electrocardiography in coronary artery disease. Circulation 55:79, 1977.

2. Beller GA, Quantitative Thallium-201 scintigraphy. Int. J. Cardiol. 5:234, 1984.

3. Berger BB, Watson DD, Taylor GJ, Craddock GB, Martin RP, Teates CD, Beller GA, Quantitative Thallium-201 exercise scintigraphy for detection of coronary artery disease. J. nucl. Med. 22:585, 1981.

4. Berman DS, Mason DT, Clinical nuclear cardiology. Grune and Stratton, New York, 1981.

5. Bulkley BH, Rouleau JR, Whitaker JQ, Strauss HW, Pitt B, The use of 201-Thallium for myocardial perfusion imaging in sarcoid heart disease. Chest 72:27, 1977.

6. Burow RD, Pond M, Schafer AW, Becker L. Circumferential profiles: A new method for computer analysis of Thallium-201 myocardial perfusion images. J. nucl. Med. 20:771, 1979.

7. Dunn RF, Freedman B, Bailey IK, Uren RF, Kelly DT, Exercise Thallium imaging: Location of perfusion abnormalities in single-vessel coronary disease. J. nucl. Med. 21:717, 1980.

8. Gutman J, Berman DS, Freeman M, Rozanski A, Maddahi J, Waxman A, Swan HJC, Time to completed redistribution of Thallium-201 in exercise myocardial scintigraphy: Relationship to the degree of coronary artery stenosis. Amer. Heart J. 106:989, 1983.

9. Hakki AH, Iskandrian AS, Segal BL, Kane SA, Use of exercise Thallium scintigraphy to assess extent of ischaemic myocardium in patients with left anterior descending artery disease. Brit. Heart J. 45:703, 1981.

10. Hör G, Kanemoto N, 201-Tl-myocardial scintigraphy: Current status in coronary artery disease, results of sensitivity/specificity in 3092 patients and clinical recommendations. Nucl. Med. 20:136, 1981.

11. Jengo JA, Freeman R, Brizendine M, Mena I, Detection of coronary artery disease: Comparison of exercise stress radionuclide angiocardiography and Thallium stress perfusion scanning. Amer. J. Cardiol. 45:535, 1980.

12. Lenaers A, Block P, Van Thiel E, Lebedelle M, Becquevort P, Erbsmann F, Ermans AM, Segmental analysis of Thallium-201 stress myocardial scintigraphy. J. nucl. Med. 18:509, 1977.

13. Massie BM, Botvinick EH, Brundage BH, Correlation of Thallium-201 scintigrams with coronary anatomy: Factors affecting region by region sensitivity. Amer. J. Cardiol. 44:616, 1979.

14. Melin JA, Piret LJ, Vanbutsele RJM, Rousseau MF, Cosyns J, Brasseur LA, Becker C, Detry JMR, Diagnostic value of exercise electrocardiography and Thallium myocardial scintigraphy in patients without previous myocardial infarction: A Bayesian approach. Circulation 63:1019, 1981.

15. Patterson RE, Horowitz SF, Eng C, Rudin A, Meller J, Halgash DA, Pichard AD, Goldsmith SJ, Herman MV, Gorlin R, Can exercise electro-cardiography and Thallium-201 myocardial imaging exclude the diagnosis of coronary artery disease? Amer. J. Cardiol. 49:1127, 1982.

16. Rigo P, Bailey IK, Griffith LSC, Pitt B, Burow RD, Wagner HN, Becker LC, Value and limitations of segmental analysis of stress Thallium myocardial imaging for localization of coronary artery disease. Circulation 61:973, 1980.

17. Ritchie JL, Myocardial perfusion imaging. Amer. J. Cardiol. 49:1341, 1982.

18. Silber S, Fleck E, Klein U, Rudolph W, Wertigkeit der Thallium-201 Belastungsszintigraphie im Vergleich zur Belastungelektrokardiographie bei Patienten mit koronarer Herzerkrankung ohne Myokardinfarkt. Herz 4:359, 1979.

19. Smalling RW, The spectrum of Thallium-201 imaging in coronary artery disease (teaching-editorial). J. nucl. Med. 24:854, 1983.

20. Albro PC, Gould LK, Westcott RJ, Hamilton GW, Ritchie JL, Williams DL, Noninvasive assessment of coronary stenoses by myocardial imaging during pharmacologic coronary vasodilatation. III. Clinical trial. Amer. J. Cardiol. 42:751, 1978.

21. Demangeat JL, Constantinesco A, Mossard JM, Chambron J, Voegtlin R, Evaluation of myocardial perfusion and left ventricular function by 201-Thallium scintigraphy after dipyridamole. Eur. J. Nucl. Med. 6:491, 1981.

22. Francisco DA, Collins SM, Go RT, Ehrhardt TC, Van Kirk OC, Marcus ML, Tomographic Thallium-201 myocardial perfusion scintigrams after maximal coronary artery vasodilatation with intravenous dipyridamole. Comparison of qualitative and quantitative approaches. Circulation 66:370, 1982.

23. Gould LK, Noninvasive assessment of coronary stenoses by myocardial perfusion imaging during pharmacologic coronary vasodilatation. I. Physiologic basis and experimental validation. Amer. J. Cardiol. 41: 267, 1978.

24. Gould KL, Westcott RJ, Albro PC, Hamilton GW, Noninvasive assessment of coronary stenoses by myocardial imaging during pharmacologic coronary vasodilatation. II. Clinical methodology and feasibility. Amer. J. Cardiol. 41:279, 1978.

25. Josephson MA, Brown G, Hecht HS, Hopkins J, Pierce CD, Peterson RB, Noninvasive detection and localization of coronary stenoses in patients: Comparison of resting dipyridamole and exercise Thallium-201 myocardial perfusion imaging. Amer. Heart J. 103:1008, 1982.

26. Leppo J, Boucher CA, Okada RD, Newell RD, Strauss HW, Pohost G, Serial Thallium-201 myocardial imaging after dipyridamole infusion: Diagnostic utility in detecting coronary stenoses and relationship to regional wall motion. Circulation 66:649, 1982.

27. Schmoliner R, Dudczak R, Kronik G, Kletter K, Hutterer B, Mösslacher H, Frischauf H, Die Aussagekraft der Thallium-Szintigraphie nach Dipyridamol in der Diagnostik der koronaren Herzkrankheit. Z. Kardiol. 69:179, 1980.

28. Schmoliner R, Dudczak R, Kronik G, Homan R, Mösslacher H, Änderungen der linksventrikulären Auswurffraktion unter Belastung und der Thallium-201-Szintigraphie nach Dipyridamol bei Koronarpatienten. Wien. Klin. Wschr. 96, 243, 1984.

29. Lebowitz E. Greene MW, Bradley-Moore P, Atkins H, Ansari A, Richard P, Belgrave E, Tl-201 for medical use. J. nucl. Med. 14:421, 1973.

30. Grosze-Heitmeyer W, Görtz P, Drüke P, Mönninghoff W, Most E, Müller U, Bender F, Dipyridamol-Test und koronare Herzkrankheit. Med. Welt 33:960, 1982.

31. Osterspey A, Jansen W, Tauchert M, Eigl J, Höpp H, Behrenbeck DW, Hilger HH, Stellenwert des Dipyridamol-Tests in der Diagnostik der koronaren Herzkrankheit. Dtsch. med. Wschr. 108:1469, 1983.

32. Schmoliner R, Slany J, Kronik G, Mösslacher H, Die Aussagekraft der Dipyridamoltests für die Diagnostik der koronaren Herzkrankheit. Wien. Klin. Wschr. 91:460, 1979.

33. Slany J. Mösslacher H, Imhof H, Bodner P, Untersuchungen zum coronary steal Phänomen bei koronarer Herzkrankheit. Verh. Dtsch. Ges. Kreislaufforschg. 40:435, 1974.

34. Slany J, Mösslacher H, Kronik G, Schmoliner R, Einflusz von Dipyridamol auf das Ventrikulogram bei koronarer Herzkrankheit. Z. Kardiol. 66:389, 1977.

35. Tauchert M, Behrenbeck DW, Hötzel J, Hilger HH, Ein neuer pharmakologischer Test zur Diagnose der Koronarinsuffizienz. Dtsch. Med. Wschr. 101:35, 1976.

36. Tavazzi L, Previtali M, Salerno JA, Chimienti M, Ray M, Medici A, Specchia G, Bobba P, Dipyridamole-test in angina pectoris: Diagnostic value and pathophysiological implications. Cardiology 69:34, 1982.

37. Afonso S, O'Brien GS, Enhancement of coronary vasodilator action of adenosine triphosphate by dipyridamole. Circulat. Res. 20:403, 1967.

38. Afonso S, Inhibition of coronary vasodilating action of dipyridamole and adenosine by aminophylline in the dog. Circulat. Res. 26:743, 1970.

39. Klabunde RE, Effects of dipyridamole on postischemic vasodilatation and extracellular adenosine. Amer. J. Physiol. 244:273, 1983.

40. Massie BM, Wisneski J, Kramer B, Hollenberg M, Gertz E, Stern D, Comparison of myocardial Thallium-201 clearance after maximal and submaximal exercise: Implications for diagnosis of coronary heart disease: Concise communication. J. nucl. Med. 23(N):381, 1982.

41. Schmoliner R, Dudczak R, Kronik G, Hutterer B, Kletter K, Mösslacher H, Frischauf H, Thallium-201-Myokardszintigraphie nach hochdosierter Dipyridamolgabe. Z. Kardiol. 70:111, 1981.

42. Gould KL, Quantitative imaging in nuclear cardiology. Circulation 66:1141, 1982.

43. Goris ML, Daspit SG, McLaughlin P, Kriss JP, Interpolative background subtraction. J. nucl. Med. 17:744, 1976.

44. Maddahi J, Garcia EV, Berman DS, Waxman A, Swan HJC, Forrester J, Improved noninvasive assessment of coronary artery disease by quantitative analysis of regional stress myocardial distribution and

washout of Thallium-201. Circulation 64:924, 1981.

45. Dudczak R, Schmoliner R, Homan R, Kletter K, Frischauf H, Serial Tl-201 images after high dose dipyridamole: Diagnostic utility of Tl-201 washout analysis. Eur. J. Nucl. Med. 9:147, 1984.

46. Wilson RA, Okada RD, Boucher CA, Guiney TE, Mc Kusick K, Pohost GM, Strauss HW, Influence of eating on serial exercise Thallium myocardial and lung clearance rates. Circulation 64:242, 1981.

47. Wilson RA, Okada RA, Strauss HW, Pohost GM, Effect of glucose-insulin-potassium-infusion on Thallium myocardial clearance. Circulation 68:203, 1983.

48. Diamond GA, Forrester JS, Analysis of probability as an aid in the clinical diagnosis of coronary artery disease. New Engl. J. Med. 300:1350, 1979.

49. Epstein SE, Implications of probability analysis on the strategy used for noninvasive detection of coronary artery disease. Amer. J. Cardiol. 46:491, 1980.

50. Schmoliner R, Dudczak R, Kronik G, Kletter K, Mösslacher H, Frischauf H, Diagnostische Wertigkeit der Thallium-201-Szintigraphie nach Dipyridamol bei Patienten mit normokinetischem Ventrikel. Z. Kardiol. 72:394, 1983.

51. Wagner HN, Bayes' Theorem: An idea whose time has come? Amer. J. Cardiol. 49:875, 1982.

52. Hlatky M, Botvinick E, Brundage B, The independent value of exercise Thallium scintigraphy to physicians. Circulation 66:953, 1982.

53. Schmoliner R, Dudczak R, Kronik C, Mösslacher H, Zangeneh M, Pollak Ch, Schurz B, Schoberwalter A, Homan R, Einflusz der Thallium-201-Szintigraphie auf die klinische Einschätzung von Brustschmerzen. In: Radioaktive Isotope in Klinik und Forschung. Gasteiner Int. Symp. 1984, 16. Band, 1. Teil, p 415.

54. Wilcken DEL, Paoloni HJ, Eikens E, Evidence for intravenous dipyridamole (Persantin) producing a "coronary steal" effect in the ischemic myocardium. Aust. N.Z.J. Med. 1:8, 1971.

55. Hintze TH, Vatner SF, Dipyridamole dilates large coronary arteries in conscious dogs. Circulation 68:1321, 1983.

56. Nott MW. The possible role of adenosine in the coronary dilator action of some pyrimidopyrimidines and pteridines. Brit. J. Pharmac. 39:287, 1970.

57. Schmoliner R, Kronik G, Dudczak R, Hutterer B, Mösslacher H, Frischauf H, Die Zuverlässigkeit der Thallium-201-Szintigraphie und der zwei-dimensionalen Echokardiographie in der Diagnostik von Infarktnarben. Med. Welt 32:264, 1981.

58. Schmoliner R, Dudczak R, Kronik G, Hutterer B, Kletter K, Mösslacher H, Frischauf H, Thallium-201 imaging after dipyridamole in patients with coronary multivessel disease. Cardiology 70:145, 1983.

59. Pichard AD, Wiener I, Martinez E, Horowitz S, Patterson R, Meller J, Goldsmith S, Gorlin R, Herman MV, Septal myocardial perfusion imaging with Thallium-201 in the diagnosis of proximal left anterior descending coronary artery disease. Amer. Heart J. 102:30, 1981.

60. Platia EV, Grunwald L, Mellits ED, Humphries JO, Griffith LSC, Clinical and arteriographic variables predictive of survival in coronary artery disease. Amer. J. Cardiol. 46:543, 1980.

61. Schmoliner R, Dudczak R, Kronik G, Kletter K, Mösslacher H, Frischauf H, Erfassung von Stenosen des Ramus interventricularis anterior mittels Thallium-201-Szintigraphie nach Dipyridamol. Herz/Kreislauf 15:3, 1983.

VISUALIZATION OF MYOCARDIAL BLOOD-FLOW CHANGES WITH
INTRACORONARY 81mKr

W.J. REMME, P.H. COX, X.H. KRAUSS, H.P.A.C.M. KRUYSSEN,
C.J. STORM, D.C. van HOOGENHUYZEN

INTRODUCTION

The decision to undertake agressive therapy of a coronary
artery lesion, be it PTCA or surgery, depends entirely on the
functional significance of the particular coronary artery
stenosis present. Although more factors than the stenosis
resistance alone determine the outcome of myocardial ischemia
(see chapter 1, this volume), this can be expected to occur
in high-grade lesions (>70% diameter stenosis). In smaller
lesions, however, the determination of regional myocardial
blood-flow may be necessary to justify a therapeutic decision.

Noninvasive myocardial perfusion studies with ^{201}Tl can
be of particular value in single vessel lesions. In multivessel disease the sensitivity to delineate the smaller lesion
may be less and overlapping of the various coronary flowbeds
may prohibit the assessment of the exact localization of
diminished myocardial perfusion.

Myocardial blood-flow studies in the intact subject can
either be performed by the thermodilution method (1,2), inert
gas washout techniques (3,4) or precordial mapping of radio-
nuclides (5-9). In the thermodilution and inert gas washout
techniques the coronary sinus has to be catheterized, which
makes it an invasive procedure, allbeit of the right side of
the heart. Although these methods allow for accurate measurements, even at high flowrates (4-10) an essential drawback is
the fact that only overall left ventricular flow is measured.
This limits its value in CAD which is essentially a regional
disease. A recent modification in the thermodilution technique now allows for 2 areas of the left ventricular outflow

to be measured (11,12). However, the specific measurement of
coronary flow through the smaller subregions of the left ventricle is not possible. In addition the obligatory positioning
of the catheter in the mid coronary sinus to prevent atrial
reflux interference with the measurements, usually precludes
proper sampling from postero-lateral regions.

Labelled microspheres of approximately 15μ in diameter
reflect transmural distribution of myocardial blood-flow very
well as has been demonstrated in animal studies (13,14).
Studies in man were carried out during heartcatheterization
with macroaggregated albumin, usually employing a dual
isotope technique. These investigations performed at rest and
after some form of stress did show the technique to be quite
reliable and safe (15-18).Obviously its potential use in
humans is however limited to only a few investigations per
patient.

Inert radioactive gases administered either directly into
the coronary circulation or non-selectively in the aortic
root have been used for the precordial mapping of coronary
blood-flow. Of these ^{133}Xe has had the widest application
(5-9). During catheterization the gas is injected in solution
as a bolus into the coronary artery and the regional wash-out
curves are measured. Several successive studies with a minimal
interval of 6-8 min can be performed (6). It has been claimed
that quantitative measurements of regional coronary blood-flow
can be made. To what extent this really is possible, when
measuring essentially 3-dimensional blood-flow changes in a
2-dimensional way is questionable. This criticism however,
applies to any kind of precordial mapping technique. Other
potential difficulties with the ^{133}Xe method is a (small)
percentage of recirculation (± 5%) and its affinity for fat
(tissue participation coeeficient(λ) in myocardium assumedly
0,72 versus λ in fat tissue of 8 (19)),which can give background
accumulation during repetitive studies. Finally its relatively
low energy spectrum (gamma rays of 81 keV 37%) facilitates
Compton scatter.

Several years ago a Krypton isotope, [81m]Kr, was introduced (20-22), which allowed the continuous measurement of

regional myocardial blood-flow changes (23-26). In this chapter our experiences with the continuous intracoronary administration of ^{81m}Kr will be discussed.

Characteristics of ^{81m}Kr

^{81m}Kr is formed by isometric transition from unstable ^{81}Rb to stable ^{81}Kr, emitting 190 keV gamma rays (65% abundance). The isotope is chemically and biologically inert and has a very short physical halflife of 13.6 sec. After intracoronary administration it diffuses readily through the capillary membranes and equilibrates rapidly with the extracellular myocardial fluid.

During continuous and constant administration ^{81m}Kr is distributed in relation to regional coronary blood-flow. Stabilization between local supply and decay of the isotope is reached within 30-60 sec after the commencement of intra-coronary administration. Any change in ^{81m}Kr distribution hereafter depends on its regional supply rate and hence on local myocardial blood-flow. When ^{81m}Kr is continuously administered at a constant rate alterations in local myocardial blood-flow can be measured as the percentage change in ^{81m}Kr distribution in relation to the control situation. Due to its very short physical halflife ^{81m}Kr is not measurable in the venous effluent in the right atrium. This together with its 190 keV radiation spectrum ensures imaging with a negligable background.

^{81m}Kr production. During our studies ^{81m}Kr was eluted from a sterile, pyrogen-free ^{81}Rb/^{81m}Kr generator. ^{81}Rb is formed during proton bombardment of natural Krypton gas, which results in a ^{81}Rb production rate of 3 mCi/μ A.h.; over 95% of which is recovered in aqueous solution (27). The ^{81}Rb/^{81m}Kr generator was calibrated to deliver 20-25 mCi at the time of the study. The unstable ^{81}Rb decays to ^{81m}Kr, which emits 190 keV gamma rays (65% abundance). Elution of the generator with 5% glucose yields a solution containing only ^{81m}Kr. Even at high perfusion rates of 25 ml/min only a negligeable break-through of ^{81}Rb occurs.

The eluate is then passed through a sterile millepore filter into the coronary artery catheter. Optimal perfusion rates from the generator in order to achieve sufficient and constant build-up of ^{81m}Kr on the ^{81}Rb column are in between 12-15 ml/min. In our studies a constant perfusion rate with 5% glucose of 13,3 ml/min was achieved with the use of a persistaltic infusion pump, resulting in 15 mCi total radio-activity per min with a 20 mCi generator.

Instrumentation. Contrary to studies with ^{133}Xe, where multicrystal cameras were preferable due to their fast count rate possibilities, the single crystal camera is better for the ^{81m}Kr studies described in this chapter. Very fast count rates as can be realized with multiple crystal cameras (up to 200.000 - 500.000 counts per sec) are unnecessary in view of the limited production of ^{81m}Kr by the generator even at a higher calibration (up to 35 mCi). On the other hand the better spatial resolution of the single crystal camera enables flow changes to be determined in relatively small areas of the left ventricle, which is less optimal with the multicrystal camera due to its poor pictorial resolution. Count rates are improved using a ½-inch crystal instead of the ¼-inch crystal gamma cameras currently used for nuclear cardiology purposes. In these studies we have tried out both crystal sizes.

Total counts over the heart/min averaged ± 250.000 for the ½ inch crystal gamma camera (General electric porta camera) and ± 180.000 for the ¼ inch (Siemens LEM portable camera) using similar data processing techniques. Data given in this chapter are obtained with the ½-inch crystal gamma camera, connected on line to a Medical Data Systems - A2 computer and energy detection set on 190 keV ± 20%. Throughout the study imaging was visualized both on a persistence scope and on a monitor connected to the computer.

Images were acquired in 15 sec frames with the camera in 45° LAO position. In some studies an additional investigation was carried out in the 30° right inferior oblique position (RIO) to achieve optimal separation between the marginal branches of the left circumflex coronary artery.

Changes in ^{81m}Kr distribution were measured in various
regions of interest. over the left ventricle, including both
normal regions and areas with CAD, over the ascending aorta,
total left heart and background regions, including the right
atrium. Areas of interest were constructed using an electronic
lightpen on the visual display unit.

Movement artefacts during the study were avoided and care
was taken that successive regions of interest did not move
out of their originally constructed areas. Further calculations were made of both total counts per area as well as of
total counts per pixel per area. In order to correct for
possible fluctuations in ^{81m}Kr delivery counts per area per
frame were always correlated with and given as percentages
of simultaneous total counts over the left heart.

Patient studies: Methodology and materials. Studies were
carried out in patients with suspected or confirmed coronary
artery disease in whom catheterization was believed necessary
either to confirm the diagnosis or to investigate the possibility of angioplasty or by-pass surgery.

Patients were studied without premedication after an
overnight fast because of concomittant metabolic investigations.

Using the Seldinger technique introducer systems were
inserted in the right femoral artery and in the right brachial
vein. This allowed the positioning of a 7F Judkins or Amplatz
left coronary artery catheter in the ostium of the left
coronary artery and a 7F Zucker bipolar pacing catheter in the
mid-coronary sinus for pacing purposes and sampling of
coronary venous blood. The length of the left coronary main
stem and the position of the catheter tip in it were then
examined in the 30° RIO position. Next, possible selective
injections in one of the branches of the left coronary artery
were studied by both slow and rapid manual injection of
contrast material in the 45° LAO and 30° RIO positions and
registered on videotape for continuous replay. When the
possibility of streaming was present different catheters and
catheter sizes were tried. Finally, any fluctuation in ^{81m}Kr

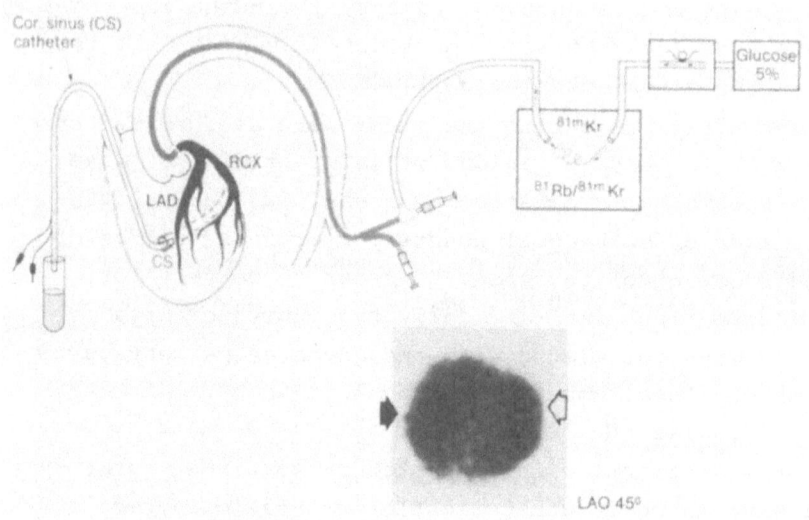

Fig. 1. Schematic representation of the study design. ^{81m}Kr is eluted in 5% glucose from the $^{81}Rb/^{81m}Kr$ generator and infused directly into the left coronary artery. At the bottom of the figure normal ^{81m}Kr distribution over the LAD and RCX area is shown in a patient without coronary artery disease. LAD = left anterior descending artery. RCX = left circumflex artery.

distribution over the left ventricle was excluded during a 10 min control period before initiation of the study.

When the possibility of streaming still existed or in the case of a short mainstem either a super-selective perfusion was carried out in the coronary branch of interest or the patient was excluded from the study altogether. A schematic representation of the investigational set-up and normal ^{81m}Kr distribution at rest is given in fig 1. A stabilization period of 20 min was allowed before initation of a stress test by way of incremental atrial pacing. During this test the heart rate was increased by 10 beats every 2 min until either anginal pain and/or atrio-ventricular block occurred. Through-out the study precordial imaging was carried out in successive 15 sec frames. Results are given for the control situations,

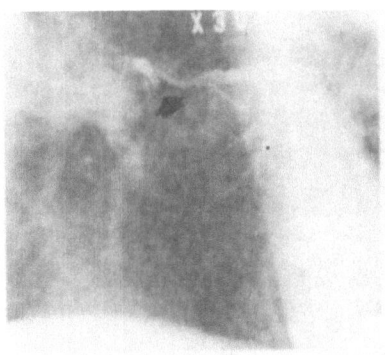
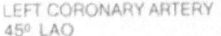
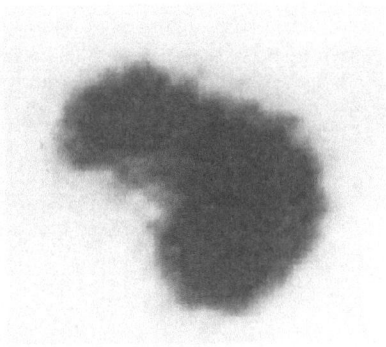

LEFT CORONARY ARTERY
45° LAO

81mKr DISTRIBUTION DURING CONTROL
45° LAO

Fig. 2. ^{81m}Kr distribution at rest in a patient with a 100% LAD occlusion (see arrow). There is diminished ^{81m}Kr perfusion over the distal LAD area and normal distribution over the RCX and proximal LAD region. LAD = left anterior descending artery. RCX = left circumflex artery.

at 100, 120, 140, 160 and 180 beats/min and during anginal pain or atrio-ventricular block, followed by determinations 15 sec, 1, 2 and 5 min after pacing. Onset and progression of anginal pain was correlated with ^{81m}Kr distribution changes in the simultaneous 15 sec imaging frames.

Results

In 2 patients a selective infusion in the diseased branch of the left coronary artery was carried out because of a short mainstem.

One patient had to be excluded due to a possible streaming artefact.

^{81m}Kr distribution changes in patients with normal coronary arteries. In 4 patients no significant coronary artery disease was present (CAD <50%). In these patients ^{81m} distribution over the left ventricle was normal during the control period and did not change during and after atrial pacing.

^{81m}Kr distribution changes in patients with CAD. In 16 patients with >50% CAD 12 areas with ≥90% and 6 areas with

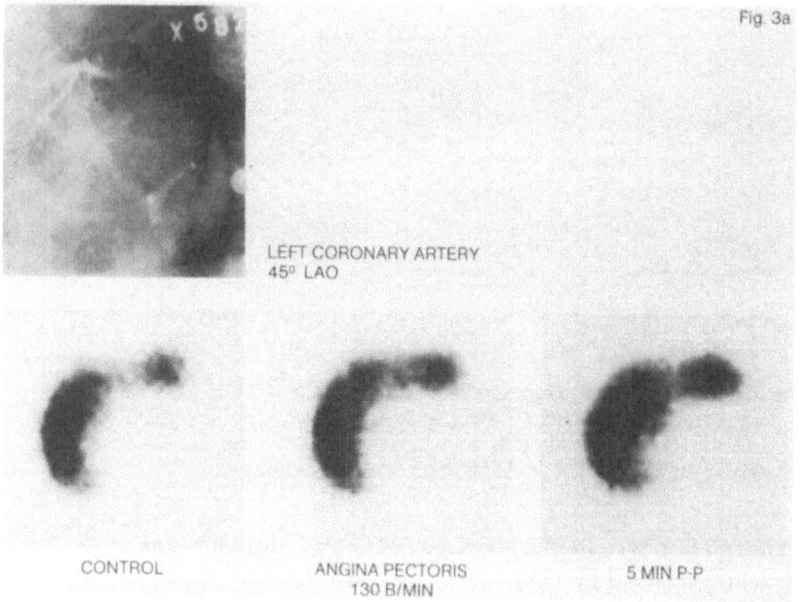

Fig. 3a. Absent ^{81m}Kr distribution in the RCX region at rest and during pacing in a patient who was catheterized twice within one week. Within this period a 99% RCX stenosis had progressed to a total occlusion without anterograde collaterals. Halfway the LAD a 50-70% stenosis is present, which however does not result in any change in ^{81m}Kr distribution in this area during pacing. LAD = left anterior descending artery. RCX = left circumflex artery.

70-90% were present. Wallmotion abnormalities during left ventriculography at rest (30° RAO and 45° LAO projections) were observed in 9 patients: 8 in ≥90% and 1 in 70-90% left CAD areas, varying from hypo- to dyskinesia. Anterograde collaterals were present in 7 areas: in 6 with ≥90% and 1 with a 70-90% stenosis.

^{81m}Kr distribution at rest. During the 10 min control period the ^{81m}Kr distribution pattern remained stable with only small fluctuations (<5%). ^{81m}Kr perfusion was normal in most areas. In only 5 an obviously diminished, however un-

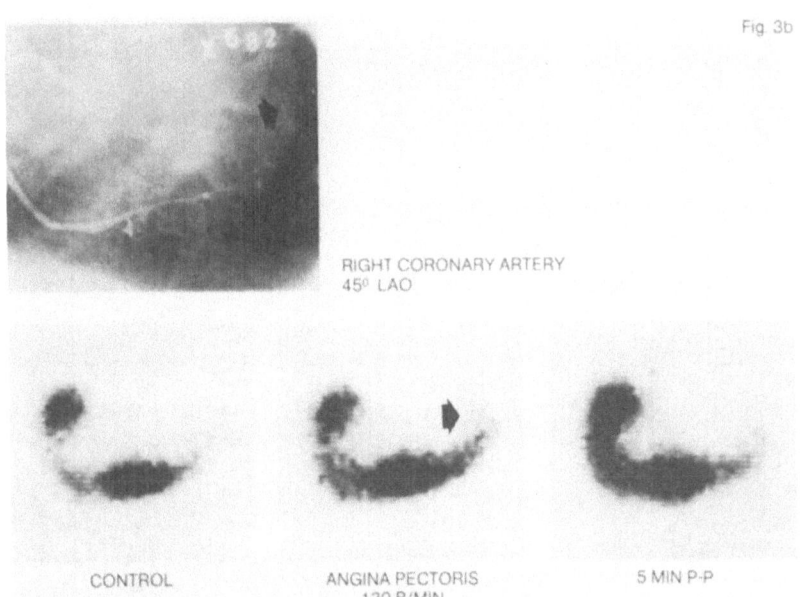

Fig. 3b

RIGHT CORONARY ARTERY
45° LAO

CONTROL   ANGINA PECTORIS   5 MIN P-P
130 B/MIN

Fig. 3b. ^{81m}Kr perfusion of the right coronary artery in the same
patient. During the interval between the two catheterizations a retrograde collateral circulation to the RCX area has developed. ^{81m}Kr
perfusion is now shown to improve markedly in the RCX area during
atrial pacing.

changed distribution was observed, all in ⩾90% left CAD
regions. In 4 of these anterograde collaterals were present
with decreased, however measurable radioactivity (fig 2). In
1 patient, who was reinvestigated within 1 week after a
previous catheterization in order to perform a Krypton study,
a 99% left marginal branch had closed without signs of a
recent infarction. However also without the formation of
anterograde collaterals (fig. 3a). No ^{81m}Kr perfusion of the
marginal area occurred, either at rest and during pacing.
Retrograde collaterals from the right coronary artery had
developed in between the 2 successive catheterizations with

Table 1. ^{81m}Kr distribution changes during and after pacing in patients with >70% L-CAD

Lesion:	control	100 b/min	120 b/min	AP	15 sec P-P	1 min P-P	5 min P-P
>90% N = 12	100%	86 ± 6*	77 ± 7*	67 ± 6.3[+*]	74 ± 6[+]	83 ± 6.2*	84 ± 6.8*
70-90% N = 6	100%	92 ± 4.6	87 ± 3.9*	80 ± 5.6*	80 ± 3.6*	88 ± 6.5*	90 ± 4.7*
normal areas	100%	112 ± 3.7*	118 ± 3*	125 ± 5.6*	120 ± 3.9*	118 ± 5.7*	110 ± 5.1

Abbreviations: L-CAD = left coronary artery disease
b/min = beats/minute
AP   = anginal pain
P-P = post-pacing
*   = p <0.05 vs control
+   = p <0.001 (AP ≥90% vs AP 70-90%)

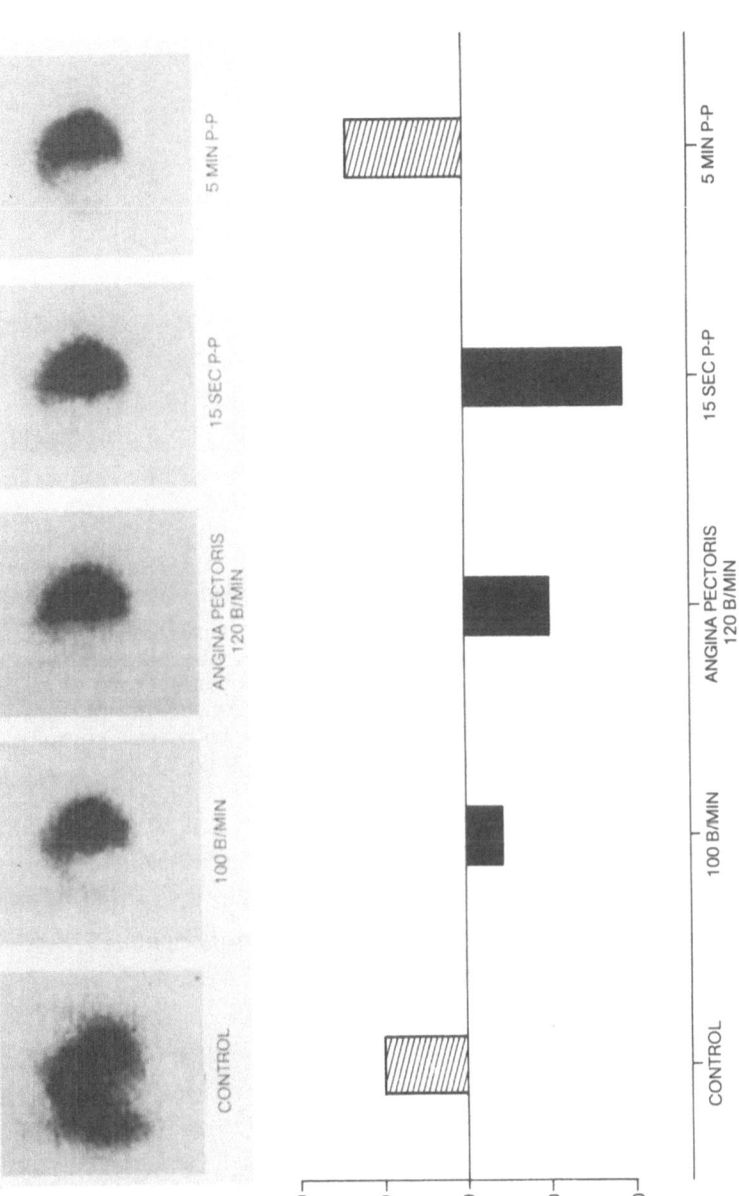

Fig. 4. Typical example of early and progressive decrease of ^{81m}Kr distribution in a 90% stenosis area (LAD). There is simultaneous increase in the normal RCX region. Changes occur before anginal pain and in this case, together with lactacte production and have not returned to control values 5 min after cessation of pacing. P-P= post pacing. B/min= beats/min. SEC= sec. RCX= left circumflex artery. LAD= left anterior descending artery.

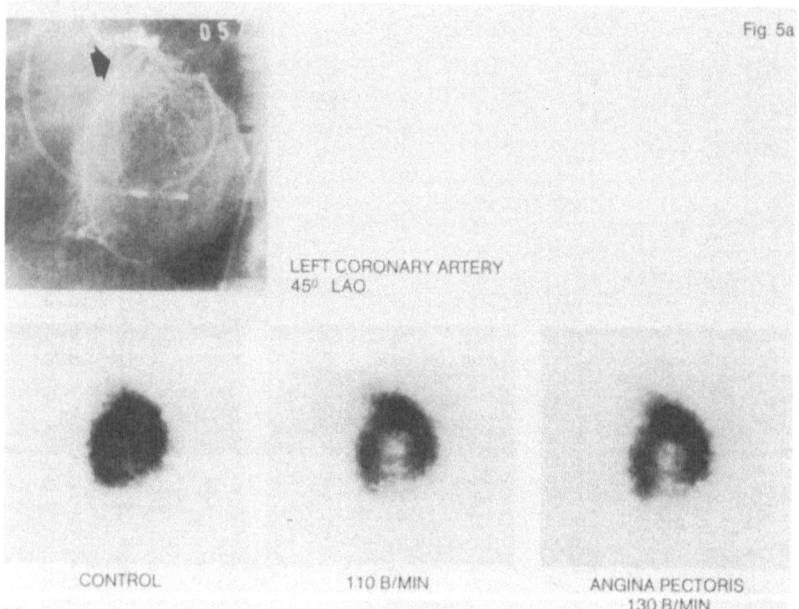

Fig. 5a. 45° LAD view of ^{81m}Kr distribution at rest and during pacing in a patient with proximal 90% lesions in the LAD (closed arrow, 5a) and obtuse marginal artery (open arrow 5b). During angina pectoris there is diminished ^{81m}Kr distribution over the LAD area, which however is not so evident in the obtuse marginal region, presumably due to normal perfusion of postero-lateral branches which in this view are partially overlying the diseased coronary artery.

some retrograde filling at rest; which however improved during the atrial pacing stress test (fig 3b). In none of the patients was the diminished ^{81m}Kr distribution at rest accompanied by signs of myocardial ischemia, such as anginal pain, ECG changes or myocardial lactate production. However, abnormal wall motion at rest was found in all and documented old myocardial infarcts in 3 patients.

^{81m}Kr distribution during pacing (table 1). During atrial pacing ^{81m}Kr distribution decreased in all >70% left-CAD areas with simultaneous increases in the normal areas. In the ≥90% lesions this fall in ^{81m}Kr perfusion developed at an

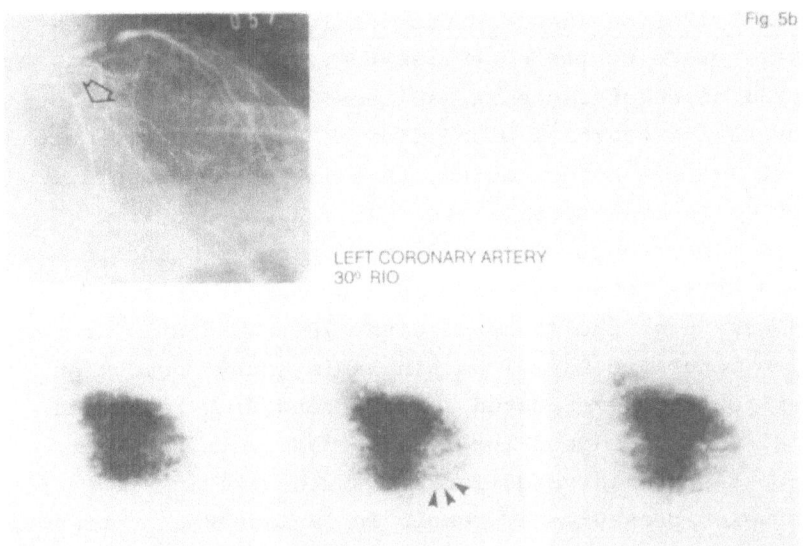

Fig. 5b

LEFT CORONARY ARTERY
30° RIO

Fig. 5b. During a second atrial pacing stress test imaging was performed
in the 30° RIO position. The obtuse marginal artery is in this view
separated from the postero-lateral branches and a ^{81m}Kr perfusion defect
is now clearly visible in this area during pacing (arrows). ^{81m}Kr distribution is still abnormal 2 min after pacing in both obtuse marginal and LAD
regions.

early stage and was progressive to the end of pacing.

An example is given in fig 4. In this patient with a
proximal 90% stenosis of the LAD artery ^{81m}Kr perfusion
diminished at an early stage before the development of anginal
pain, however, together with lactate production. During anginal
pain an impressive shift in ^{81m}Kr distribution from the diseased
to the normal area is seen. This progressive decrease of ^{81m}Kr
perfusion of early onset was found in all ⩾90% lesions. In the
70-90% stenosis group a change in ^{81m}Kr distribution usually
only occurred halfway or towards the end of pacing.

Further, the magnitude of the changes differ between the
2 groups with significantly lower ^{81m}Kr perfusion during anginal
pain, 67 ± 6.3% of control in the >90% lesions as compared to

a decrease to 80 ± 5.6% in the 70-90% stenosis group (p<0.001). The fact that ^{81m}Kr changes are found in all >70% areas and not in the <50% lesions indicates its possible use to discriminate between significant and non-significant CAD.

^{81m}Kr distribution changes after pacing. In our studies usually late return to the control situation was found long after general signs of ischemia had subsided. Given the fact that the overall myocardial blood-flow is back to normal within the first 1-2 min after pacing, this implies an absolute flow reduction in the ischemic area. As can be seen from table 1 this flow reduction lasted more than 5 min and in some patients was still found to exist as long as 15 min after pacing. In only 6 of the 18 areas with >70% CAD did ^{81m}Kr distribution return to normal within 5 min after pacing. An explanation for this unexpected long-lasting flow reduction after atrial pacing induced ischemia is difficult to give. Prolonged post-stenotic vasodilatation with lowering of peripheral perfusion pressure may result in an increase in stenotic resistance and a reduction in regional flow (28). A continuing adenosine release from the ischemic area is likely in view of the fact that myocardial venous hypoxanthine levels are still increased 5 min after pacing in analogue studies (29). Regional myocardial blood-flow which is still abnormal 15 min after pacing is possibly the reason for a non-reproducible lactate pattern during repetitive atrial pacing stress tests with this interval (30).

Repetitive ^{81m}Kr distribution imaging in various positions. ^{81m}Kr imaging in our studies was always started in the 45° LAO position, separating the LAD and RCX regions. In addition perfusion studies of the right coronary artery were performed from this angle. This than allows a clear view of the right coronary perfusion areas in the infero-apical and postero-lateral regions (fig 3) without the problems of overprojection of the left coronary artery blood-supply in these areas. In single vessel lesions and in most of the patients with multi-vessel disease one left coronary artery in the 45° LAO view study was usually sufficient to obtain all the information

needed. However, in some instances a second study was necessary
from a different imaging angle in order to separate the branches
of the left circumflex artery. The 30° right inferior oblique
position was chosen for this purpose separating the various
marginal branches of this artery. The second study was performed
after a 30 min interval. An example is given in fig 5. This
patient had both a >90% stenosis of the LAD and of the obtuse
marginal branch. During atrial pacing in the 45° LAO projection
there is an obvious decrease of ^{81m}Kr distribution over the
LAD area, however, not so apparent over the RCX area (fig 5a).
Due to overprojection of the normal postero-lateral branch
over the stenotic obtuse marginal artery a decrease in ^{81m}Kr
perfusion in the latter could be compensated by hyperemia and
an increase in ^{81m}Kr activity in the normal postero-lateral
area.

The functional significance of the obtuse marginal stenosis
is now demonstrated in the second study with the gamma camera
in the 30° RIO position (fig 5b). The marginal branches and their
perfusion area are now separated and diminished ^{81m}Kr distrubu-
tion is clearly seen in the peripheral obtuse marginal region,
as well as in the LAD area.

Selective intra-coronary ^{81m}Kr infusion versus nonselective
administration. Due to its very short half-life ^{81m}Kr must be
administered either directly into the coronary artery (selective) or in the immediate vicinity of the coronary artery ostia
(non-selective). Though the possibility of a streaming artefact with the intracoronary method, imposes an important theoretical drawback to the procedure its occurence is in our
experience easily recognizable and preventable.

In the great majority of patients this type of study can
be carried out without streaming artefacts after selection of
the appropriate type of catheter. Also a change in catheter-
tip position during pacing and fast heart rates, giving rise to
a more superselective infusion and hence a distribution artefact, is unlikely in view of the fact that in most patients
^{81m}Kr distribution did not return to the control situation
immediately after cessation of pacing, which would be expected
in case of artefacts. The consistent observation of a decreased

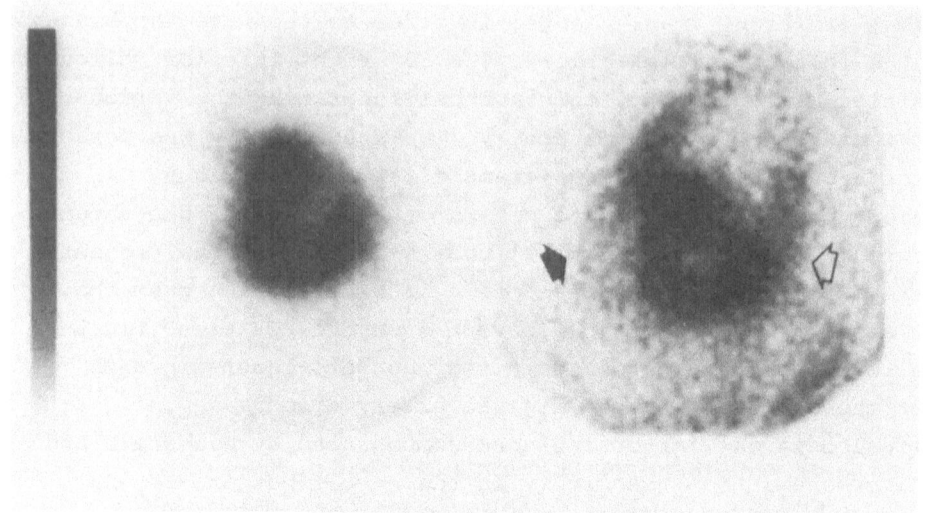

Fig. 6. Direct intracoronary administration of ^{81m}Kr (left image) compared with an infusion of the same amount into the aortic sinuses (right image). The difference in activity over the heart is obvious. Also, perfusion of the right coronary bed can be seen (closed arrow), which may overlap in the infero-apical region. The same problem may occur in the RCX area by counts from the descending aorta (open arrow) during intra-aortic administration. RCX = left circumflex artery.

^{81m}Kr perfusion pattern during episodes of spontaneous anginal pain and normal resting heart rates found in the same areas as during pacing induced ischemia is also a strong argument against streaming artefacts (data not given in this chapter).

In our experience the selective intracoronary infusion of ^{81m}Kr provided acceptable information about the functional significance of the coronary artery disease present.

On the other hand we were unable to obtain reliable data when applying nonselective methods of administration of ^{81m}Kr in the aortic root and/or aortic sinuses both with "normal" or specially designed catheters.

Invariably the total amount of counts over the heart was far too low to allow proper statistical analysis. This is not surprising taking into consideration the relatively small portion of cardiac output which enters the coronary circulation. Even using special catheters, designed for delivery of ^{81m}Kr directly in the coronary sinuses, the total amount of

of radioactivity over the left ventricle is proportionally
small compared with the direct intracoronary administration.
An example of the best nonselective ^{81m}Kr imaging we were
able to manage is shown in fig 6 as well as an intracoronary
study in the same patient. The difference in activity is obvious.
Also demonstrated is the obligate simultaneous perfusion of
the right coronary artery with overprojection in the infero-
apical region. Both this overprojection and the relatively
high background activity of the descending aorta, usually
underlying the circumflex area present problems defining ^{81m}Kr
perfusion changes in these regions. Problems were not encountered with the direct intracoronary administration.

Clinical implications

As the investigation is necessarily invasive it is not
suitable for use as a routine procedure. However, valuable
information can be derived from this kind of study especially
with reference to the functional significance of the various
lesions in multivessel disease. This information is not always
available from conventional, noninvasive techniques.

Due to the short half-life of ^{81m}Kr a multitude of successive studies can be performed in the same patient without
extra exposure to radiation other than that necessary for the
instantaneous study. The effect of repetitive stress tests and
pharmaceutical intervention on regional myocardial blood-flow
and myocardial ischemia can be evaluated. Further, the localization of perfusion disturbances during spontaneous anginal
attacks or ergonovine-induced coronary spasm can be investigated
as well as the influences of vaso-active drugs in these situations. Presumably the most important reason however, to subject
the patient to this kind of investigation will be the situation
where a moderate coronary artery lesion of 50-70% exists and
the decision whether to perform surgery or angioplasty is
debatable. The clinical significance of this stenosis will be
adequately demonstrated during an atrial pacing stress test
with continuous intracoronary administration of ^{81m}Kr.

REFERENCES

1. Ganz W, Tamura K, Marcus HS et al, Measurement of coronary sinus blood-flow by continuous thermodilution in man. Circulation 44:181, 1971.

2. Weisse AB, Regan IJ, A comparison of thermodilution, coronary sinus blood-flows and Krypton myocardial blood-flows in the intact dog. Cardiovasc. Res. 8:526, 1974.

3. Rau G, Messung der Koronardurchblutung mit der Argon-Fremdgasmethode. Arch. Kreisl-Forsch. 58:322, 1969.

4. Tauchert M, Kochsiek K, Heiss HW et al, Technik der Organdurchblutungs-messung mit der Argonmethode. Z. Kreisl-Forsch. 60:871, 1971.

5. Cannon PJ, Measurement of regional myocardial perfusion by intra-coronary injection of Xenon-133. In: Clinical Nuclear Cardiology, Berman DS, Mason DT (eds), Grune Stratton, New York, p 119, 1981.

6. Engel HJ, Assessment of regional myocardial blood-flow by the pre-cordial ^{133}Xenon clearance technique. In: The pathophysiology of myocardial perfusion. Schaper W (ed), Elsevier/North-Holland Bio-medical Press, Amsterdam.

7. Holman BL, Cohn PF, Adams DF et al, Regional myocardial blood-flow during hyperemia induced by contrast agent in patients with coronary artery disease. Amer. J. Cardiol. 38:416, 1976.

8. Schmidt DH, Weiss MB, Casarella WJ et al, Regional myocardial perfu-sion during atrial pacing in patients with coronary artery disease. Circulation 53:807, 1976.

9. Maseri A, l'Abbate A, Pesola A et al, Regional myocardial perfusion in patients with atherosclerotic coronary artery disease at rest and during angina pectoris induced by tachycardia. Circulation 55:423, 1977.

10. Tauchert M, Kochsiek K, Weiss HW et al, Measurement of coronary blood-flow in man by the argon method. In: Myocardial blood-flow in man. Maseri A (ed), Minerva Medica, Turin, p. 139, 1972.

11. Pepine CJ, Mehta J, Webster WW et al, In vivo validation of a thermo-dilution method to determine regional left ventricular blood-flow in patients with coronary disease. Circulation 58:795, 1978.

12. Feldman RL, Pepine CJ, Whittle JL et al, Coronary hemodynamic findings during spontaneous angina in patients with variant angina. Circulation 64:76, 1981.

13. Domenech RJ, Hoffmann JJE, Noble MJM et al, Total and regional coronary blood-flow measured by radioactive microsphere in consious and anaesthetized dogs. Circulat. Res. 25:581, 1969.

14. Winkler B, The tracer microsphere method. In: The pathophysiology of myocardial perfusion. Schaper W (ed), Elsevier/North-Holland Bio-medical Press, Amsterdam, p. 13, 1979.

15. Ashburn WL, Braunwald E, Simon AL et al, Myocardial perfusion imaging with radioactive labeled particles injected directly into the coronary circulation of patients with coronary artery disease. Circulation 44:851, 1971.

16. Weller DA, Adolph RJ, Wellman HN et al, Myocardial perfusion scinti-
    graphy after intracoronary injection of Tc-99m labeled human albumin
    microspheres. Circulation 46:963, 1972.

17. Kirk GA, Adams R, Jansen C et al, Particulate myocardial perfusion
    scintigraphy: Its clinical usefulness in evaluation of coronary
    artery disease. Sem. Nucl. Med. 7:67, 1977.

18. Ritchie JL, Hamilton GW, Gould KL et al, Myocardial imaging with
    Indium-113m and Technetium-99m-macroaggregated albumin. Amer. J.
    Cardiol. 35:380, 1975.

19. Conn HL jr, Equilibrium distribution of radioxenon in tissue:
    Xenon-hemoglobin association curve. J. Appl. Physiol. 16:1065, 1961.

20. Jones T, Clark JC, A cyclotron produced ^{81}Rb-^{81m}Kr generator and
    its uses in gamma camera studies. Brit. J. Radiol. 42:237, 1969.

21. Clark JC, Horlock PL, Watson IA, Krypton-81m generators. Radiochem.
    Radioanalyt. Letters 25:245, 1976.

22. Kaplan E, Mayron LW, Evaluation of perfusion with the ^{81}Rb-^{81m}Kr
    generator. Sem. Nucl. Med. 6:163, 1976.

23. Remme WJ, Krauss XH, Hoogenhuyze Van DCA et al, Continuous determina-
    tion of regional myocardial blood-flow with intracoronary Krypton-
    81m. In preparation.

24. Selwyn AP, Steiner R, Kivisaari A et al, Krypton-81m in the physiologic
    assessment of coronary artery stenosis in man. Amer. J. Cardiol.
    43:547, 1979.

25. Remme WJ, Cox PH, Krauss XH, Continuous myocardial blood-flow
    distribution imaging in man with Krypton-81m intracoronary
    (Abstract). Amer. J. Cardiol. 49,979, 1982.

26. Remme WJ, Kruyssen HA, Cox PH et al, Assessment of functionally
    significant coronary artery disease during continuous intracoronary
    administration of Krypton-81m. Eur. Heart J. (suppl E) 4:32, 1983.

27. Remme WJ, Cox PH, Krauss XH et al, Continuous myocardial blood-flow
    imaging Krypton-81m selective intracoronary. In: Radioisotopes in
    cardiology. Salvatore M, Porta E (eds), 1983.

28. Guillaume M, Richard R et al, Krypton-81m generator for ventilation
    and perfusion. Dosimetry, routine production, methodology for
    medical applications. Monographic, Institut National Radioéléments,
    Fleurus, Belgium, 1982.

29. Schwartz JS, Carlyle PF, Cohn JN, Decline in blood-flow in stenotic
    coronary arteries during increased myocardial energetic demand in
    response to pacing-induced tachycardia. Amer. Heart J. 101:435, 1981.

30. Remme WJ, Jong De JW, Verdouw PD, Effects of pacing-induced myocardial
    ischemia on hypoxanthine efflux from the human heart. Amer J. Cardiol.
    40:55, 1977.

31. Remme WJ, Hoogenhuyze Van DH, Storm CS et al, Lactate extraction
    pattern during repeated ischemia in the human heart (Abstract).
    J. Mol. Cell. Cardiol. (suppl I) 13:76, 1981.

Tc^{99m}-DMPE, A POTENTIAL SUBSTITUTE FOR ^{201}TL CHLORIDE?

C. SCHÜMICHEN, P. BERGMANN, M. HALL

INTRODUCTION

In contrast to Tc^{99m} "tagged" radiopharmaceuticals, in which Technetium is bound to large molecules, the Tc^{99m} "essential" complexes, where the Technetium centre provides the structural frame-work and the charge of the whole complex, have received little attention in the past. Technetium forms anionic as well as cationic co-ordinative complexes (1). By using o-phenylene bisdimenthylarsine DIARS) (=L) as the ligand, complexes of the type $[Tc(II)Cl_2L_2]$, $[Tc(III)Cl_2L_2]Cl$ and $[Tc(V)Cl_4L_2]ClO_4$ have been prepared by Fergusson and Nyholm in 1959 (2,3).

Because of their potential use as myocardial imaging agents, Tc^{99m}-DIARS and various other cationic complexes have been synthetized under "no carrier added" conditions and quantitatively evaluated in a dog model by Deutsch and co-workers (4). Tc^{99m}-DIARS complexes successfully imaged the dog myocardium, but were not soluble in water. More recently a water soluble compound, bis (1,2 dimethylphosphino)ethane or $(CH_3)_2P$-CH_2CH_2-$P(CH_3)_2$, hereafter refered as DMPE, was developed by the same group (5). The cationic Technetium-99 complex trans- $[Tc$-$99(DMPE)_2Cl_2]^+$ was prepared and its chemical structure characterized by single-crystal, X-ray structural analysis. The Tc^{99m} analog, Tc^{99m}-DMPE, most likely of the same structure, proved to be a very promising myocardial imaging agent in the dog (5,6). The similar kinetics of Tc^{99m}-DMPE compared to ^{201}Tl in the dog suggested its usefulness in the evaluation of ischemic heart disease also in man (7).

However, further investigation clearly demonstrated, that the biodistribution of Tc^{99m}-DMPE is strongly species dependent

(8). Unfortunately unsatisfactory results were obtained in man (9). Hence the continuing research for Tc^{99m} labelled myocardial imaging agents has to be focussed on the mechanism of myocardial uptake as well as on the origin of the species differences in the biokinetics of these agents.

Preparation

DMPE was obtained from Strem Chemicals, Newburyport in Massachusetts. It is a flammable liquid, highly air sensitive and because of this stored under argon. It is a powerful reductant, able to reduce (Tc(VII) to Tc(III) when the temperature is raised to 145°. Since DMPE is not water soluble, all preparations have to be made in alcoholic solution. The pH in the preparation has to be adjusted to 7-9, at high pH a complex without myocardial uptake and at low pH $(Tc^{99m}\text{-DMPE})^+$ with delayed uptake in the myocardium is formed (8).

A convenient mode of preparation was reported at the Third World Congress for Nuclear Medicine and Biology in Paris 1982 (10):

1 ml pertechnetate
1 ml ethylalcohol
0,25 ml 0,2 m HCl
0,3 ml DMPE

An even better heart-liver-ratio is obtained, when 1,0 M HCl instead of 0,2 M HCl is used. In all results shown here the preparation was kept free of oxygen by purging with N_2 and was heated up to 145°C for two hours. The preparation was diluted with isotonic and other dilution media (oxygen-free), before a constant volume of 0,5 ml was injected into a tail vein of the rat.

The labelling yield obtained with the method of described preparation above, was excellent and no further chromatographic purification was necessary. The excess of DMPE in the preparation can only be extracted in part by acetone or CCL_4. Because of potential toxic side effects of DMPE this mode of preparation can only be recommended for animal experiments. For clinical use much lower DMPE concentrations in the preparation can

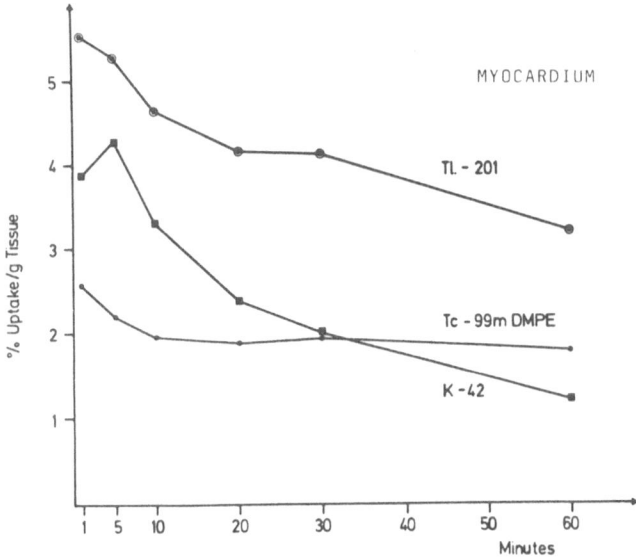

Figs 1-3: Biokinetics of Tc^{99m}-DMPE compared with ^{42}K and ^{201}Tl chloride in the rat (male Wistar rats 180 g, 3 mg DMPE/kg bodyweight, n=10 each).

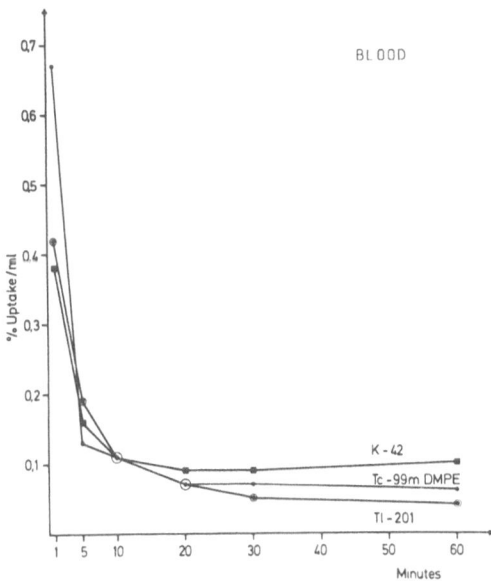

Fig. 2.

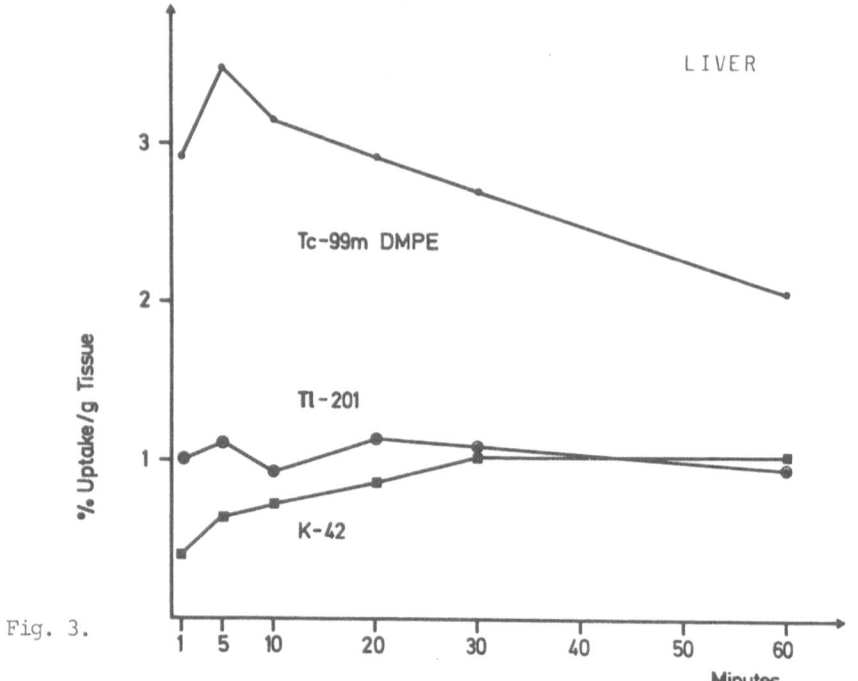

Fig. 3.

be used, under optimized reaction conditions a radiochemical yield of greater than 95% Tc[99m]-DMPE could be achieved (11).

Electrical charge

The charge of Tc[99m]-DMPE was determined by means of "carrier-free" electrophoresis. This was carried out in a glastube, filled with purified seasand to avoid heat circulation. No other carrier was used to minimize absorptive effects (12). The migration of Tc[99m]-DMPE, observed with a gamma camera, was found to be opposite to that of Tc[99m]-pertechnetate. By this the cationic character of Tc-[99m]-DMPE is definitely proved.

Biokinetics compared to [42]K and [201]Tl

The biodistribution of Tc[99m] was compared with [42]K and ^{201}Tl chloride in the rat, 3 mg DMPE/kg bodyweight was injected in 0,5 ml (male Wistar rats, 160-180 g n= 10 each point). The most relevant results are shown in figs 1-3. Initial uptake of Tc[99m]-DMPE in the myocardium was lower than that of other agents, but 60 min after injection the myocardial uptake of Tc^{99m}-DMPE was superior to that of ^{42}K (fig 1). ^{201}Tl uptake in the myocardium exceeded that of ^{42}K at any time. The clearance rate from the myocardium was the highest in the case of $42K$ and the lowest in the case of $Tc99m$-DMPE.

The blood-clearance rate of all three agents was essentially the same (fig 2) whereas the liver uptake of Tc^{99m}-DMPE exceeded that of the other agents considerably (fig 3).

In vitro and in vivo stability

Tc^{99m}-DMPE proved to be extremely stable, in 0,2 M aquaous NaCl no hydrolysis or decomposition over period of three weeks was detectable (6). Even when the DMPE concentration in the preparation injected was lowered to $10^{-7}M$, the biodistribution in the rat remained unchanged. It can be concluded, that Tc^{99m}-DMPE is much more stable than most Tc^{99m} tagged radio-pharmaceuticals used in nuclear medicine hitherto.

Species differences in biodistribution

The well known species differences in the biodistribution of Tc^{99m}-DMPE were evaluated quantitatively in a rat model, results are shown in table 1. The Tc^{99m}-DMPE preparation was diluted prior to injection in various media, such as 0,9% NaCl, phosphate buffer pH 7,4, rat plasma and human plasma. All preparations were kept oxygen-free through purging with N_2; for maintenance of pH phosphate buffer was added to rat and human plasma.

In general, the biodistribution was not changed significantly, regardless if Tc^{99m}-DMPE was diluted in isotonic saline, phosphate buffer pH 7,4 or rat plasma pH 7,4. However, if dilution was made in human plasma pH 7,4, myocardial uptake was lowered and liver uptake increased by factor 2 each. Uptake in the other organs remained unchanged. These changes are well in accordance with the observations made in man (8).

Protein binding

Relative protein binding of Tc^{99m}-DMPE in rat and human

Tab. 1:   **1 hr Biodistribution of Tc-99m DMPE in the Rat**

Dilution of Tc-99m DMPE in various media prior to injection.

Final DMPE concentration 3×10^{-6}M, 0.5 ml injected (male Wistar rats, 160-180 g, n = 18 each)

Whole organ	0.9% NaCl	Phosphate buffer pH 7.4	Rat plasma 50% buffer	Human plasma 50% buffer
Blood	0.66 + 0.08	0.65 + 0.08	0.96 + 0.25	0.56 + 0.07
Myocardium	**0.98** + 0.17	**1.11** + 0.14	**1.12** + 0.14	**0.66** + 0.19
Liver	**18.1** + 4.6	**15.9** + 6.22	**16.2** + 3.75	**32.5** + 2.49
Spleen	1.17 + 0.24	1.37 + 0.42	1.06 + 0.38	1.25 + 0.30
Stomach	1.49 + 0.23	1.61 + 0.26	1.72 + 0.31	1.11 + 0.18
Kidneys	10.4 + 2.00	10.2 + 2.29	11.0 + 1.58	9.09 + 0.97
Muscle	15.1 + 3.41	17.4 + 4.82	19.6 + 5.26	13.2 + 1.69
Bone (avg.)	4.90 + 0.79	4.87 + 0.66	5.70 + 0.76	4.93 + 0.74
Urine	1.38 + 0.48	1.34 + 0.32	1.24 + 0.30	1.07 + 0.37

Tab. 2: **Relative Protein Binding of Tc-99m DMPE**
in Rat and Human Plasma (%)
(50% phosphate buffer, pH 7.4, O_2-free)

	Total	Albumin	Globulins
Rat	99.9 %	12.7 %	87.3 %
Man	99.9 %	98.8 %	1.2 %

Tab. 3: **Electrophoresis of Plasma**
(50% phosphate buffer, pH 7.4)

	Albumin	a1	a2	ß	y
Rat	48.5	18.5	6.6	17.3	8.9
Man	63.6	2.6	6.0	9.2	18.4

Tabl. 4: **Toxicity of Tc-99m DMPE**
(toxic concentrations in blood calculated
from in vivo studies in the rat and in vitro
studies in human blood, safety factor 10 is
introduced because of an in homogeneous
distribution of DMPE in aqueous solutions)

$0.3 \cdot 10^{-6}$ hemolysis
$3 \cdot 10^{-6}$ hemoglobinuria
$100 \cdot 10^{-6}$ thrombosis

Upper Safety Level of DMPE
0.3 mg/kg body weight in $3 \cdot 10^{-6}$ M

plasma was evaluated by means of the ammonium sulphate method, previously described (10). Results are shown in table 2. The DMPE concentration in blood was adopted to that achieved in vivo after injection of 3mg DMPE/kg body weight. Both in rat and human plasma the total relative protein binding of Tc^{99m} was nearly 100%. Because of the very fast blood-clearance it can be assumed, that Tc^{99m}-DMPE is only loosely bound to plasma proteins. On the other hand, plasma protein binding might be (in part) responsible for the low renal excretion rate of Tc^{99m}-DMPE.

By fractional protein precipitation with ammonium sulphate it can be shown, that in the rat most activity is bound to globulins, whereas in man the activity is mainly bound to albumin. Electrophoresis of plasma revealed significant species differences, rat plasma contains less albumin and more globulins than human plasma (table 3).

Toxic side effects

The Tc^{99m}-DMPE agent was not believed to be in any way toxic (5), but it was recommended that extensive toxicity studies should be performed. In our studies severe hemolytic side effects of DMPE were observed. These toxic side effects of Tc^{99m}-DMPE were studied in vitro in rat and human blood and in vivo in the rat.

1. In vitro: immediate coagulation and hemolysis of rat and human blood after addition of small amounts of the Tc^{99m}-DMPE preparation.
2. In-vivo: Direct relationship between hemolysis and DMPE amount administered to the rat. 30 mg DMPE/kg body weight caused hemolysis and hemo-globinuria in all animals, 3 mg DMPE/kg in 10%.

Hemoglobin was measured quantitatively in plasma and urine. Hemoglobinuria was assumed if more than 0,1 ml/dl was assessed. The hemolytic rate remained unchanged when DMPE alone in alcoholic solution was injected, when DMPE was oxidized by purging with O_2 or when the preparation was not heated up before injection or when the temperature was raised to 200°C for two hours.

Also, the oxidized and like Tc^{99m}-DMPE water soluble form of DMPE, of unknown chemical structure, shows hemolytic activity. For this reason hemolytic side effects may also occur, when the excess of DMPE in the preparation is removed by extraction. Furthermore hemoglobin is obviously chemically altered by DMPE and further toxicity studies have to be performed for more quantitative details. The preliminary toxic levels of Tc^{99m}-DMPE are shown in table 4.

Conclusions

The systematic search for Tc^{99m} labelled myocardium imaging agents by Deutsch and co-workers resulted in a series of monocationic Tc99m complexes of known chemical structure. Of these agents Tc^{99m}-DMPE appears to be the most promising one, because it is water - soluble. Kinetic studies clearly show, that neither ^{201}Tl nor Tc^{99m}-DMPE are real analogs of K^{+}. Hence, the myocardial uptake mechanism of both agents needs further clarification. On the other hand, the kinetics of Tc^{99m}-DMPE in the myocardium are similar to that of ^{201}Tl and by this reason Tc^{99m}-DMPE may serve as a substitute for ^{201}Tl. The use of this agent in man however, is limited by two effects:

1. DMPE is a toxic agent and care has to be taken that the toxic levels shown in table 4 are not exceeded.

2. The biodistribution of Tc^{99m}-DMPE is less favorable in man than in the rat and dog, due to differences in plasma protein binding.

It has already been pointed out (4), that the cationic character of Tc^{99m} complexes by itself is essential for myocardial uptake but not sufficient to ensure it. It is now clear, that a Tc^{99m} labelled myocardial imaging agent has to be especially designed for use in man. For this purpose the rat model shown here may be useful.

REFERENCES

1. Colton R, Peacock RF, An outline of technetium chemistry. Quart. Chem. Soc. 16:239, 1962.

2. Fergusson JE, Nyholm RS, New oxidation states of technetium (Letter to the editor). Nature 183:1039, 1959.

3. Fergusson JE, Nyholm RS, Pentavalent technetium. Chem. Ind. (London) pp 347-348, 1960.

4. Deutsch E, Glavan KA, Sodd VC, Nishiyama H, Ferguson DL, Lukes SJ, Cationic Tc-99m complexes as potential myocardial imaging agents. J. nucl. Med. 22:897, 1981.

5. Deutsch E, Bushong W, Glaven KA, Elder RL, Sodd VJ, Scholz KL, Fortman DL, Lukes SJ, Heart imaging with cationic complexes of technetium. Science 214:85, 1981.

6. Nishiyama H, Deutsch E, Adolph RJ, Sodd VJ, Libson K, Saenger EL, Gerson MC, Gabel M, Lukes SJ, Vanderheyden JL, Fortman DL, Scholz KL, Grossman LW, Williams CC, Basal kinetic studies of Tc-99m DMPE as a myocardial imaging agent in the dog. J. nucl. Med. 23:1093, 1982.

7. Nishiyama H, Adolph RJ, Deutsch E, Sodd VJ, Libson K, Gerson MC, Saenger EL, Lukes SJ, Gabel M, Vanderheyden JL, Fortman DL, Effect of coronary blood flow on uptake and washout of Tc-99m DMPE and Tl-201. J. nucl. Med. 23:1102, 1982.

8. Vanderheyden JL, Deutsch E, Libson K, Ketring AR, Synthesis and characterization of 99m Tc-(dmpe)$^+$, a potential myocardial imaging agent. J. nucl. Med. 24:9, 1983.

9. Dudczak R, Angelberger P, Homan R, Kletter K, Schmoliner R, Frischauf H, Evaluation of 99m Tc-Dichloro bis (1,2-Dimethylphosphino) ethane (99m Tc-DMPE) for myocardial scintigraphy in man. Eur. J. Nucl. Med. 8:513, 1983.

10. Sodd VJ, Deutsch A, Nishiyama H, Adolph RJ, Grossman LW, Scholz KL, Libson K, Fortman DL, Vanderheyden JL, Saenger EL, Development and use of a new 99mTc myocardial perfusion agent - DMPE. In: Nuclear Medicine and Biology II. Raynaud C (ed), Pergamon Press, France, Paris, pp 2255-2260, 1982.

11. Angelberger P, Wagner-Löffler M, Hruby E, Dudczak R, Synthesis, radiochromatography and biodistribution of Tc-99m-dimethylphosphino-ethane (DMPE). Third Int. Symp. on Radiopharmacology, Freiburg, p 6, 1983 (abstract).

12. Schümichen C, Koch K, Kraus A, Kuhlicke G, Weiler K, Wenn A, Hoffmann G, Findings of technetium-99m to plasma proteins: Influence on the distribution of Tc-99m phosphate agents. J. nucl. Med. 21:1080, 1980.

IV. IMAGING WITH FATTY ACIDS, INFARCT IMAGING

IMAGING WITH ^{123}I LABELLED FATTY ACIDS

R. DUDCZAK

INTRODUCTION

Thallium-201 scintigraphy and radionuclide ventriculography with Tc^{99m}-labelled albumin are now routinely used in the diagnosis of a variety of cardiac disorders, to provide information which is mainly directed to morphologic and functional aspects of disease. However, interest in cardiac metabolism has increased as a result of growing concern of the fundamental aspects of heart disease. In the metabolic chain for the production of adenosine triphosphate by the myocardial cell the preferential use of fatty acids as substrate is well established (1-4,9). An additional diagnostic approach is the use of ^{123}I labelled fatty acids.

Several radiopharmaceuticals emerged that are supposedly specific for myocardial metabolic studies (5-9) and preliminary clinical results were reported (10-15). Also fatty acid analogues were produced, with tellurium incorporated into the fatty acid chain as a means of inhibiting their metabolism (16-18). The feature of these compounds is their prolonged myocardial retention. The myocardial uptake of these compounds is related to blood-flow and these radiopharmaceuticals were proposed to evaluate myocardial perfusion (16-18).

With respect to heart disease, it is likely that non-invasive assessment of myocardial fatty acid metabolism will result in an improvement of diagnostic as well as prognostic implications and complement the results of other radionuclide procedures (19). The aim of the present report is to describe clinical results obtained with radioiodinated aromatic and aliphatic fatty acids. The radiopharmaceuticals used in our patient were ^{123}I labelled p-phenylpentadecanoic acid (p-IPPA) and ^{123}I labelled heptadecanoic acid (HDA).

Radiopharmaceutical preparation

^{123}I produced by the ^{127}I (p,5n) ^{123}Xe reaction was supplied from IRE Fleurus, Belgium. Labelling of p-IPPA with ^{123}I was per-formed according to Machulla[9] by electrophilic aromatic substi-tution. Separation and purification was effected by high pressure liquid chromatography (HPLC), which resulted in a carrier free preparation [20]. HDA was labelled by nucleophilic substitution [8] of the Br-substituted compound; purification was done by HPLC, which again resulted in a nearly carrier free preparation [20]. After vacuum evaporation the HPLC eluents of p-IPPA and HDA were taken up in ethanol and dissolved in 5% albumin solution. Sterilization was done by membrane filtration.

Patients

In clinical studies 66 patients were investigated (p-IPPA: n=11; HDA: n=55). The patients were classified according to ECG, hemodynamic parameters and coronary angiography. The latter was performed in all of them using the Judkins technique. Luminal narrowing of 70% or greater was described as critical. Infarction scars were assumed in the presence of ventricular asynergies and corresponding coronary artery stenosis and typical ECG pattern indicative of a transmural myocardial infarction (MI) or a documented history of MI. By coronary angiography a total of 63 narrowed vessels (p-IPPA: n=12; HDA n=51) were identified, 20 of these corresponding to old infarctions (p-IPPA: n=4; HDA: n=16).

In all patients with CAD myocardial perfusion was assessed by ^{201}Tl scintigraphy after dipyridamole stress and 3-4 hours later in the redistribution period [21]. Visual interpretation and computerized mapping of circumferential profiles of thallium perfusion images was used to locate and size defects, thereby attempting to identify CAD and the number of vessels involved [22,23]. In the scintigrams 4 hours after dipyridamole stress redistribution was believed to indicate coronary artery disease, but viable myocardium [24].

p-IPPA studies included 3 controls and 8 patients with coronary artery disease (CAD).

HDA studies were done in 9 controls and 31 patients with CAD (one vessel disease, n=20, St.p.MI., n=9: two vessel disease, n=2; three vessel disease, n=9, St.p.MI., n=7). 15 patients with cardiomyopathy were evaluated including 9 with congestive (dilatative) cardiomyopathy (COCM) and 6 with hypertrophe cardiomyopathy (HCM; non-obstructive; n=3; obstructive: n=3). According to the NYHA classification patients with COCM were stage III, and patients with HCM stage I-II.

11 patients, 1 control, 9 patients with single vessel disease and one with three vessel disease underwent in a repeated study symptom limited bicycle exercise testing. HDA was given at peak work load, and the patients were asked to continue to exercise for 0.5 to 1 minute.

Myocardial scintigraphy with ^{123}I labelled p-IPPA and HDA

Patient preparation. Patients were studied after an overnight fast, supine, in the LAO 45° position. For thyroid blockade patients received potassium iodide 1 h prior to i.v. HDA. In p-IPPA studies no premedication was given.

Procedure. Radionuclide studies were done with a LFOV gamma camera interfaced to a computer using a high sensitivity low energy parallel hole collimator. Data aquisition was started and continued for 100 min in p-IPPA and for 70 min in HDA studies, respectively, simultaneously with the intravenous injection of 74-111 mBq p-IPPA or HDA. Data were stored as 64x64 digitized images with a frame rate of 1/min.

Scintigraphic analysis. The regional distribution of the ^{123}I labelled fatty acids was assessed visually and supplemented with a semiquantitative analysis to estimate regional fatty acid uptake by the myocardium. Anatomically oriented regions of interest were outlined and the fatty acid uptake within those regions was averaged and expressed as a ratio of background corrected regional myocardial activity to background activity. As representative of blood background the vena cava superior region was chosen. In patients with CAD three regions corresponding to the circulation area of a main coronary artery (septal, posterolateral, and inferior) were utilized. In patients with COCM and HCM the heart was divided in five consecutive segments which consisted of the inferior wall and the upper and lower part of the septal and posterolateral wall.

Myocardial time activity curve analysis. Regional myocardial time activity curves were generated. The background (V. cava superior region) corrected regional myocardial time activity curves could be described by two exponentials. Accordingly, they were fitted with a biexponential function and the elimination half time of the initial (t_a 1/2) and second component (t_b 1/2) was expressed in minutes. A correlation coefficient (r) was obtained from the regression line between counts and time for characterization of the second phase of the fatty acid time activity curve. In p-IPPA and HDA studies the r value for the second component was 0.88±0.03 and 0.90±0.04 respectively.

By back extrapolation of the monoexponential slope of each component to zero the relative size of each component was evaluated, and the relation of the initial to the second component was expressed by its ratio (C_a/C_b). This should provide an estimate of the relative contribution of the initial and second component on the entire myocardial ^{123}I fatty acid utilization.

In 24 HDA studies myocardial time activity curves were also generated utilizing ^{123}I NaI for background correction (10,11). This procedure was proposed to correct for catabolically released iodide. ^{123}I NaI was given i.v. 70 min after i.v. HDA and counts were monitored for additional 10 min. Using this procedure for background correction, such curves were subsequently analysed as described before. However, it is sufficient to use the vena cava superior region for background correction (25). The results derived with both methods for background corrected myocardial time activity curves compared favourably for calculated elimination half times (r=0.97; p <0.001). The mean % difference in elimination half time of the initial component was 1.76% with a SD of 6.7%. This shows that backdiffusion of catabolically released iodide in the myocardial cell is of minor importance.

Clinical findings in patients with coronary artery disease

Comparable scintigraphic findings were found with both fatty acids. The maximum myocardial uptake occured at 7-15 min after tracer administration. In normal myocardium the uptake was homogenous. The myocardium to background ratio was 2.11±0.22 and 2.33±0.28 in p-IPPA and HDA studies, respectively. These findings were correlated to the ^{201}Tl myocardium/background ratio in normal myocardium (r=0.81; p<0.001).

In regions supplied by stenosed vessels (n=63) already at rest in 35 a reduced fatty acid uptake was found. The decrease in regional activity was more pronounced in infarcted regions. Sequential scintigrams appeared useful to estimate differences in regional myocardial activity retention as shown in example in fig 1 in a p-IPPA study.

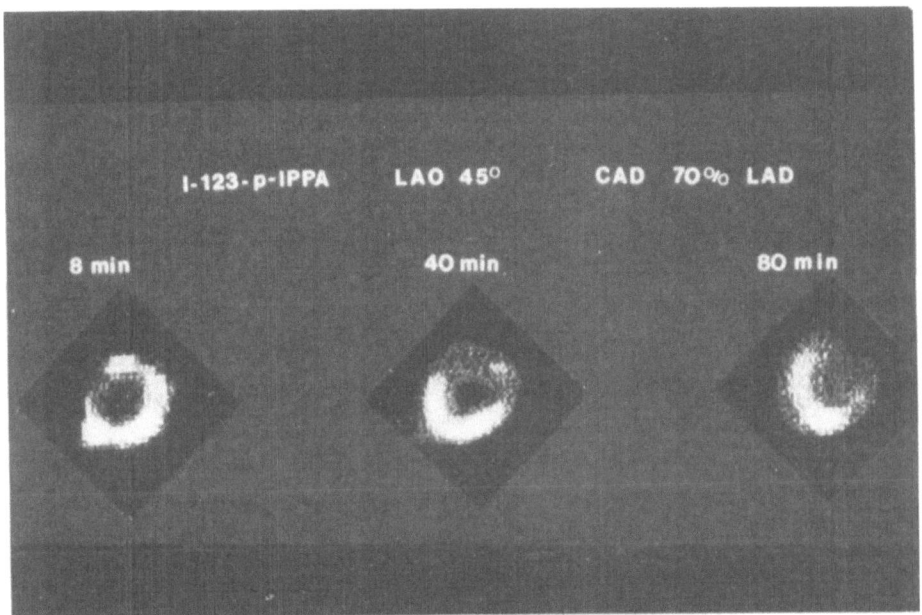

Fig. 1. Sequential myocardial scintigrams in a patient with single vessel disease (70% LAD stenosis) after intravenous administration of 111 MBq 123I p-IPPA. 8 min p.i. a reduced tracer accumulation is seen in the septal region. Later scintigrams indicate a delayed regional clearance of p-IPPA from the septal wall. The regional time activity curves of this patient are shown in fig 2.

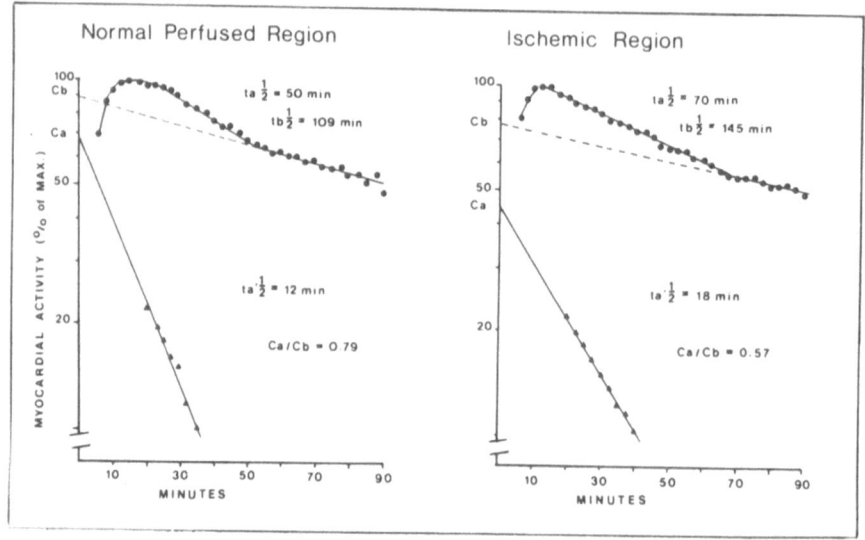

Fig. 2.   Regional myocardial time activity curves in a patient with CAD
(70% LAD stenosis) after intravenous injection of ^{123}I p-IPPA.

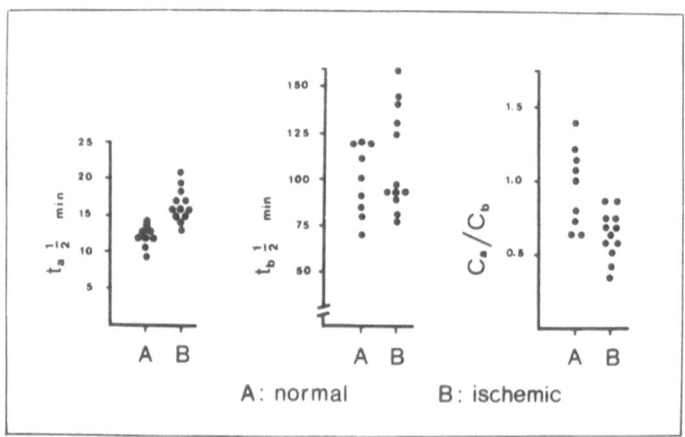

Fig. 3. Elimination half time of the initial phase (t_a 1/2, min) and second
phase (t_b 1/2 min) and component ratio (C_a/C_b) from normal perfused myocardium
(A) and myocardial regions supplied by stenosed vessels (B) in p-IPPA studies.

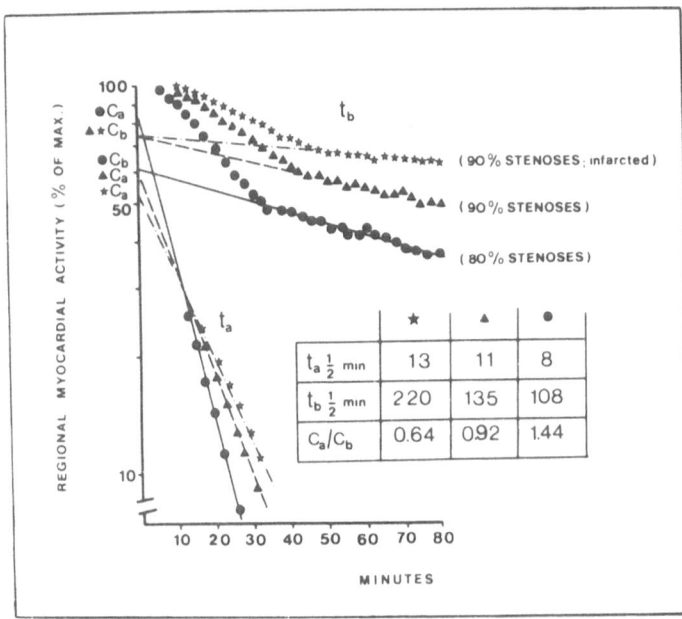

Fig. 4. Example of regional myocardial time activity curves after intravenous injection of 111 MBq ¹²³I HDA in a patient with three vessel disease
and previous myocardial infarction. Corresponding to the degree of myocardial
damage the elimination half time of the initial phase is prolonged and the
component ratio reduced.

However, the evaluation of regional turnover rates may add the
information of a semiquantitative analysis to the qualitative data
The myocardial time activity curve after intravenous administration of p-IPPA in this patient with CAD is shown in fig 2. The
initial component was monoexponential between 10-55 min, the
second component prominent from 50-65 min after if p-IPPA
demonstrated a slower elimination half time. A delayed clearance
of p-IPPA is seen in the region supplied by the stenosed vessel.

For normal myocardium (n=9) the elimination half time of the
initial phase (t_a 1/2) was 12.2±1.79 min, the elimination half
time of the second phase (t_b 1/2) 99.2±18.7 min and the component
ratio (C_a/C_b) 0.95±0.27. The elimination half time of the initial
phase was faster by 32% (p<0.005) in normal myocardium than in
diseased myocardial regions (n=12; t_a 1/2: 16.2±2.26 min; C_a/C_b:
0.69±0.14). No differences were found in the elimination half
time of the second component between normal regions and those

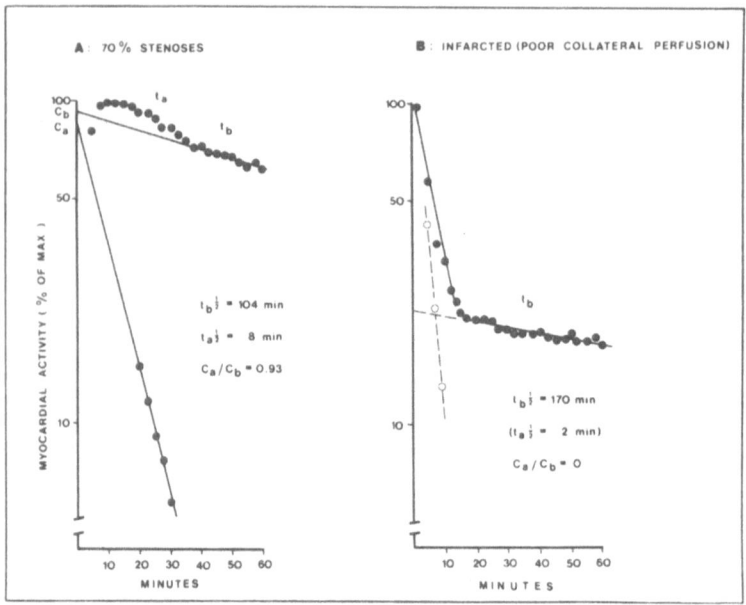

Fig. 5. Example of regional myocardial time activity curves in a patient with three vessel disease and previous myocardial infarction following i.v. HDA. Coronary angiography indicated poor collateral perfusion of the infarcted region.

supplied by stenosed vessels (t_b 1/2: 110.8±29.6 min) (fig 3).

A similar biphasic behaviour in the time course of myocardial activity was observed after i.v. HDA, which was however, significantly faster than for p-IPPA ($p<0.005$). An example of a myocardial time activity curve in a patient with three vessel disease is shown in fig 4. This demonstrates that according to the degree of myocardial damage the elimination half time of the initial component is prolonged. This is further accompanied by a decrease in the size of the initial component, while the contribution of the second component on the myocardial utilization of HDA increases, as expressed by the decreased component ratio.

In 5 patients no component ratio could be calculated, from either 3 infarcted regions or in 2 patients for even the entire myocardium. In 3 infarcted regions corresponding to totally occluded vessels and poor collateral perfusion a very fast initial phase was found in the time course of the myocardial activity.

Table 1 Elimination half time of the initial phase (t_a 1/2 min) and second phase (t_b 1/2 min), and the component ratio (C_a/C_b) in controls (n=9) and patients with coronary artery disease (n=31) in studies with ^{123}I heptadecanoic acid

	t_a 1/2 min	t_b 1/2 min	C_a/C_b
A controls	8.96 ± 1.73 n = 9	48.7 ± 19.4 n = 9	1.52 ± 0.64 n = 9
B normal perfused myocardium	9.55 ± 1.43 n = 22	54.9 ± 18.2 n = 20	1.39 ± 0.59 n = 20
C "normal" myocardium (best vessel in patients with 3 vessel disease)	9.73 ± 1.58 n = 9	68.0 ± 26.5 n = 9	1.32 ± 0.49 n = 9
D "chronic" ischemic myocardium (70%-90% coronary artery stenosis)	11.55 ± 1.75[b] n = 25	61.7 ± 24.4 n = 25	1.02 ± 0.49[e] n = 25
E infarcted myocardium	13.20 ± 1.75[a] n = 13	86.1 ± 41.6[c] n = 14	0.85 ± 0.21[d] n = 11

significant different from controls: a: p<0.0005; b: p<0.001; c: p<0.005; d: p<0.01; e: p<0.05

This possibly reflects backdiffusion of unmetabolized HDA from the infarcted region. This very rapid phase was followed by a slow component, fig 5. From this it may be assumed that in these regions the fatty acid utilization was associated with an enhanced cytosolic esterification of the labelled compound.

In 2 patients studied 3 weeks after a transmural infarction the myocardial count rate exhibited a monoexponential decline. The elimination half time was 8 and 9 min for the normal perfused region and 12 and 14 min for the infarcted area. The underlying mechanism is unclear. If in these patients a diminished availability of alpha-glycerophosphate could account for this finding, as possible adaptive mechanism to prevent ATP wasting, is unknown (26).

Table 1 summarizes the elimination half times and the com-

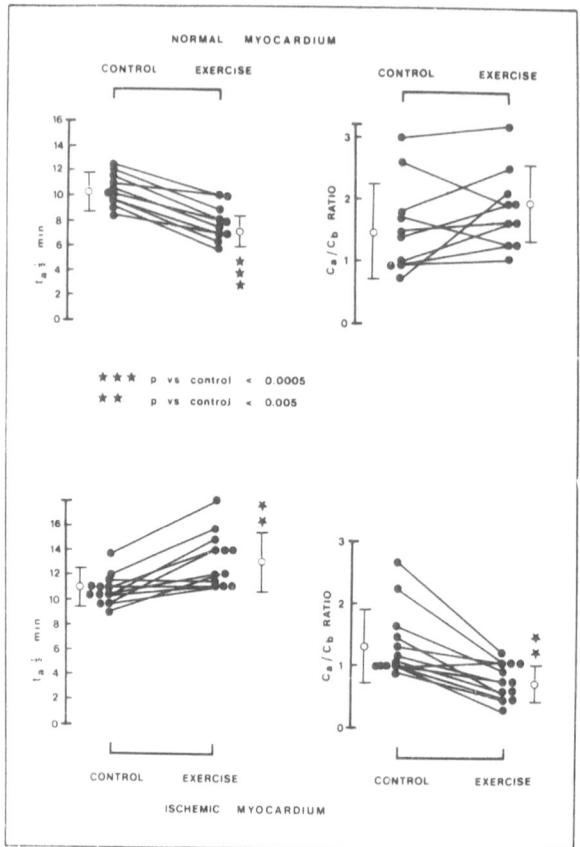

Fig. 6. Elimination half time of the initial phase (t_a 1/2, min) and component ratio (C_a/C_b) before and after symptom limited bicycle exercise stress testing in HDA studies. The findings in normal perfused myocardium are given in the upper panel and those from the ischemic regions in the lower panel.

ponent ratio obtained in all patients with CAD. No differences were found between controls and the normal perfused regions of patients with CAD, as well as the best region of patients with three vessel disease. It is however apparent, that in the remaining regions coronary artery stenosis induced in non infarcted and infarcted regions a prolongation in t_a 1/2 by 29% (p<0.001) and 47% (p<0.0005), and T_b 1/2 by 30% and 76% (p<0.005), respectively. Compared to controls the component ratio was reduced by 33% in noninfarcted regions (p<0.05) and by 45% in infarcted myocardium (p<0.01).

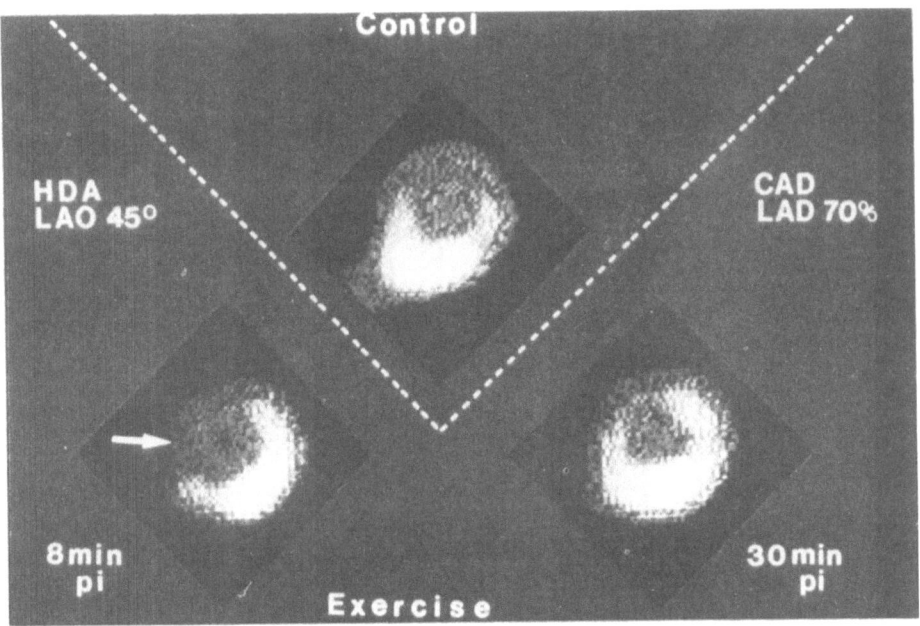

Fig. 7. Myocardial scintigrams in a patient with single vessel disease (70% LAD stenosis). The scintigrams recorded at rest show a homogenous activity distribution of intravenously injected HDA. However, after exercise the septal region demonstrates initially (8 min p.i.) a reduction in tracer accumulation in the septal region, whereas at 30 min p.i. nearly no regional differences are seen, due to a delayed HDA clearance from the septal wall.

In exercise stress studies we evaluated the ability of the heart for the metabolic usage of ^{123}I HDA at an increased myo-cardial energy demand. 11 Patients underwent in a repeated study symptom limited exercise stress testing. Uptake and elimination of HDA was homogenous in the control and persisted following exercise. In the control but also in normal perfused myocardium of patients with CAD the t_a 1/2 decreased from 10.3±1.25 min at rest to 7.95±1.36 min after exercise (p<0.005). Exercise caused an increase in the component ratio from 1.48±0.8 to 1.88±0.68, which was however, yet not significant (fig 6).

Following exercise HDA uptake was reduced in 10 of 12 regions supplied by stenosed vessels. In 5 regions a normal rest image became abnormal with exercise (fig 7), which was accompagnied by an increase in t_a 1/2 by 23.6±8.9%. In 5 patients

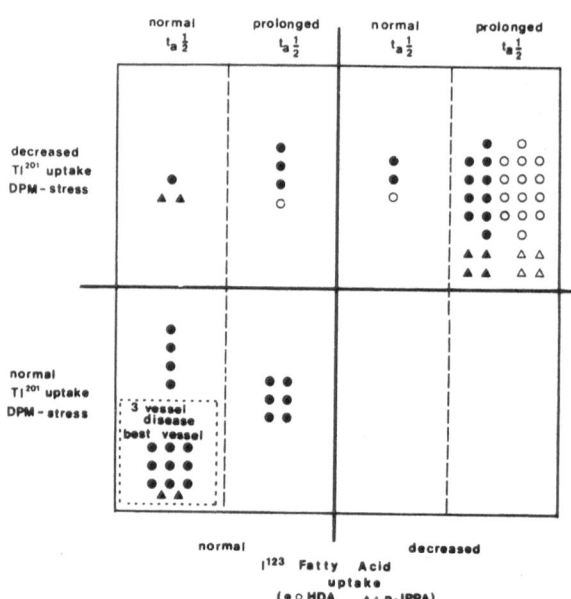

Fig. 8. Comparison of the findings of ^{201}Tl (dipyridamole stress) scintigrams and studies using ^{123}I HDA (•,o) and ^{123}I p-IPPA (▼,v) for myocardial scintigraphy in patients with coronary artery disease. The open symbols (o,v) indicate infarcted regions. The filled symbols (•,▼) mark those regions which were supposed to represent viable myocardial regions, as indicated by ^{201}Tl stress and redistribution scintigrams.

who demonstrated an increased regional deficit in tracer accumulation after exercise, as compared to the rest study, the t_a 1/2 increased by 33.2±9.7%.

All regions supplied by stenosed vessels showed at rest a t_a 1/2 of 11.04±1.21 min and a component ratio of 1.33±0.6. Exercise caused an increase in t_a 1/2 to 13.3±2.35 min (p<0.005) and a decrease in C_a/C_b to 0.72±0.26 (p<0.005) (fig 6). It is interesting to note that in the patient with three vessel disease an increase in the elimination half time was seen in all 3 myocardial regions after exercise.

Myocardial scintigraphy with ^{123}I labelled fatty acids give different information to that obtained with ^{201}Tl and assessment of myocardial viability might be enhanced by using both tracers, since fatty acids assess primarily metabolism and ^{201}Tl perfu-

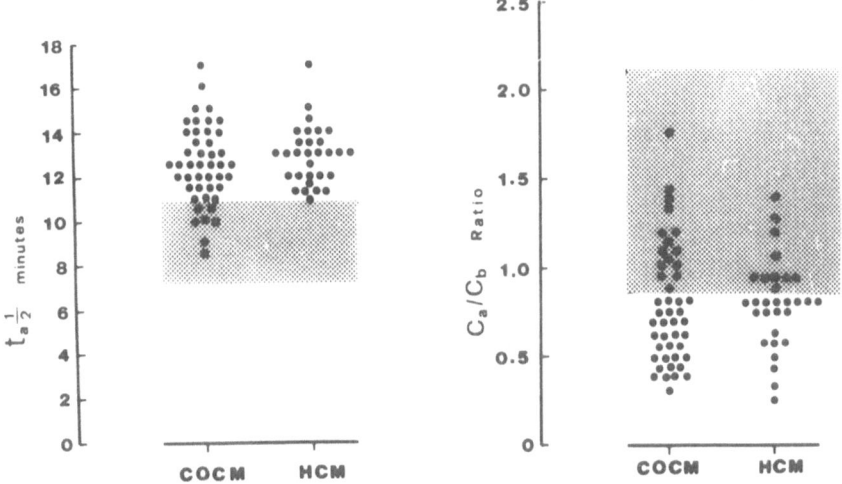

Fig. 9. Elimination half time of the initial phase (t_a 1/2, min) and component ratio (C_a/C_b) in patients with COCM (n=9) and HCM (n=6). In each patient 5 myocardial regions were evaluated. The shaded area indicates the findings in controle ($\bar{x} \pm$ SD).

sion. [201]Tl scintigraphy proved to be a clinical tool with high sensitivity (89%) to predict in our patients CAD, yet it showed less sensitivity (64%) to predict the number of stenosed vessels. A regional decrease in activity accumulation occured more frequently by ^{201}Tl stress scintigraphy than in ^{123}I fatty acid studies done at rest. From the ^{201}Tl findings the fatty acid behaviour neither in its uptake nor in its myocardial clearance could be predicted. The myocardial regions supplied by stenosed vessels can be arranged by their uptake pattern in ^{201}Tl stress and redistribution scintigrams. These findings may be further classified according to the results of ^{123}I fatty acid scintigraphy. Thus, e.g., an ischemic, but supposedly viable myocardial region, as identified by ^{201}Tl, may be associated with either a normal or pathological fatty acid uptake and turnover rate (fig 8). The possible abnormal fatty acid finding would then indicate a higher degree of myocardial damage.

Clinical findings in patients with cardiomyopathy

The scintigraphic appearance of HDA showed a different pattern in patients with COCM than with HCM. In COCM activity distribution was heterogenous, and deficits in tracer uptake were, unlike to patients with CAD, not related to the circulation area of main coronary artery. The myocardial uptake as estimated from the myocardium/background ratio was less in patients with COCM (1.77 ± 0.24) than in patients with HCM (2.2 ± 0.56) ($p<0.05$). Sequential scintigrams in patients with COCM indicated that myocardial activity retention was also heterogenous, which did however, not correspond to the scintigram at accumulation peak time. It should be noted, that regional findings were erratic in COCM but not in HCM. In patients with HCM activity distribution appeared normal. Analysis of the myocardial time activity curves demonstrated, that compared to controls in patients with cardiomyopathy the elimination half time of the initial phase was prolonged. ($p<0.01$) and the component ratio decreased ($p<0.01$. In patients with COCM and HCM the average regional T_a 1/2 was 12.5 ± 1.77 min and 12.9 ± 1.29 min, respectively. The component ratio was 0.78 ± 0.33 in COCM and 0.81 ± 0.23 in HCM (fig 9).

Discussion

[123]I labelled fatty acids provide a new diagnostic tool to evaluate non-invasively myocardial tissue function and to identify metabolically compromised myocardium. After the introduction of ^{123}I long chain fatty acids as tracers for myocardial studies, considerable interest was focused on the clinical findings in patients with heart disease. In the course of these studies a variety of ^{123}I aliphatic fatty acids were used to evaluate myocardial fatty acid metabolism, most of which have employed quantification of the results using the evaluation of myocardial turnover rates (10-15).

The data presented corroborate the results of others in the scintigraphic findings, showing a decreased uptake of radioiodinat fatty acids in regions supplied by stenosed vessels (10-15). However, because of a longer study performance a more extensive interpretation of the data for the myocardial time activity curve seems possible. In earlier studies with aliphatic fatty acids counts were accumulated for 30-40 min following intravenous administration of the radioiodinated tracer. The decline in the myocardial count rate that could be followed there was monoexponential. By applying an approach as proposed in our patient studies the time course of myocardial activity shows a biphasic slope (27-29). Thus the evaluated elimination half times calculated earlier from the monoexponential slopes are considerably longer than those found by us. It appears feasible to assume that analysis of data derived from myocardial fatty acid clearance curves which fit to a biexponential function provide a more detailed information on myocardial fatty acid utilization.

Most of the data available on p-IPPA deal with animal experiments, which demonstrate its incorporation into myocardial lipids and its metabolic degradation, as final catabolite bencoic acid is found (28,30-32). It also was shown that the rate of production of C-14 O_2 as the end product of oxidation of C-14 palmatic acid paralleled the formation rate of bencoic acid (31). Studies in mice have also shown that HDA is incorporated into triglyzerides (11,30). These animal experiments support the use of p-IPPA and HDA as metabolic tracers for myocardial studies.

The positive correlation between the myocardial uptake of ^{123}I labelled fatty acids and ^{201}Tl in our patients is in agreement with the assumption that in normal myocardium the uptake of fatty acids is dependent on blood-flow. But additional control mechanisms located in cell membranes or in the intracellular compartment have to be taken into account (3,34). This could explain the occurance of accumulation defects with p-IPPA and HDA at rest in CAD patients whose ^{201}Tl perfusion scintigraphy at rest was normal, as well as diffusely reduced HDA uptake in patients with COCM and normal coronary morphology.

In our patients we found a slower myocardial elimination half time for p-IPPA in comparison to HDA. This could be due to a delayed myocardial utilization of p-IPPA and/or to a slower release of its lipophilic catabolites from the myocardial tissue. In addition, the amount of p-IPPA utilized via the initial component was smaller than for HDA.

The myocardial clearance of ^{123}I labelled fatty acids is affected by their metabolic usage and washout of labelled catabolites. In previous studies we could demonstrate that the time course of myocardial activity could be influenced by infusion of insulin-glucose (27). As flow was undoubtedly not changed during the pharmacologic intervention these data suggested that under conditions of insulin-glucose infusion, the washout of labelled degradation products does not appear to be the rate limiting step influencing HDA elimination from the myocardium. This finding was also in line with in vitro experiments, which have shown that insulin-glucose provided an increased amount of alpha-glycerophosphate for cytosolic esterification of fatty acids and decreased the availability of carnitine (35,36). These data support the assumption, that the delayed clearance of HDA observed in these studies reflect its decreased utiliza tion induced by insulin-glucose.

The biphasic appearance of the time course of myocardial activity of radioiodinated fatty acids in man from regions with normal or reduced uptake are in agreement with findings reported for C-11 palmitate in dogs (37-41). In C-11 palmitate studies the initial component was referred to immediate β-oxidation of the labelled compound and the second component to a slower turnover of tri-glyzerides (38,39). It was further demonstrated that myocardium rendered ischemic exhibited a decreased tracer uptake and a decreased rate of β-oxidation (39-41).

Small differences in the elimination half time of p-IPPA and HDA in patients and those given in studies with C-11 palmitate in dogs might be due to the different species studied (37-41). Also the intracellular fate of the radioiodinated fatty acids may be different compared to C-11 palmitate. One can speculate that the utilization of p-IPPA and HDA involveq several triglyzeride pools. Probably p-IPPA utilization undergoes metabolic degradation via slower mobilizable triglyzeride pools than HDA. In in-vitro experiments various triglyzeride pools were identified (42-44). Also other sites of transient binding of the radioiodinated compounds to intracellular proteins may be possible (45).

Studies with ^{123}I labelled fatty acids may have potential to allow an estimation on the grade of myocardial viability in

patients with CAD, and thus extend information gained by ^{201}Tl.
A transient defect in serial ^{201}Tl myocardial images suggests
viable myocardium in the presence of coronary artery stenosis (23,
24). Such a ^{201}Tl finding may be associated with a normal regional fatty acid uptake and elimination rate. Also seemingly normal
elimination rates from regions with reduced uptake were found sometimes. This shows that coronary artery stenosis must not be accompagnied by alterations in fatty acid utilization in studies done
at rest. Interposition of normal myocardium may contribute to
these results. Moreover, various grades of prolonged elimination
rates from regions with normal as well as reduced fatty acid uptake were observed from noninfarcted and infarcted regions supplied
by stenosed vessels; the prolongation appeared to be more pronounced in the latter. Possibly the delayed clearance of ^{123}I p-IPPA
and ^{123}I HDA is related to a decreased rate in myocardial fatty
acid metabolism (1-4, 43,46). In addition, the amount of ^{123}I fatty
acids utilized via the slow turnover phase is greater than that
associated with the rapid turnover phase as indicated by the reduced component ratio. The changes in HDA and p-IPPA kinetics in
noninfarcted regions supplied by stenosed coronary arteries already at rest is rather surprising. However, in the course of the
disease ischemia may occur in waves and redistribution of blood-
flow can combat for some of its effects. This behaviour may be
referred to as "chronic ischemia", which may cause disturbances
in fatty acids metabolism. This is feasible, as also in chronic
ischemia the activity of transferase enzymes may be reduced (47).
It seems conceiveable, that alterations in fatty acid utilization
might be found in parallel to the frequency and severity of transient ischemic attacks occuring in the course of the disease. Those
viable myocardial regions as identified by ^{201}Tl stress scintigraphy, which were exposed to less severe transient ischemic attacks
or subjected to them for a shorter period of time may not show
disturbances in ^{123}I fatty acid utilization at rest. Presumably
changes in myocardial fatty acid utilization, similar to those
found in severely damaged tissue may occur in myocardial tissue
also after a longer time interval by moderate and frequent ischemic
attacks.In patients who manifest an abnormal ^{201}Tl finding in

association with an impairment in ^{123}I fatty acid utilization at rest, the degree of myocardial damage is probably a greater one. Thus, studies with p-IPPA and HDA might provide a means to assess to some extent the degree of myocardial viability, and to identify a subgroup of patients who are at increased risk for irreversible myocardial damage (48,49).

Additional stress studies may be useful, foremost in patients with normal ^{123}I fatty acid findings at rest. This could provide a more subtle information in myocardial viability, by grading the findings as to what extent the stress applied induce alterations in uptake and the metabolic usage of ^{123}I fatty acids at an increased energy demand of the heart.

In agreement with others were our results in patients with COCM (12,13), which demonstrated disturbances in HDA utilization. Similar findings were also reported in p-IPPA studies (28,48,49). A similar delayed elimination of HDA was found in patients with HCM. However, in contrast to patients with COCM the uptake of HDA was not reduced and mostly an even distribution of the tracer was found within the myocardium. Thus the findings differed in the uptake pattern and distribution of the elimination rate of HDA, which was heterogenous in COCM, but not in HCM. Yet patients with COCM were clinically in stage III NYHA and patients with HCM were in class I-II. However, there was no discrepancy between the degree in the impairment in HDA utilization, which manifested in a delayed elimination and an altered compartmentalisation of the labelled compound. The application of ^{123}I labelled fatty acids provide useful information in demonstrating disturbances in the metabolic usage of fatty acids by the myocardium. It is probable that these studies may be used as a mean of separating groups of patients with heart disease.

Our data show that comparable clinical findings may be gained by the use of either aliphatic or aromatic radioiodinated fatty acids.

An advantage of p-IPPA as compared to radioiodinated aliphatic fatty acids is the absence of free halide arising as a degradation product (8,10,11). Thus the possibility of super position of stomach activity is eliminated, which might interfere sometimes

with the regional interpretation of scintigrams. Yet, for evaluating the dynamic behaviour of fatty acid turnover rates the studies
are more time consuming than those with aliphatic fatty acids.
From the above it appears, that depending on the equipment available
one may prefer p-IPPA if only sequential scintigrams are to be
performed. However, if computer assisted analysis of myocardial
turnover rates can be done, to provide semiquantitative data on
^{123}I fatty acid utilization, studies with aliphatic fatty acids
appear to be more practicable, because they are less time consuming.

Conclusions

The use of p-IPPA and HDA as metabolic tracers was substan-
tiated by animal experiments demonstrating their incorporation
in cardiac lipids; as final catabolites ^{123}I-bencoic acid and
^{123}I-NaI, respectively, were found (10,30,31); yet by pharmacological induced blockade of β-oxidation no free kalide arose in
HDA studies (50). In addition, this assumption was confirmed
in man, by the fact, that pharmacologic interventions as well
as a diminished blood-supply were effective modulators of ^{123}I
fatty acid utilization (51,52). Studies with radioiodinated
fatty acids have several advantages as they can be performed
with conventional gamma camera equipments which is readily
available. Certain limitations are given by super position of
normal myocardium that may mask the detection of metabolically
compromised myocardium, and quantification of the results is
limited. However, the possibility to evaluate the myocardial
metabolic function in man noninvasively may add a complementary diagnostic tool in the clinical follow-up of patients with
heart disease.

REFERENCES

1. Bing RJ, Cardiac Metabolism. Physiol. Rev. 45:171, 1965.

2. Opie LH, Metabolism of the heart in health and disease. Part I. Amer. Heart J. 76:685, 1968.

3. Neely JR, Rovetto MJ, Oram JF, Myocardial utilization of carbohydrate and lipids. Progr. cardiovasc. Dis. 15:289, 1972.

4. Neely JR, Morgan HE, Relationship between carbohydrate and lipid metabolism and the energy balance of heart muscle. Ann. Rev. Physiol. 34:413, 1974.

5. Evans JR, Gunton RW, Baker RG et al: Use of radioiodinated fatty acid for photoscans of the heart. Circulat. Res. 16:1, 1965.

6. Robinson GD, Lee AW, Radioiodinated fatty acids for heart imaging: Iodine monochloride addition compared with iodide replacement labelling. J. nucl. Med. 16:17, 1975.

7. Poe ND, Robinson GD, Graham LS et al, Experimental basis for myocardial imaging with ^{123}I-labeled hexadecanoic acid. J. nucl. Med. 17:1077, 1976.

8. Machulla HJ, Stöcklin G, Kupfernagel CH et al, Comparative evaluation of fatty acids labelled with C-11, CI-34m, Br-77 and I-123 for metabolic studies of the myocardium: Concise communication. J. nucl. Med. 19:298, 1978.

9. Machulla HJ, Marsmann M, Dutschka K, Biochemical concept and synthesis of a radioiodinated phenylfatty acid for in vivo metabolic studies of the myocardium. Eur. J. Nucl. Med. 5:171, 1980.

10. Freundlieb Ch, Höck A, Vyska K et al, Myocardial imaging and metabolic studies with (17-123I) iodoheptadecanoic acid. J. nucl. Med. 21:1043, 1980.

11. Vyska K, Höck A, Freundlieb C et al, Stoffwechseluntersuchung am Herzen mit [123]J-Fettsäuren und ^{11}C-Methylglukose. Nuklearmedizin 20:148, 1981.

12. Höck A, Freundlieb Ch, Vyska K et al, Myocardial imaging and metabolic studies with (17-123I) iodoheptadecanoic acids in patients with idiopathic congestive cardiomyopathy. J. nucl. Med. 24:22, 1983.

13. Feinendegen LE, Vyska K, Freundlieb Ch et al, Non invasive analysis of metabolic reactions in body tissues, the case of myocardial fatty acids. Eur. J. Nucl. Med. 6:191, 1981.

14. Van der Wall EE, Den Hollander W, Heidendal GAK et al, Dynamic myocardial scintigraphy with 123I-labeled free fatty acids in patients with myocardial infarction. Eur. J. Nucl. Med. 6:383, 1981.

15. Van der Wall EE, Heidendal GAK, Den Hollander W et al, Metabolic myocardial imaging with 123I-labeled heptadecanoic acid in patients with angina pectoris. Eur. J. Nucl. Med. 6:391, 1981.

16. Knapp FF, Ambrose KR, Callahan AP et al, Effects of chain length and Tellurium position on the myocardial uptake of Te-123m fatty acids. J. nucl. Med. 22:988, 1981.

17. Elmaleh DR, Knapp FF, Yasuda T et al, Myocardial imaging with 9-(Te-123m) Telluroheptadecanoic acid. J. nucl. Med. 22:994, 1981.

18. Goodman MM, Knapp FF, Callahan AP, et al, A new, well retained myocardial imaging agent: Radioiodinated 15-(p-Iodophenyl)-6-Tellurapentadecanoic acid. J. nucl. Med. 23:904, 1982.

19. Dudczak R. Höfer R, Myocardial scintigraphy with I-123 labeled fatty acids. Summary of a Round Tabel Discussion. J. Radioanal. Chem. 79:329, 1983.

20. Angelberger P, Wagner-Löffler M, Dudczak R et al, I-123(131) labeled aliphatic and aromatic fatty acids: optimized preparation and biodistribution. In: Radioaktive Isotope in Klinik und Forschung, Vol. 15. Höfer R, Bergmann H (eds), H. Egermann, Vienna, pp 249, 1982.

21. Schmoliner R, Dudczak R, Kronik G et al, Thallium-201-Myokardszintigraphie nach hochdosierter Dipyridamolgabe, Z. Kardiol. 70:111, 1981.

22. Vogel RA, Quantitative aspects of myocardial perfusion imaging. Seminars Nucl. Med. 10:146, 1980.

23. Botvinick EH, Dunn RF, Hattner RS et al, A consideration of factors affecting the diagnostic accuracy of thallium 201 myocardial perfusion scintigraphy in detecting coronary artery disease. Seminars Nucl. Med. 10:157, 1980.

24. Pohost GM, Alpert NM, Ingwall JS et al, Thallium redistribution: Mechanisms and clinical utility. Seminars Nucl. Med. 10:70, 1980.

25. Dudczak R, Schmoliner R, Angelberger P et al: Myocardial perfusion and metabolism as assessed by Tl-201 and I-123 heptadecanoic acid (HDA) scintigraphy. Nuklearmedizin suppl. 19:540, 1982.

26. Opie IH, Metabolism of free fatty acids, glucose and catecholamines in acute myocardial infarction. Amer. J. Cardiol. 36:938, 1975.

27. Dudczak R, Schmoliner R, Derfler K et al, Effect of ischemia and pharmacological interventions on the myocardial elimination of I-123 heptadecanoic acid. J. nucl. Med. 23:P34, 1982.

28. Dudczak R, Schmoliner R, Angelberger P et al, Myocardial studies with I-123-p-phenyl-pentadecanoic acid in patients with coronary artery disease (CAD) and cardiomyopathy (CMP). J. nucl. Med. 23:P34, 1982.

29. Dudczak R, Kletter K, Frischauf H et al, Myocardial turnover rates of I-123 heptadecanoic acid (HDA) and I-123 p-phenyl-pentadecanoic acid(p-IPPA). In: Radioaktive Isotope in Klinik und Forschung, Vol. 15. Höfer R, Bergmann H (eds), H. Egermann, Vienna, pp 685, 1982.

30. Reske SN, Sauer W, Machulla HJ et al, 15(p(^{123}I) iodophenyl) pentadecanoic acid as tracer of lipid metabolism: Comparison with (1-^{14}C) palmitic acid in murine tissues. J. nucl. Med. 25:1335, 1984.

31. Reske SN, Machulla HJ, Winkler C, Metabolism of 15-p (I-123-phenyl)-pentadecanoic acid in hearts of rats. J. nucl. Med. 23:P10, 1982.

32. Coenen HH, Harmand MF, Kloster G et al, 15-(p-75-Br bromo-phenyl) pentadecanoic acid: Pharmacokinetics and potential as heart agent. J. nucl. Med. 22:891, 1981.

33. Weiss ES, Hoffman EJ, Phelps ME et al, External detection and visualization of myocardial ischemia with 11-C-substrates in vitro and in vivo. Circulat. Res. 39:24, 1976.

34. Oram JF, Bennetch SL, Neely JR, Regulation of fatty acid utilization in isolated perfused rat hearts. J. Biol. Chem. 248:5299, 1973.

35. Gordon RS, Cherkes A, Gates H, Unesterified fatty acid in human blood plasma. II. The transport function of unesterifie fatty acid. J. clin. Invest. 36:810, 1957.

36. Fisher RB, Williamson JR, The effects of insulin, adrenaline and nutrients on the oxygen uptake of the perfused rat heart. J. Physiol. 158:102, 1961.

37. Schelbert HR, Henze E, Phelps ME, Emission tomography of the heart. Seminars Nucl. Med. 10:355, 1980.

38. Schön HR, Schelbert HR, Robinson G et al, C-11 labeled palmitic acid for the noninvasive evaluation of regional myocardial fatty acid metabolism with positron-computed tomography. I. Kinetics of C-11 palmitic acid in normal myocardiu Amer. Heart J. 103:532, 1982.

39. Schön HR, Schelbert HR, Najafi A et al, C-11 labeled evaluation of regional myocardial fatty acid metabolism with positron-computed tomography. II. Kinetics of C-11 palmitic acid in acutely ischemic myocardium. Amer. Heart J. 103:548, 1982.

40. Lerch RA, Bergmann SR, Ambos HD et al, Effect of flow-independent reduction of metabolism on regional myocardial clearance of ^{11}C-palmitate. Circulation 65:731, 1982.

41. Lerch RA, Ambos HD, Bergmann SR et al, Localization of viable, ischemic myocardium by positron-emission tomography with C-11 palmitate. Circulation 64:689, 1981.

42. Stein O, Stein Y, Lipid synthesis, intracellular transport and storage. III Electron microscopic radioautographic study of the rat heart perfused with tritiated oleic acid. J. Cell. Biology 36:63, 1968.

43. Idell-Wenger JA, Grotyohann LW, Neely JR, Coenzyme A and carnitine distribution in normal and ischemic hearts. J. biol. Chem. 253:4310, 1978.

44. Crass MF, McCaskill ES, Shipp JC et al, Metabolism of endogenous lipids in cardiac muscle: Effect of pressure development. Amer. J. Physiol. 220:428, 1971.

45. Gloster J, Harris P, Fatty acid binding to cytoplasmic proteins of myocardium and red and white skeletal muscle in the rat. A possible new role for myoglobin. Biochem. biophys. Res. Commun. 74:506, 1977.

46. Whitmer JT, Idell-Wenger JA, Rovetto MJ et al, Control of fatty acid metabolism in ischemic and hypoxic hearts. J. biol. Chem. 253:4305, 1978.

47. McMillin Wood J, Sordahl LA, Lewis RM et al, Effect of chronic myocardial ischemia on the activity of carnitine palmitylcoenzyme. A transferase of isolated canine heart mitochondria. Circul. Res. 32:340, 1973.

48. Dudczak R, Schmoliner R, Kletter K et al, Clinical evaluation of 123I-labeled p-phenylpentadecanoic acid (p-IPPA) for myocardial scintigraphy. J. nucl. Med. & Biol. 27:267, 1983.

49. Dudczak R, Myokardszintigraphie mit I-123 markierten Fettsäuren. Wien. Klin. Wschr. 95:Suppl. 143, pp 1-35, 1983.

50. Lerch RA, Myocardial kinetics of C-11 palmitate and ^{123}I-heptadecanoic acid: Similarities and differences. Workshop on radiolabeled free fatty acids. Amsterdam 6.7.1984.

51. Dudczak R, Kletter K, Frischauf H et al, The use of ^{123}I-labeled heptadecanoic acid (HDA) as metabolic tracer: preliminary report. Eur. J. Nucl. Med. 9:81, 1984.

52. Dudczak R, Homan R, Zangeneh A et al, Myocardial metabolic studies in patients with cardiomyopathy. J. nucl. Med. 24:P20, 1983 (abstr).

MYOCARDIAL INFARCT IMAGING WITH TECHNETIUM-99m (Sn)
PYROPHOSPHATE

J. DRESSLER, G. HÖR

INTRODUCTION

Myocardial imaging can be classified into acute infarct
("hot spot") scintigraphy and myocardial perfusion ("cold
spot") scintigraphy. Unlike cold spot imaging techniques, in
which radioactive indicators (201Tl, radiolabelled fatty acids)
distribute in proportion to blood-flow and where altered myocardial segments are seen as regions with reduced or absent
activity, in infarct scintigraphy the acutely damaged tissue is
visualized by the uptake of infarct avid tracers. Early reports
on radiotracers which accumulate in myocardial infarcts (1)
date back more than 20 years and most of the radiopharmaceuticals
listed in table 1 are mainly of historical interest. Since
Bonte et al (2) and Parkey et al (3) discovered the potential
Tc^{99m}-(Sn) pyrophosphate (PYP) which was initially introduced
as a bone scanning agent, this tracer is, at the present time,
the radiopharmaceutical of choice for recognition of acute
myocardial necrosis. Although hot spot scanning has become
widely accepted for clinical use this test is not routinely
performed to establish the presence of acute myocardial infarction. Nevertheless there are some advantages in comparison
to the utilization of ^{201}Tl myocardial perfusion imaging. The
intent of this report is to review some details concerning the
uptake of Tc^{99m}-pyrophosphate, the technical aspects of the
procedure, the interpretation of imaging and the indication
and limitation of this imaging technique.

Mechanism of uptake

To date the mechanism of uptake and fixation of PYP has
not been completely clarified. The accumulation of PYP (and

Table 1. Infarct-avid radiopharmaceuticals

^{203}Hg - Chlormerodrine
^{203}Hg - Fluoresceine
^{131}I / Tc^{99m} Tetracycline
^{67}Ga
Tc^{99m} - Glucoheptonate
Tc^{99m} - DMSA
Tc^{99m} - Labelled compounds of phosphate
Tc^{99m} - Heparin
Tc^{99m} - Colloids
^{111}In - White blood-cells or platelets
^{131}I - Antimyosin antibodies
$^{18}Fluorine$

other labelled diphosphonates) is depending at least on 3
factors:
a) the severity of tissue damage
b) a residual collateral blood-flow into this area
c) the time elapsed after the onset of necrosis prior to
   application of PYP.

The flow dependency of the accumulation of PYP has been
demonstrated in numerous animal experiments (4-9) using the
microsphere technique, the distribution of ^{201}Tl and histo-
morphologic staining. The PYP concentration was highest in
segments with flow reductions of 60-70% below control but fell
as flow decreased further toward the centre of experimental
induced infarctions with greater reduction in flow. This
observation is consistent with the frequent clinical finding
of the "doughnut" pattern where accumulation of PYP is most
intense in the periphery of the infarction.

The presence of intramitochondrial dense bodies in irreversibly damaged myocardium has been well established (9,10). It
is thought, that these hydroxy-apatite like deposits are

indeed the binding site of PYP (11,12). The assumption of flow dependency of PYP accumulation is further supported by observations in experiments with permanent and transient coronary occlusion (13,14,15).

On the other hand the hypothesis of a PYP binding to intramitochondrial calciumphosphate has been challenged by evidence indicating that PYP attaches to denatured protein (16) and that fixation of the agent to irreversibly damaged myocardium occurs even in the absence of calcium (17). It is conceivable that both calcium phosphate and protein molecules are the major binding sites. Moreover, while PYP may to some extent accumulate in transiently or reversibly injured cells, most of the evidence support the hypothesis that the agent primarily binds to irreversibly damaged myocardial cells.

Methodological consideration

In experimental animals with fixed coronary occlusion (18) and in patients with myocardial necrosis (19) scintigrams become positive within 10 to 12 hours after acute infarction and show increasing contrast over the first 24 to 72 hours. Only a few instances have been reported where positive studies were obtained as early as 4 hours after the onset of acute symptoms (20). In the majority of the patients the scintigrams will become normal after the first 1 or 2 weeks.

Scintigrams are usually made with a gamma camera equipped with a low energy, high resolution, parallel hole collimator. At least 300.000 counts should be recorded per image. Imaging is commenced about 2 hours after injection in the straight anterior, the 45° left anterior oblique and the left lateral projection. Occasionally additional views may be needed and repeat images are recommended if there is a diffuse uptake suggesting a "blood-pool" scintigram.

Since Parkey's original report (3) on Tc^{99m}-PYP scintigrapy numerous studies have indicated that other Tc^{99m}-labelled phosphates such as methylene-diphosphonate (21,22,23), polyphosphate (24,25) and imido-diphosphonate (26,27) may also be used for infarct imaging.

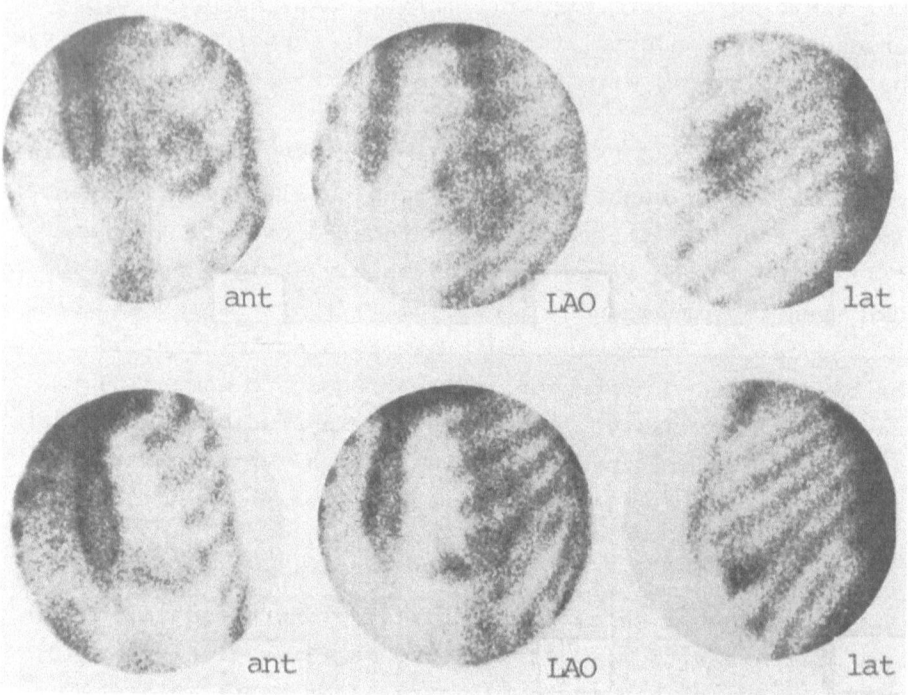

Fig. 1. Positive infarct scintigraphy with Tc^{99m}-PYP. Upper row: "Doughnut" sign in large anterior wall infarction. Lower row: inferior myocardial infarction. Intensity of uptake is graded 3+.

The absorbed radiation dose per study resulting from these tracers is nearly the same. When injecting 15 mCi Tc^{99m}-PYP it is just about 200 mrd to the gonades and 130 mrd to the whole body, whereas the radiation exposure to the urinary tract may be about ten times higher.

Image interpretation

Normally the bone structures are visualized only, whereas a scintigram is considered positive if abnormal activity is present in the region of the heart. The intensity with which an acute myocardial infarction is visualized does not appear to be strictly related to size or extent of myocardial injury.

For interpretative purposes a classification describing the activity has been proposed (3,28):

0 intensity - no visible uptake

1+ intensity - uptake lower than in the ribs

2+ intensity - uptake equal to that of the ribs

3+ intensity - uptake higher than in the ribs

4+ intensity - uptake equal to or higher than in the sternum

Grade zero is obviously negative, grade 1+ is usually considered equivocal, especially when the uptake is diffuse. Grade 2+
to 4+ indicates positive scans, especially when the uptake is
discrete. For purpose of diagnostic accuracy it is important
to identify the abnormal uptake in at least 2 projections and
to define clearly its location in the myocardium (fig 1).

Image interpretation is difficult when the uptake in the
myocardium is diffuse. This pattern is frequently observed
in patients with acute nontransmural infarctions, but it is
considered nonspecific because it also occurs in patients
without evidence of cardiac disease. Diffuse uptake distinctly
differs from discrete uptake with the latter accumulation of
Tc-PYP occuring in a well defined segment of the left ventricle.
A specific form of discrete uptake is the so called doughnut
pattern, i.e., the agent accumulates predominantly in the periphery of the infarct. This pattern is consistent with large
anterior, antero-lateral or antero-septal infarction and
suggests a poor prognosis (29).

Most investigators have indicated, that abnormal myocardial
uptake can be adequately detected on analog scintigrams, although
Berger et al (30) have pointed out, that computer techniques
may slightly improve the overall sensitivity.

Accuracy of infarct scintigraphy

If performed within the optimal time interval (i.e. 1-7 days
after onset of symptoms) scintigraphy with PYP permits detection and aging of an acute myocardial infarction with a high
degree of sensitivity. In most reports the sensitivities range
from 85 to 100%. Compiling the results of 15 studies that include a total of 1057 patients with proven acute myocardial
infarction yields an overall sensitivity of 90% (table 2).
According to Cowley et al (31) the technique is better in

Table 2. Results of infarct scintigraphy with PYP

Patients with		Positive scans		Patients without AMI	Negative scans	Reference
AMI	SE	AMI	SE			
31	17	31	17	67	36	Ahmad et al (32)
55	25	52	24			Berger et al (30)
81	18	76	7	126	87	Bermann et al (28)
26	22	24	18			Campeau et al (24)
80		68		16	14	Coleman et al (33)
56	13	53	12	125	96	Cowley et al (31)
59	12	47	12	41	25	Holman et al (20)
249		237		82	23	Lessem et al (34)
42		40		59	57	Okada et al (35)
16	15	16	13	28	15	Poliner et al (36)
26		25		120	100	Prasquier et al (37)
43	31	29	16	40	36	Massie et al (38)
6	16	3	7	58	38	Walsh et al (39)
101	17	96	17	71	71	Willerson et al (19)
			.	101	92	Willerson et al (40)
871	186	807	143	934	690	Total

AMI = acute myocardial infarction (transmural)

SE = subendocardial infarction

detecting anterior than inferior myocardial infarction. The reason is probably related to the proximity of the anterior wall to the gamma camera in all projections. Photons originating from the more distant posterior and inferior wall are subjected to a higher degree to attenuation and are imaged with poorer resolution. Table 2 includes results obtained in 934 patients without an acute myocardial infarction. Of these 690 had negative scans which results in an overall 74% specifity of PYP imaging. The reported sensitivities in patients with acute subendocardial infarctions are lower (77%) and differ from 40 to 100%. This wide range can be related to the different image interpretation. Thus in some series the diffuse uptake of 1+ and 2+ intensity was judged as a positive scintigram. For the cumulative patient population listed in the table the overall sensitivity with 77% decreases to 22% when discrete uptake only is considered abnormal. In order to preserve the specifity of the test Bermann et al (28) therefore proposed to consider diffuse uptake even of 2+ intensity as equivocal. The reason for the prevalence of diffuse uptake in acute subendocardial infarction has been the subject of many discussions but thus far remains uncertain.

Sizing of acute myocardial infarction

Although the intensity of PYP is not strictly related to the mass of infarcted myocardiun, there is sufficient evidence from animal as well as from clinical studies, that the planimetered area of PYP uptake can indeed be used as an index of the size of infarction (15,43,47). Expressed in square centimaters this estimate correlates with post mortem measurements of infarct size in animal experiments or with biochemical (enzyme) estimates of infarct weight in patients, i.e. the area under the complete serum CK curve (29,44,45,46,47). At present however these correlations (r= 0,87 - 0,92) apply only to patients with anterior myocardial infarctions, whereas sizing of inferior localized infarcts has remained unsatisfactory (29). In a clinico-pathological study infarcts of less than 3 gram in size could not be recognized (44). Dual

Table 3. Abnormal Tc^{99m}-phosphate images in the absence of acute myocardial infarction

---

A. UPTAKE IN CARDIAC STRUCTURES / PROCESSES

   Unstable and stable angina pectoris

   Old myocardial infarction

   LV-aneurysm

   Myocardiopathy

   Cardiac contusion, cardioversion

   Calcified cardiac valves

   Pericarditis, endocarditis

   Regional wall motion abnormalities

   Chemotherapy (Adriamycin-cardiomyopathy)

B. UPTAKE IN NON-CARDIAC STRUCTURES / PROCESSES

   Trauma, inflammation or tumour of ribs, skin
      or soft tissue

   Calcified rib cartilage

   Uptake of gastric mucosa, breast tissue
      or lymph nodes

   Irradiation

   Hyperhidrosis

   Blood-pool activity

   Metastatic calcification
      (secondary hyperparathyrioidism)

   Hot kidneys (tubular necrosis)

---

imaging (PYP/201Tl) has been advocated for a more precise sizing of necrosis versus periinfarct ischemia (53). The development of three dimensional imaging techniques (48,49) may improve the potential of infarct imaging for determination of infarct size in future.

Differential diagnosis

Reports on specifity of PYP imaging (table 2) suggest that PYP uptake occurs also in a number of conditions other than acute myocardial infarction (table 3). Discrete uptake is occasionally noted long after acute infarction with or without left ventricular aneurysm (41). While in acute myocardial

Table 4. Clinical applications of acute infarct scintigraphy with Tc99m-PYP

---

1. Clinically suspected myocardial infarction in the presence of non-diagnostic ECG and enzyme changes

2. Detection of right ventricular infarction

3. Diagnosis of AMI after resuscitation

4. Diagnosis of perioperative infarction

5. Detection of cardiac trauma

6. Prognosis of future morbidity and mortality

7. Detection of cardiotoxicity of chemotherapeutics

---

infarction the discrete uptake pattern prevails many patients with stable or unstable angina present with diffuse uptake (42). Uptake may also be caused by cardiac contusion, calcified cardiac valves, peri- and endocarditis (for references see 23).

Occasionally, PYP concentrates in non-cardiac structures adjacent to the heart, which can be readily recognized if scintigrams are performed in at least 3 projections. The sites of uptake may be inflammatory changes of soft tissues, trauma or metastasis in ribs overlaying the cardiac regions of calcified cartilage. Uptake may be due to surgical incisions, breast tissue or cardioversion. Finally break down of the radiopharmaceutical can result in excretion of ionic Tc^{99m}-pertechnetate by the gastric mucosa. Binding of Tc^{99m} to red blood-cells may present a blood-pool scintigram simulating a diffuse cardiac uptake.

Clinical applications

Scintigraphy with PYP can not be recommended as a routine test in myocardial infarction as long as the diagnosis is readily established by conventional means such as typical history, characteristic electrocardiography and serum enzyme changes. Unfortunately in situations, where the diagnosis can not be achieved definitively by standard techniques, the sensitivity of the scintigraphic approach frequently also yields

negative or equivocal results. Nevertheless additional clinically useful information can be expected in situations as listed
in table 4. Infarct scintigraphy can be of value in patients
surviving the acute phase and being admitted several days
later to hospital, when enzymes and ECG are no longer diagnostic.
If the test is performed within 7 days with positive result and
the study becomes negative on later controls a recent infarction
is to be confirmed.

Myocardial infarctions of the inferior wall are known to be
often associated with right ventricular involvement. This
condition is frequently missed by standard techniques including
scintigraphy with ^{201}Tl. If there is reduced right ventricular
function, both radionuclide ventriculography and PYP scintigraphy will establish the correct diagnosis and influence the
therapeutic regimen.

In patients with cardiac arrest, who are successfully resus-
citated, the diagnosis of an acute myocardial infarction may
be obscured. Imaging in these instances can provide the diagnosis.
Similar problems arise in the diagnosis of perioperative infarctions and acute trauma to the heart, where the value of
standard diagnostic techniques is limited. Several reports
have suggested the use of PYP scintigraphy for monitoring the
cardiotoxity of chemotherapeutics. Further investigations are
necessary to clarify the diffuse cardiac uptake of activity in
this conditions.

The potential value of serial imaging with PYP in patients
with myocardial infarction for prognostication of subsequent
morbidity and mortality has been emphasized (41,50,51). Those
patients with persistently positive studies have a generally
poorer prognosis with a significantly higher incidence of angina,
arrhythmias of left ventricular failure during follow-up than
those with negative scintigrams at the time of discharge. Furthermore, patients with persistently positive scans had a significantly higher mortality within the first 1-2 years (52). Additionally to the intensity the extent of uptake can be a strong prognostic index. Perez-Gonzalvez et al (51) used the measured infarct sizes from PYP scintigrams and ^{201}Tl scintigrams as an

indicator of the late prognosis after AMI. Both early scintigraphic parameters appeared more accurate than other clinical
laboratory results for prediction of favorable or unfavorable
evolution after myocardial infarction.

Conclusions

Of the wide range of radiopharmaceuticals which accumulate
in acutely infarcted myocardium PYP has proven clinically
practicable for the scintigraphic detection of acute myocardial
infarction. However, in contrast to myocardial perfusion scintigraphy with ^{201}Tl the current state of infarct imaging is inadequate during the early phase of an infarction and just adds
additional clinical value if conventional techniques fail to
establish the diagnosis. In this early stage serial examinations
of global and regional left ventricular function using radionuclide ventriculography are more important. The combination
with ^{201}Tl scintigraphy is useful in differentiating right
ventricular and remote from acute infarction. Furthermore it
can enhance the sensitivity of infarct detection. Although an
intense, discrete cardiac uptake strongly suggest an irreversibly damaged myocardium, it is not specific for infarction and
other causes must be ruled out. When using conventional planar
scintigraphy an accurate sizing of infarct weight seems possible
just in anterior wall infarction. On the other hand the infarct
scintigraphy with PYP is easily performed, cheep and suitable
for follow-up studies. There is strong evidence that the persis-
tance and extense of uptake is an excellent prognostic parameter
of future morbidity and mortality in patients after an acute
myocardial infarction.

REFERENCES

1. Holman BL, Infarct-avid radiopharmaceuticals for the evaluation of acute myocardial necrosis. Clin. Nucl. Cardiol. Grune and Stratton, New York pp 144-153, 1981.

2. Bonte FJ, Parkey RW, Graham KD, A new method for radionuclide imaging of myocardial infarction. Radiology 110:473, 1974.

3. Parkey RW, Bonte FJ, Meyer SL, A new method for radionuclide imaging of acute myocardial infarction in humans. Circulation 50:540, 1974.

4. Zaret BL, DiCola VC, Donabedian RK, Dual radionuclide study of myocardial infarction. Relationships between myocardial uptake of Potassium-43, Technetium-99m stannous pyrophosphate, regional myocardial blood flow and creatine phosphokinase depletion. Circulation 53:422, 1976.

5. Bruno FP, Cobb FR, Rivas F, Evaluation of ^{99m}Technetium stannous pyrophosphate as an imaging agent in acute myocardial infarction. Circulation 54:71, 1976.

6. Marcus ML, Tomanek RJ, Erhardt JC, Relationships between myocardial necrosis and Technetium-99m pyrophosphate uptake in dogs subjected to sudden occlusion. Circulation 54:647, 1976.

7. Kronenberg MW, Ettiger UR, Wilson GA, A comparison of radiotracer and biochemical methods for the quantitation of experimental myocardial infarct weight: In vitro relationships. J. nucl. Med. 20:224, 1979.

8. Dressler J, Schmahl W, Hör G, Distribution of Thallium-201 and Tc-99m labelled phosphates in experimental infarction. Trans. Eur. Soc. Cardiol. 1:17, 1978.

9. Shen AC, Jennings RB, Kinetics of calcium accumulation in acute myocardial ischemic injury. Amer. J. Path. 67:441, 1972.

10. D'Agostino AN, An electron microscopic study of cardiac necrosis produced by 9 a-fluorocortisol and sodium phosphate. Amer. J. Path. 45:633, 1964.

11. Jennings RB, Herdson PB, Sommers HM, Structural and functional abnormalities in mitrochondria isolated from ischemic dog myocardium. Lab. Invest. 20:548, 1969.

12. Buja LM, Parkey RW, Dees JH, Morphologic correlates of Technetium-99m stannous pyrophosphate imaging of acute myocardial infarcts in dogs. Circulation 52:595, 1975.

13. Coleman RE, Klein MS, Ahmed SA, Mechanisms contributing to myocardial accumulation of Technetium-99m stannous pyrophosphate after coronary arterial occlusion. Amer. J. Cardiol. 39:55, 1977.

14. Izquierdo C, Devous MD, Nicod P, A comparison of infarct identification with Technetium-99m pyrophosphate and staining with triphenyl tetrazolium chloride. J. nucl. Med. 24:492, 1983.

15. Bianco JA, Kemper AJ, Taylor A, Technetium-99m pyrophosphate in ischemic and infarcted dog myocardium in early stages of acute coronary occlusion: Histochemical and tissuecounting comparisons. J. nucl. Med. 24:485, 1983.

16. Dewanjee MK, Localization of skeletal-imaging ^{99m}Tc chelates in dead cells in tissue culture: Concise communication. J. nucl. Med. 17:993, 1976.

17. Schelbert H, Ingwall J, Sybers H, Uptake of Tc-99m pyrophosphate and calcium in irreversibly damaged myocardium. J. nucl. Med. 17:534, 1976.

18. Buja LM, Tofe AJ, Kulkarni PV, Sites and mechanisms of localization of Technetium-99m phosphorus radiopharmaceuticals in acute myocardial infarcts and other tissues. J. clin. Invest. 60:724, 1977.

19. Willerson JT, Parkey RW, Bonte FJ, Acute subendocardial myocardial infarction in patients. Its detection by Technetium-99m stannous pyrophosphate myocardial scintigrams. Circulation 51:436, 1975.

20. Holman BL, Lesch M, Alpert JS, Myocardial scintigraphy with Technetium-99m pyrophosphate during the early phase of acute myocardial infarction. Amer. J. Cardiol. 41:39, 1978.

21. Kahn P, Aldor E, Blazek G, Negative und positive Darstellung der Herzinfarktes. J. nucl. Med. 16:63, 1977.

22. Kelly RJ, Chilton H, Hackshaw BT, Comparison of Tc-99m-pyrophosphate and Tc-99m-methylene diphosphonate in acute myocardial function. J. nucl. Med. 20:402, 1979.

23. Dressler J, Szintigraphie des akuten Myokardinfarktes mit Tc-99m-Phosphat-Verbindungen. Herz 5:93, 1980.

24. Campeau RJ, Gottlieb S, Chandarlapaty SKC, Accuracy of Technetium-99m labelled phosphates for detection of acute myocardial infarction (abstract). J. nucl. Med. 16:518, 1975.

25. Gould LA, Perez LA, Hayt DB, Clinical experience with Technetium-stannous-polyphosphate for myocardial imaging. Brit. Heart J. 38:744, 1976.

26. Joseph SP, Ell PJ, Ross P, ^{99m}Tc-imidodiphosphonate: A superior radiopharmaceutical for in vivo positive myocardial infarct imaging. II. Clinical data. Brit. Heart J. 40:234, 1978.

27. Cook DJ, Makar LJ, Chatterton BE, ^{99m}Tc-Imidodiphosphonate: A better tracer for infarct-avid imaging. Eur. J. Nucl. Med. 7:207, 1982.

28. Berman DS, Amsterdam EA, Hines HH, A new approach to the interpretation of Technetium-99m pyrophosphate scintigraphy in the detection of acute myocardial infarction: Clinical assessment of diagnostic assurancy. Amer. J. Cardiol. 39:341, 1977.

29. Henning H, Schelbert HR, Righetti A, Dual myocardial imaging with Technetium-99m pyrophosphate and Thallium-201 for detecting, localizing and sizing acute myocardial infarction. Amer. J. Cardiol. 40:147, 1977.

30. Berger HJ, Gottschalk A, Zaret BL, Dual radionuclide study of acute myocardial infarction. Ann. Intern. Med. 88:145, 1978.

31. Cowley MJ, Manke JA, Rogers WJ, Technetium-99m stannous pyrophosphate myocardial scintigraphy. Reliability and limitations in assessment of acute myocardial infarction. Circulation 56:192, 1977.

32. Ahmad M, Dubiel JP, Logan KW, Limited clinical diagnostic specificity of Technetium-99m-stannous pyrophosphate myocardial imaging in acute myocardial infarction. Amer. J. Cardiol. 39:50, 1977.

33. Coleman RE, Klein MS, Roberts R, Improved detection of myocardial infarction with [99m]-pyrophosphate and serum MB CPK. Amer. J. Cardiol. 37:732, 1976.

34. Lessem J, Johansson BW, Nosslin B, Myocardial scintigraphy with Tc-99m pyrophosphate in patients with unstable angina pectoris. Acta Med. Scand. 203:491, 1978.

35. Okada RD, Woolfenden JM, Raessler KL, Technetium-99m stannous pyrophosphate myocardial scintiphotos in patients admitted to rule out acute myocardial infarction. Cardiology 62:305, 1977.

36. Poliner L, Parkey RW, Bonte FJ, Technetium-99m-stannous pyrophosphate myocardial scintigrams to recognize acute subendocardial myocardial infarcts in patients (abstract). Amer. J. Cardiol.37:162, 1976.

37. Prasquier R, Tavadask MR, Botvinick EH, The specificity of the diffuse pattern of cardiac uptake in myocardial infarction imaging with Technetium-99m stannous pyrophosphate. Circulation 55:61, 1977.

38. Massie BM, Botoinick EH, Werner JA, Myocardial scintigraphy with Technetium-99m stannous pyrophosphate: An intensive test for nontransmural myocardial infarction. Amer. J. Cardiol. 43:186, 1979.

39. Walsh W, Lessem J, Fill H, Value of ^{99m}Tc-pyrophosphate myocardial scintigraphy in patients with suspected myocardial infarction (abstract). Amer. J. Cardiol. 37:180, 1976.

40. Willerson JT, Parkey RW, Bonte FJ, Technetium-99m stannous pyrophosphate myocardial scintigrams in patients with chest pain of varying etiology. Circulation 51:1046, 1975.

41. Olson HG, Lyons KP, Dronow WS, Prognostic value of a persistently positive Technetium-99m stannous pyrophosphate myocardial scintigram after myocardial infarction. Amer. J. Cardiol. 43:889, 1979.

42. Abdulla AM, Canedo MI, Cortez BC, Detection of unstable angina by ^{99m}Technetium pyrophosphate myocardial scintigraphy. Chest 69:2, 1976.

43. Stokely EM, Buja M, Lewis SE, Measurement of acute myocardial infarcts in dogs with 99m-Tc-stannous pyrophosphate scintigrams. J. nucl. Med. 17:1, 1976.

44. Poliner LR, Buja LM, Parkey RW, Clinicopathologic findings in 52 patients studies by Technetium-99m stannous pyrophosphate myocardial scintigraphy. Circulation 59:257, 1979.

45. Botvinick EH, Shames D, Lappin H, Noninvasive quantitation of myocardial infarction with Technetium-99m pyrophosphate. Circulation 52:909, 1975.

46. Sharpe DN, Botvinick EH, Shames DM, The clinical estimation of acute myocardial infarct size with ^{99m}Tc pyrophosphate scintigraphy. Circulation 57:307, 1978.

47. Silber S, Fleck E, Gehrke S, Klinische Infarktgrössen-bestimmung mit 99m-Technetium-pyrophosphat: Korrelation zum CK(MB)-Verlauf. Z. Kardiol. 5:152, 1978.

48. Keyes JW, Leonard FF, Brody SL, Myocardial infarct quantification in the dog by single photon emission computed tomography. Circulation 58:227, 1978.

49. Lewis SE, Stokely EM, Devous MD, Quantitation of experimental canine infarct size with multipinhole and rotating slanthole tomography. J. nucl. Med. 22:1000, 1981.

50. Aldor E, Heeger H, Kalm P, Prognostic significance of follow-up scintigraphy with ^{99m}Tc-pyrophosphate in myocardial infarction. Z. Kardiol. 67:717, 1978.

51. Perez-Gonzalvez J, Botvinick EH, Dunn R, The late prognostic value of acute scintigraphic measurement of myocardial infarction size. Circulation 66:960, 1982.

52. Holman BL, Chiskolm RJ, Braunwald E, The prognostic implications of acute myocardial infarct scintigraphy with ^{99m}Tc-pyrophosphate. Circulation 57:320, 1978.

53. Wackers FJTH, Myocardial imaging in the coronary care unit. Martinus Nijhoff Publishers, The Hague, 1980.

V. TOMOGRAPHIC TECHNIQUES

SINGLE PHOTON EMISSION COMPUTED TOMOGRAPHY (SPECT) IN
NUCLEAR CARDIOLOGY

H.J. BIERSACK, C. WINKLER

INTRODUCTION

Tomographic techniques using single photon (SP) emitters
have gained increasing importance in nuclear cardiology during
the last few years. First clinical experiences by Holman et
al (1) demonstrated the feasibility of the assessment of myocardial perfusion by means of ^{201}Tl and transaxial SPECT performed by the CLEON 711 body imager. In a more recent study
Burdine et al (2) used a rotating double-headed gamma camera
system for ECG-gated imaging of cardiac blood-pool. In 1979
Vogel et al (3) reported on myocardial imaging with the aid
of a seven-pinhole (camera) collimator; another approach to
longitudinal emission tomography was the application of slanthole collimators (4-8) which has, however, not gained widespread acceptance.

The most important SP tomographic myocardial imaging techniques and respective clinical results can be summarized as
follows:

SPECT of the myocardium

Multidetector scanning system. An early approach for sec-
tional myocardial scanning with ^{201}Tl was the Multidetector
Scanning System (CLEON 711 body imager). This device consists
of a ring-shaped gantry assembly in which 10 scanning detectors
at 36-degree intervals are mounted. The effective field of
view is limited to the central 50 cm. The gantry can be tilted
through an angle of ± 15° to the vertical allowing image sections of various angles. The respective algorithms include
filters for collimator correction, smoothing, and empirical
attenuation correction (1). A complete 4-section study takes

about 20 min, each transaxial slice containing 200,000 to 350,000 counts. FWHM is about 17 mm for Tc^{99m}.

Initial clinical results obtained by Holman et al (1) showed that myocardial defects in patients with prior infarction were clearly separated from anatomic structures such as cardiac chambers and normally perfused myocardium. The images yielded high contrast ratios permitting prompt and easy identifications of myocardial infarcts. Kirsch et al (9) used a double isotope technique (^{201}Tl, Tc^{99m}-pyrophosphate) to estimate the infarct size in an experimental study. The SPECT results and the real infarct sizes revealed excellent correlation (r= 0.94) in 16 animals. Possible sources of error like motion of the beating heart and blurring respiration as well as attenuation effects had no apparent gross influence on the accuracy of this method.

Pinhole tomography. In 1978 Vogel et al (10) introduced pinhole tomography in nuclear cardiology. This method uses a wide-field gamma camera and a seven-pinhole collimator. Through pinholes (5.5 mm ∅) scintigraphy data are simultaneously acquired from different angles and the myocardium is projected onto 7 independent regions of the crystal. Multiple planes (up to 12) are reconstructed from the set of data by use of a computerized addition-multiplication algorythm and variation of the superimposition relationships among the projected views. The planes are processed iteratively. Plane resolution (FWHM) is 1 cm and depth resolution comes to 1.5 cm.

The first clinical results achieved with this imaging technique appeared to be excellent: among 42 patients with angiographically proven coronary artery disease, there were only 31 in whom abnormalities could be established by conventional scintigraphy whereas in 40 of these cases perfusion defects were demonstrated tomographically. From these results it was concluded that pinhole tomography is highly sensitive to the presence of coronary artery disease using stress Thallium imaging. A multicenter study performed in 1980 seemed to verify these promising results (11). However, one year later, Ritchie et al (12) reported on rather unfavourably experiences when using seven-pinhole tomography in patients with prior myo-

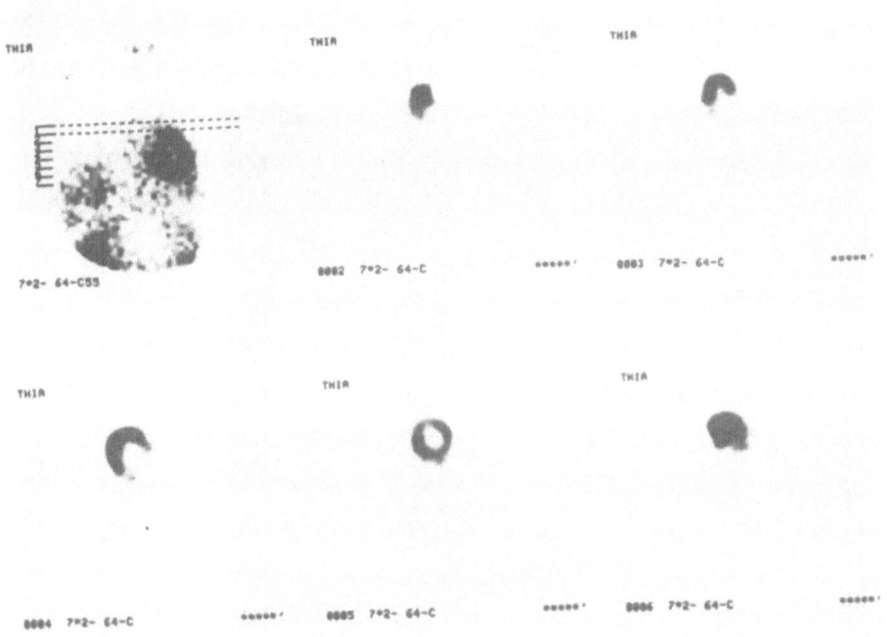

Fig. 1. Normal SPECT of the
myocardium (^{201}Tl).
a) Transverse sections.
b) Scheme left lateral.
c) Sagittal sections.
d) Scheme anterior
e) Coronar sections.

cardial infarction. The authors were unable to ascertain statistical significant differences in either sensitivity or specificity between the planar and tomographic approaches. They then
concluded that seven pinhole tomography has no real advantage
over standard planar imaging. In phantom studies it was shown
that a small area of decreased activity - geometrically 3 cm
in depth - was seen throughout all 12 of the tomographic
slices. Thus it was pointed out that there is no depth localization possible by means of pinhole tomography (12). These
disappointing results were confirmed subsequently by Tamaki
et al (13) who evaluated seven-pinhole tomography in comparison
to rotating gamma camera investigations. In their study the

340

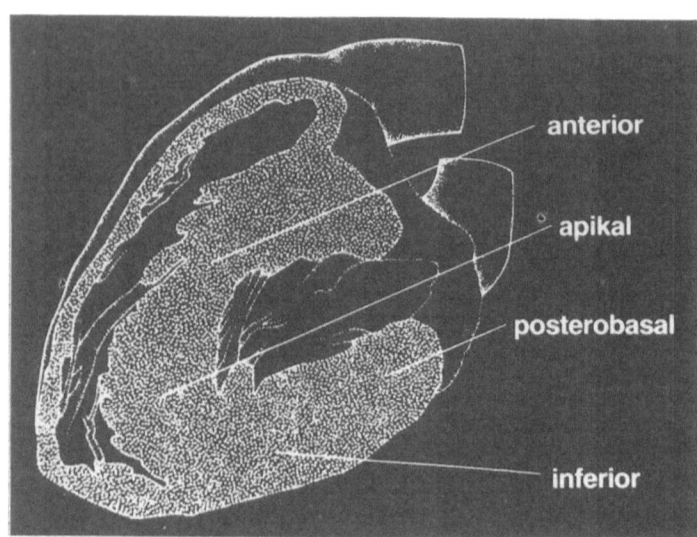

anterior

apikal

posterobasal

inferior

Fig. 1b

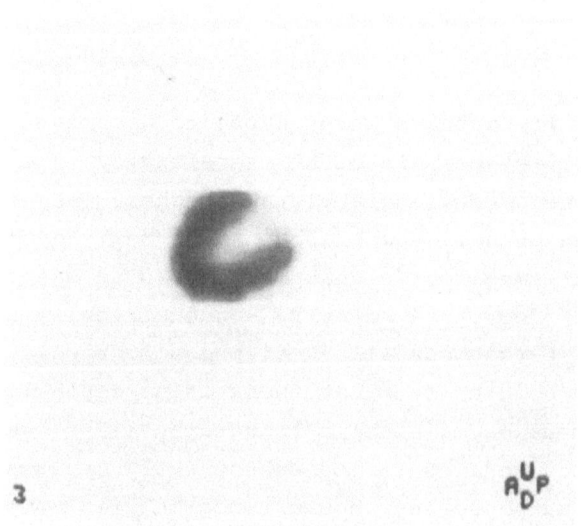

Fig. 1c

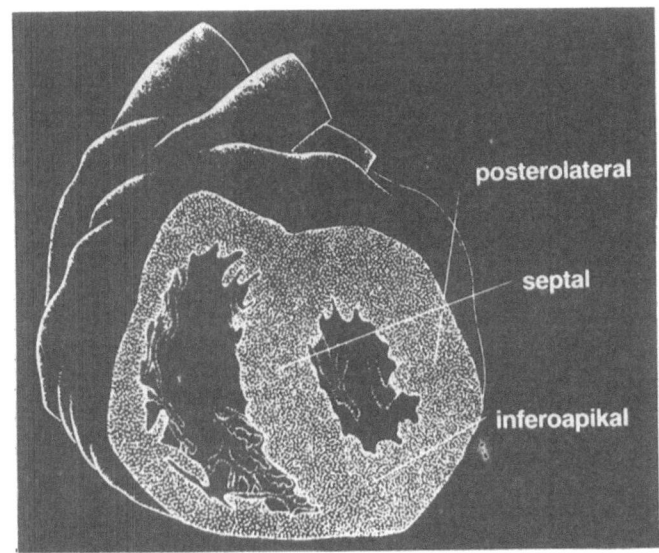

Fig. 1d

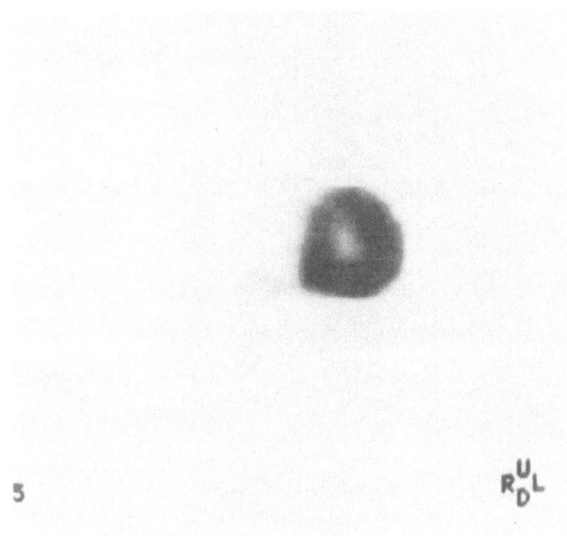

Fig. 1e

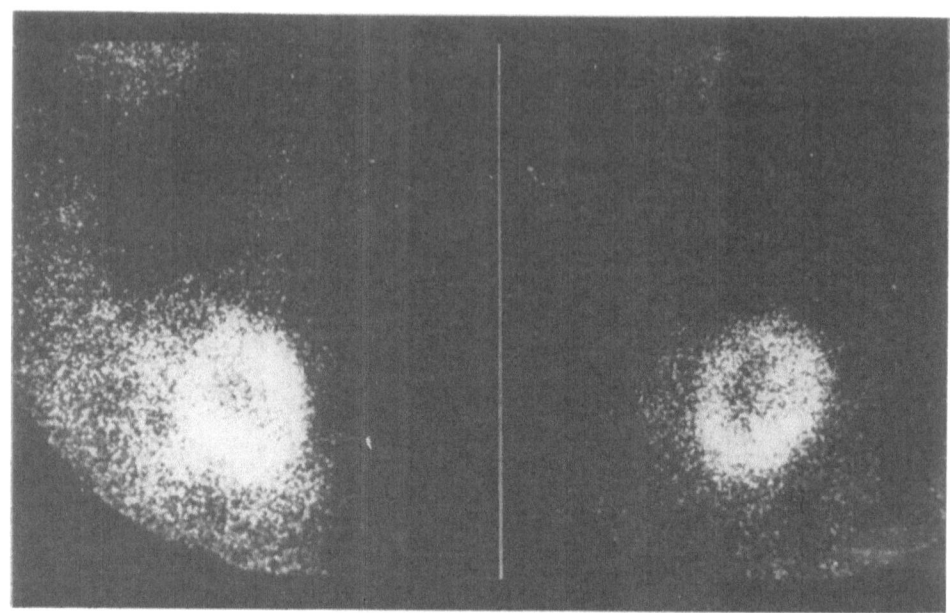

Fig. 2. SPECT of a patient with coronary artery disease and lesions in the anterior wall and septum; the anterior wall lesion is only visualized by the (transverse) sections of SPECT.
a) Biplanar scintigraphy with ^{201}Tl (left = left lateral, right = 45° LAO).
b) Transverse sections of SPECT.

Fig. 2b

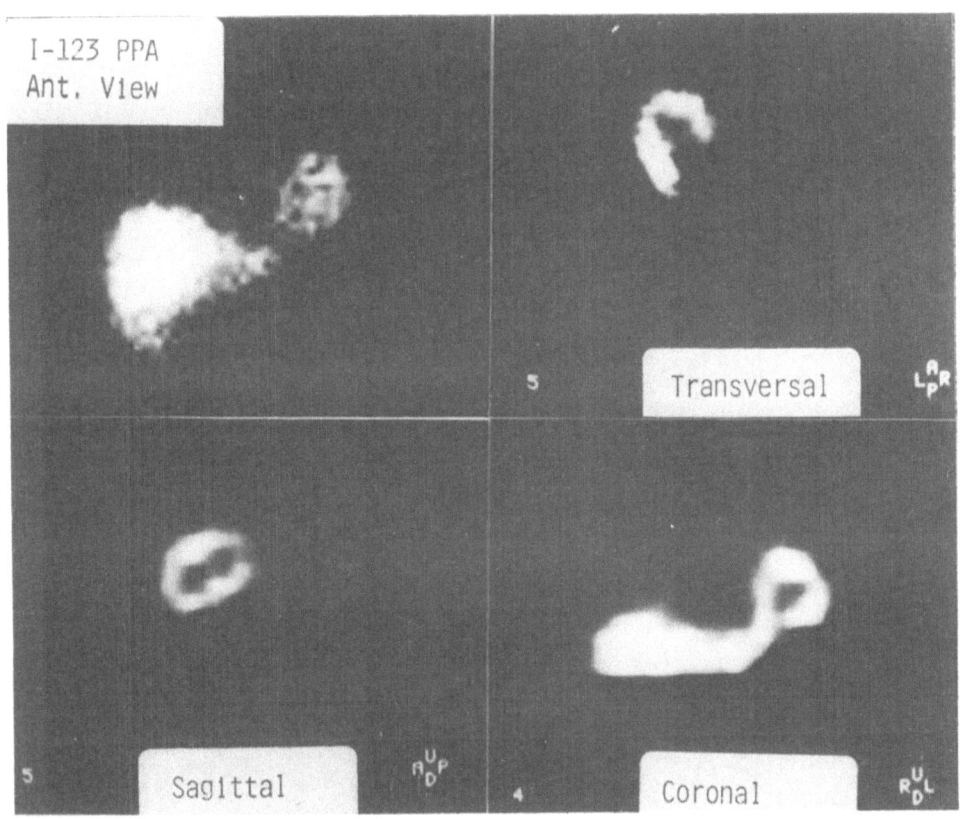

Fig. 3. SPECT of the myocardium with ^{123}IPPA in a healthy subject; note the high liver uptake of IPPA in anterior projection!

overall accuracy was 81% in planar scintigraphy, 83% in seven-pinhole tomography, and 94% in rotating gamma camera tomography.

Rotating gamma camera (fig 1,2). The experiences of Tamaki and others point to the fact that conventional biplanar Thallium scintigraphy may be oftentimes not adequate to determine exactly the extent of tissue injury. A main limitation of biplanar scintigraphy for myocardial imaging is that decreased activity due to the left ventricular cavity must be differentiated from impaired myocardial uptake. Furthermore,

344

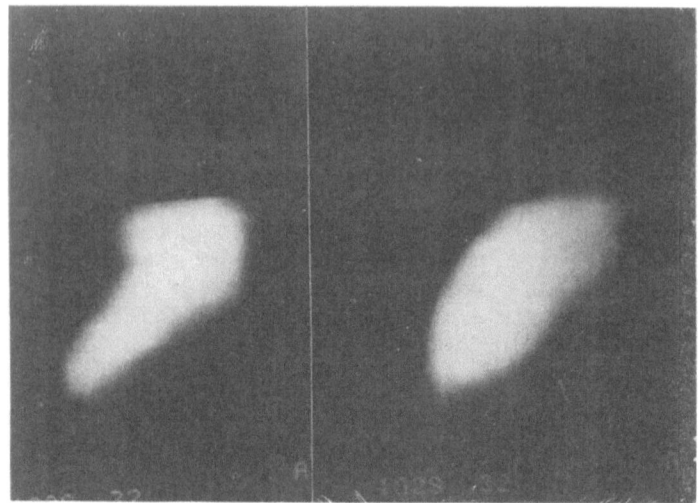

Fig. 4a

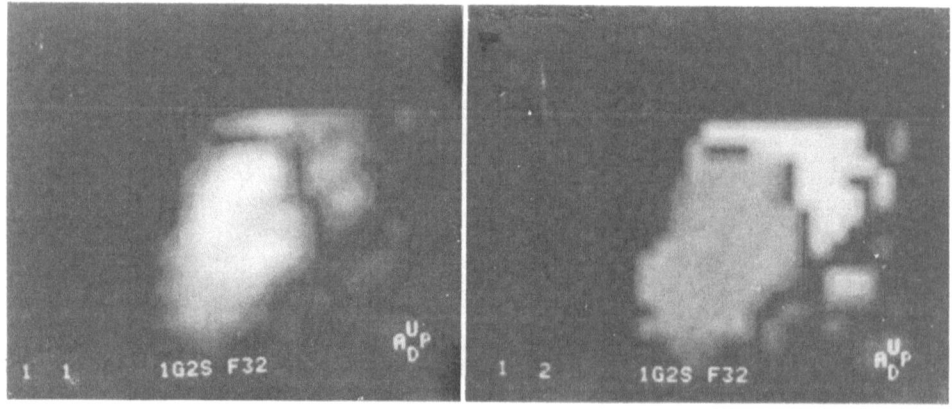

Fig. 4b   Fig. 4c

Fig. 4. Normal SPECT of the gated cardiac blood-pool (Tc^{99m}-HSA).
a) Endsystolic (left) and enddiastolic (right) image (sagittal section).
b) Amplitude image (sagittal).
c) Phase image (sagittal).

345

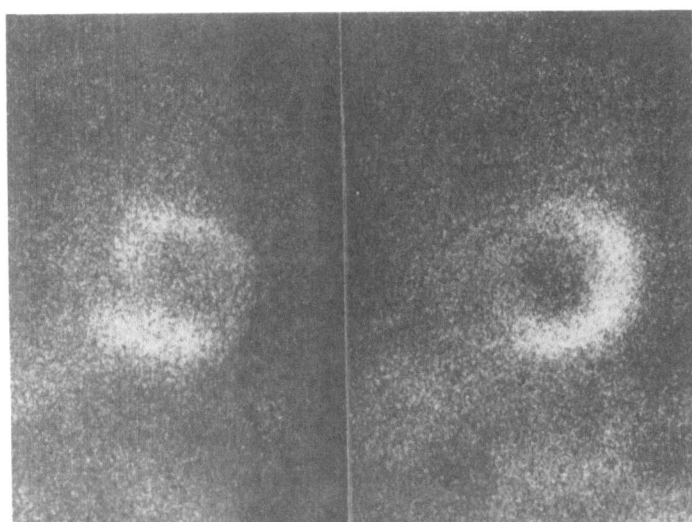

Fig. 5a

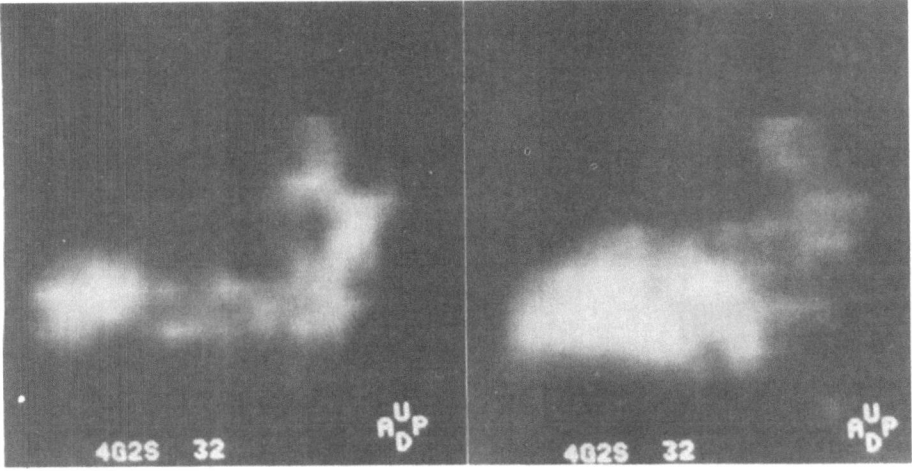

Fig. 5b

Fig. 5. Gated cardiac blood-pool (SPECT) (Tc^{99m}-HSA) of a patient with myocardial infarction and lesions antero-septal; SPECT of the blood-pool exhibits a huge aneurysm of anterior wall and apex. The involvement of the middle part of the anterior wall can only be established by SPECT but not by the conventional 45° LAO study.
a) Biplanar scintigraphy with ^{201}Tl (left = left lateral, right = 45° LAO).
b) Endsystolic (left) and enddiastolic (right) image of the gated blood-pool (SPECT).
c) Phase image of the gated blood-pool SPECT (sagittal).
d) Conventional 45° LAO gated blood-pool study.

346

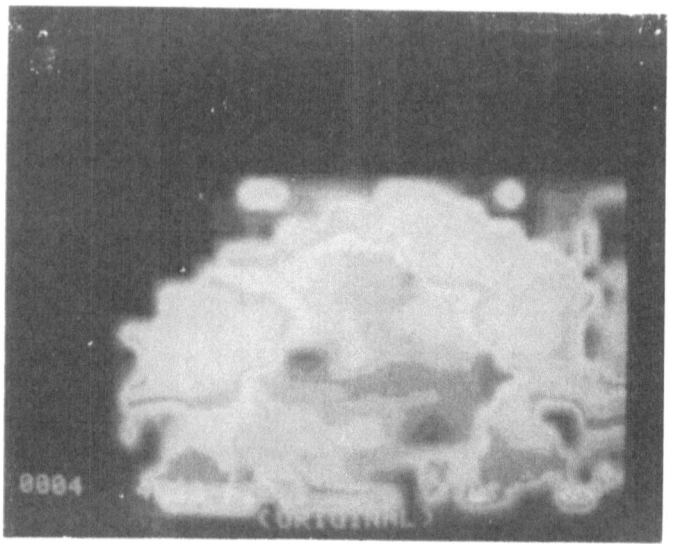

Fig. 5c

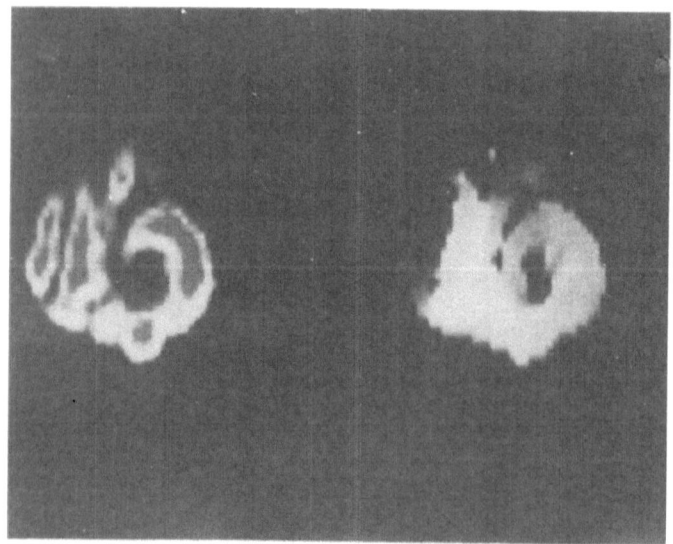

Fig. 5d

superimposition of normally perfused myocardium over hypoperfused regions as well as wall motion abnormalities may cause
difficulties in estimating the extent and degree of perfusion
deficits. Thus, the correlation between determination of
infarct size from conventional two-dimensional scintigraphy
and the results of postmortem examination has been only fair
(14). Therefore it appeared to be desirable to develop a
reliable method for cross-sectional myocardial imaging.

Initial experiences with a stationary gamma camera and
the patient rotating on a chair were described by Bundinger
et al (15). But the imaging and reconstruction time were too
long for routine clinical applications. In 1981 Maublant et
al (16) as well as our group (17) have reported on the use
of a rotating gamma camera system for SPECT of the myocardium
and the early results were confirmed one year later in a
larger series of patients (18,19). Maublant et al (18) established an increase of sensitivity from 89% (conventional scintigraphy) up to 98% (SPECT) with no difference of specificity
(93%). These excellent results were verified by Tamaki et al
(13) who found a significantly improved overall accuracy
(conventional scintigraphy: 81% vs SPECT: 94%). In our investigations, however, there appears to be no considerable difference
between SPECT and conventional scintigraphy in regard to
demonstration of existing lesions (19). Nevertheless, in many
cases the extent and localization of infarctions or scars can
be estimated more accurately by SPECT. On the basis of an
experimental model we studied the extent to which even small
intramural myocardial ischemia can be demonstrated by SPECT.
For this purpose, ligation of the ramus interventricularis
anterior or the left circumflex artery was performed in dogs
to produce myocardial lesions of the anterior or posterior
wall. CAT served as a control method showing that even small
intramural lesions with a volume of about 1 ml could be
detected (20). Furthermore, a comparison of stress and redistribution ^{201}Tl imaging with a rotating gamma camera allows
a more clearcut delineation of stress induced myocardial
ischemia (21,22).

SPECT with a rotating gamma camera is usually performed after injection of 2 mCi ^{201}Tl chloride. The study time is about 20 min, and 64 frames (4k matrix) during one 360° rotation are acquired, the total count rate being about 2 to 4 x 10^6. After reconstruction of transversal slices, additional sagittal and coronal slices are obtainable within a short processing time using array processors. (It should be mentioned that sagittal slices are most helpful for evaluation of the posterior wall). As determined through phantom studies, a resolution between 12 and 14 mm - depending on the distance from a defect from the rotation axis - could be obtained (23) when extensive quality control was performed (24).

The paper of Tamaki et al (25) first raised the question of 180° and 360° data collection: the 180° image - although requiring only half the investigation time - revealed clearer perfusion defects due to less background noise in comparison with the 360° image. Another paper by Coleman et al (26) dealt with the probability of myocardial ^{201}Tl SPECT, using the data from only 180° rotation as opposed to the 360° rotation data collection usually employed. Tamaki et al (25) concluded that 180° data collection is a more effective technique in the clinical evaluation of coronary artery disease because lesion contrast is higher and the study time required is shorter. Coleman et al (26), however, pointed out that for their double-headed SPECT system, the 360° collection permits attenuation correction, has less variability in counting statistics, and gives contrast ratios similar to those of 180° collection. Hoffman (27) summarized the results of these 2 papers and pointed out that the 180° SPECT scans with ^{201}Tl may be partially justifiable, but mainly because the low energy of the gamma emission of Thallium causes problems of attenuation, scatter, and scatter rejection. With the 180° collection, however, practicable attenuation correction and also quantitative assessment of myocardial ^{201}Tl uptake is not feasible. With the use of Tc^{99m} or ^{123}I-labelled tracers, the net attenuation of the radiation will be about 50% less across the body, the scatter fraction is considerable smaller, and spatial resolu-

lution will be superior to ^{201}Tl imaging (27). It may be anticipated that with the introduction of the mentioned tracers
180° data collection will become out of date.

Future perspectives. Myocardial SPECT with fatty acids
(fig 3). Until recently, studies of cardiac metabolism in man
have been limited to assessment of arteriovenous differences
of myocardial substrates using arterial and coronary-sinus
sampling techniques. Without mentioning that these procedures
are invasive it has to be realized that they can only determine global cardiac metabolism. Contrary to this fatty acids
can be used for metabolic imaging and SPECT renders possible
non-invasive determination of regional myocardial metabolism.
Reske et al (28,29) were the first to achieve metabolic SPECT
images using ^{123}I-paraphenylpentadecanoic acid (IPPA) as a
tracer. In these studies a rotating gamma camera system
served for emission tomographic myocardial imaging, and high
quality transsectional pictures of the canine heart with
clear delineation of left ventricular walls were obtained.
Myocardial infarcts were visualized as areas of deficient
radioactivity uptake. IPPA disappearance rate from non-infarcted
myocardial regions turned out to be significantly prolonged
when compared with unaffected controls - as was established
by sequential SPECT (6 studies during 1 hour). Hence it could
be proved that besides of the absence of free fatty acid uptake
in infarcted areas there is also a general metabolic impairment in the entire heart muscle. It may be emphasized in
principle that ^{123}I-labelled fatty acids offer 2 advantages
as tracers for cardiac imaging when compared to ^{201}Tl: one
higher amounts of radioactivity can be used, and two attenuation is less due to higher gamma energy. Thus, myocardial
SPECT with radioiodinated fatty acids may "herald a new way of
thinking about clinical disorders where characterization of
the metabolic disorders produces new modes of therapy designed
to restore normal metabolism" (30). In view of the use of
^{123}I as a label the problem of ^{124}I - the decay product of
^{123}I with its unprofitable high gamma energy - has yet to be
considered e.g. when long transportation ways delay prompt

delivery of the radiopharmaceutical.

Myocardial SPECT with Tc[99m]-DMPE. A new promising imaging agent is Tc[99m]-labelled dichlorbis (1,2-dimethylphosphino) ethane (DMPE) (31,32). Blood-clearance of ^{201}Tl and Tc[99m]-DMPE are essentially the same but the latter agent shows faster overall kinetics and higher heart-to-lung ratios. The similar conduct of this radiopharmaceutical compared to ^{201}Tl suggest its usefulness in the evaluation of ischemic heart disease. Thus, Tc[99m]-DMPE may one day replace 201Tl with its problems (low gamma energy, high radiation load) for SPECT of myocardial perfusion.

SPECT of the gated cardiac blood-pool (fig 4,5).

Gated blood-pool scintigraphy is nowadays a routine tool in non-invasive nuclear cardiology. The investigation is usually carried out in 45° LAO projection to avoid superimposition through right ventricular activity. However, this procedure is limited to the visualization of septal, apical, and posterolateral wall motion while the contraction of the anterior wall cannot be assessed. To overcome this disadvantage, bilateral collimators (33) as well as first pass techniques (34,35) are used in order to additionally get information about the anterior wall. However, in dual projection heart studies image degradation is caused due to overlying right ventricular activity and first pass studies comprise only a few heart beats and selection of a "representative heart cycle" is not possible.

Because of these disadvantages SPECT with a rotating gamma camera was introduced into cardiac blood-pool investigation. Already in 1979 Burdine et al (2) pointed at the principal feasibility of ECG-gated cardiac blood-pool imaging by SPECT. Since then a series of further reports has been published concerned with this new imaging technique (36-41). At present, 64 frames (4k matrix) during one full rotation of 360° are usually acquired within 20 min (42) after an equilibrium of 15 to 25 mCi Tc[99m]-labelled RBC's or HSA is achieved. Each heart beat is divided into 8 (up to 16) time increments.

After reconstruction of transverse slices additional sagittal
and coronar slices can also be obtained within short processing
time. For evaluation of the cardiac wall motion cine display
as well as endsystolic and enddiastolic images are used (36,
37,39). A new approach for visualization of the myocardial
contraction pattern are Fourier phase and amplitude images.
It appears essential however, that 3-dimensional Fourier
analysis is performed because of perpendicular movement of
the transversal cardiac sections during the heart beat. Respective algorithms were reported by Brunol and Nuta (43). It
may be emphasized that reconstruction of sagittal slices
facilitates considerably the evaluation of left ventricular
wall motion because in 1 or 2 slices the anterior wall, the
apex, and the posterior wall are visualized. The hereby obtained results can easily be interpreted and resemble the 30°
RAO projection of X-ray laevocardiography. The ability to see
the cardiac chambers separately in motion permits evaluation
of both ventricles unimpeded by superimposition of other
structures and points at potentials for calculating ventricular
volumes. Comparative studies of Eilles et al (36) yielded a
close correlation of ejection fractions estimated by conventional blood-pool scintigraphy and SPECT. (Maximal ejection
and filling rates, however, should preferently be calculated
from conventional techniques due to their higher timely resolution of 20 to 50 frames per heart cycle.

On the basis of clinical experiences from our group (42)
it can be stressed that SPECT of the gated cardiac blood-pool
permits accurate information concerning anterior wall motion.
All patients with radiologically proven contraction abnormalities of this region yielded positive SPECT results whereas
the conventional LAO technique was failing. Moreover, analysis
of the contraction pattern (hypo-, a-, and dyskinesia) was
rendered possible by means of parametric (Fourier phase and
amplitude) SPECT. To sum up and in conclusion it may be stated
that combined examination with the aid of gated conventional
(45° LAO) imaging and SPECT of the cardiac blood-pool (including parametric techniques) comprehensive information concerning
regional contraction patterns of the entire left and right
ventricle can be obtained for representative heart cycles.

REFERENCES

1. Holman BL, Hill TC, Wynne J et al, Single-photon transaxial emission computed tomography of the heart in normal subjects and in patients with infarction. J. nucl. Med. 20:736, 1979.

2. Burdine JA, Murphy PH, DePuey EG, Radionuclide computed tomography of the body using routine radiopharmaceuticals. II. Clinical applications. J. nucl. Med. 20:108, 1979.

3. Vogel RA, Kirch DL, LeFree MT et al, Thallium-201 myocardial perfusion scintigraphy: Results of standard and multi-pinhole tomographic techniques. Amer. J. Cardiol. 43:787, 1979.

4. Lewis SE, Stokely EM, Devous MD et al, Quantitation of experimental canine infarct size with multi-pinhole and rotating-slant-hole tomography. J. nucl. Med. 22:1000, 1981.

5. Shosa DW, O'Connell JW, Hattner RS, Motivation for the rotating slant hole approach to scintillation camera tomography. J. nucl. Med. 21:27, 1980.

6. Pavel D, Byrom E, Meyer-Pavel C et al, Cardiac tomography using a rotating slant hole collimator and a portable camera. J. nucl. Med. 21:27, 1980.

7. Herfkens RJ, Shoes DW, Hattner RS et al, Clinical applications of rotating slanthole tomography to cardiovascular nuclear medicine. J. nucl. Med. 21:70, 1980.

8. Gottschalk SC, Smith KA, Wake RH, Comparison of 7 pinhole and rotating slanthole tomography of a cardiac phantom. J. nucl. Med. 21:27, 1980.

9. Kirsch CM, Darsee JR, Hill TC et al, In-vivo Bestimmung der Infarktgrösse des Myocardinfarkts mit der Single Photon Emissions-Computertomographie. 19th Int. Ann. Meeting Soc. Nucl. Med. (Europe) Bern, abstracts p. 178, 1981.

10. Vogel RA, Kirch D, LeFree M et al, A new method of multiplanar emission tomography using a seven pinhole collimator and an Anger scintillation camera. J. nucl. Med. 19:648, 1978.

11. Vogel RA, Alderson P, Berman D et al, A multicenter comparison of standard and seven pinhole tomographic Tl-201 scintigraphy. Results of quantitative interpretation of tomograms. J. nucl. Med. 21:70, 1980.

12. Ritchie JL, Williams DL, Caldwell JH et al, Seven-pinhole emission tomography with Thallium-201 in patients with prior myocardial infarction. J. nucl. Med. 22:107, 1981.

13. Tamaki N, Mukai T, Ischii Y et al, Clinical evaluation of Thallium-201 emission myocardial tomography using a rotating gamma camera: Comparison with seven-pinhole tomography. J. nucl. Med. 22:849, 1981.

14. Wackers FJT, Becker AE, Samson G, Location and size of acute transmural myocardial infarction estimated from Thallium-201 scintigrams. A clinical pathological study. Circulation 56:72, 1977.

15. Budinger TF, Gullberg GT, Mayer BR, Transverse section imaging of the myocardium. J. nucl. Med. 17:551, 1976.

16. Maublant J, Cassagnes J, Jourde M et al, Myocardial emission tomography with Thallium-201: Value of multiple and orthogonal sections in the study of the myocardial infarction. Eur. J. Nucl. Med. 6:289, 1981.

17. Biersack HJ, Reske SN, Simon H et al, Emissions-Computertomographie (Single Photon) des Myocards mit [201]Tl. In: Nuclearmedizin: Computer assisted functional analysis. Schmidt HAE, Roesler H (eds) Schattauer Verlag, Stuttgart, New York, p 245, 1982.

18. Maublant J, Cassagnes J, LeJeune JJ et al, A comparison between conventional scintigraphy and emission tomography with Thallium-201 in the detection of myocardial infarction: Concise communication. J. nucl. Med. 23:204, 1982.

19. Biersack HJ, Reske SN, Knopp R et al, Single-Photon Emission-Computer-tomographie des Myocards. Dtsch. med. Wschr. 107:476, 1982.

20. Biersack HJ, Lackner K, Eichelkraut W et al, SPECT (^{201}Tl) des Myo-kards nach experimentellem Infarkt. Nucl. Med. 21:254, 1982.

21. McIntyre WJ, Go RT, Cook SA et al, Comparison of stress and redistribu-tion [201]-Thallium planar imaging with a single photon transaxial tomographic technique. In: Nucl. Med. and Biol. Proc. IIIrd World Congress Nucl. Med. and Biol. Raynaud C (ed), Pergamon, p 1281, 1982.

22. Büll U, Kirsch CM, Roedler HD et al, Die 201-Tl-Emissionscomputer-tomographie des linken Ventrikels. Nuklearmediziner 4:267, 1982.

23. Biersack HJ, Knopp R, Franken T et al, Emissions-Computertomographie (Single Photon) mit einem rotierenden Gammakamera-System (Gammatone). NucComp. 11:256, 1980.

24. Todd-Pokropek A, Single photon emission computerised tomography (SPECT): Quality control and assurance. In: Radioaktive Isotope in Klinik und Forschung. Höfer R, Bergmann H (eds), Egermann Wien, p 539, 1983.

25. Tamaki N, Mukai T, Ischii Y et al, Comparative study of Thallium-emission myocardial tomography with 180° and 360° data collection. J. nucl. Med. 23:661, 1982.

26. Coleman RE, Jaszcak RJ, Cobb FR, Comparison of 180° and 360° data collection in Thallium-201 imaging using single-photon emission computerized tomography (SPECT): Concise communication. J. nucl. Med. 23:655, 1982.

27. Hoffman EJ, 180° compared with 360° sampling in SPECT. J. nucl. Med. 23:745, 1982.

28. Reske SN, Machulla HJ, Biersack HJ et al, Nicht-invasive Erfassung des regionalen myocardialen Stoffwechsels von omega-J-123-para-phenylpentadecansäure durch single photon Tomographie. In: Nuclearmedizin: Computer assisted functional analysis. Schmidt HAE, Roesler H (eds) Schattauer Verlag, Stuttgart, New York, p 258, 1982.

29. Reske SN, Biersack HJ, Lackner K et al, Assessment of regional myo-cardial uptake and metabolism of omega-(p-1231-phenyl) pentadecanoic acid with serial single-photon emission tomography. Nucl. Med. 21:249, 1982.

30. Goldstein RA, Myocardial metabolic imaging: A new diagnostic era. J. nucl. Med. 23:641, 1982.

31. Deutsch E, Glaven KA, Sodd VJ et al, Cationic Tc-99m complexes as potential myocardial imaging agents. J. nucl. Med. 22:897, 1981.

32. Nishiyama H, Deutsch E, Adolph RJ et al, Basal kinetic studies of Tc-99m DMPE as a myocardial imaging agent in the dog. J. nucl. Med. 23:1093, 1982.

354

33. Knopp R, Biersack HJ, Schmidt H et al, Erfahrungen mit dem Einsatz einer "Bilateral-Collimators" bei der Herzfunktionsszintigraphie. NucComp. 11:256, 1980.

34. Hecht H, Mirell SG, Rolett EL et al, Left ventricular ejection fraction and segmental wall motion by peripheral first-pass radionuclide angiography. J. nucl. Med. 19:17, 1978.

35. Büll U, Knesewitsch P, Kleinhans E et al, Die erste Radionuklid-Passage mit der Einkristall-Gammakamera. Nucl. Med. 20:109, 1981.

36. Eilles C, Strauss P, Gerhards W et al, Klinische Wertigkeit der EKG-getriggerten Single-Photon-Emissionscomputertomographie (GA-SPECT) des Herzbinnenraums. In: Radioaktive Isotope in Klinik und Forschung. Höfer R, Bergmann H (eds), Egermann Wien, Vol. 15/II, p 675, 1982.

37. Eilles C, Gerhards W, Strauss P et al, EKG-getriggerte Emissions-Computertomographie der Herzbinnenräume. Methoden und klinische Ergebnisse. Nuklearmediziner 5:275, 1982.

38. Shields RA, Testa HJ, Lwason RS et al, Emission computer tomography of the heart using a gamma camera. Eur. J. Nucl. Med. 5:49, 1980.

39. Moore ML, Murphy PH, Burdine JA et al, ECG-gated emission computed tomography of the cardiac blood pool. Radiology 137:233, 1980.

40. Maublant J, Bailly P, Mestas D et al, Feasibility of gated single-photon emission transaxial tomography of the cardiac blood pool. Radiology 146:837, 1983.

41. Philippe L, Itti R, Lorgeron JM et al, Tomographic measurement of left ventricular ejection fraction and comparison with conventional projections. In: Nucl. Med. and Biol. Proc. IIIrd World Congress Nucl. Med. and Biol. Raynaud C (ed), Pergamon, p 1285, 1982.

42. Biersack HJ, Reichmann K, Reske SN et al, Erste klinische Erfahrungen mit der parametrischen SPECT des Herzbinnenraums. NucComp. 14:36, 1983.

43. Brunol J, Nuta V, GEGAT: Gated cardiac emission computed axial tomography. NucComp. 13:260, 1982.

POSITRON EMISSION TOMOGRAPHY (PET) OF THE MYOCARDIUM

K. VYSKA, L.E. FEINENDEGEN

The most important nuclear medical contributions to cardiology developed in the past ten years are without doubt the
non-invasive determination of the cardiac ejection fraction
by the method of ECG-gated blood-pool analysis, the non-
invasive investigation of cardiac wallmotion, and myocardial
scintigraphy by means of Tl^{201} (1-7).

Whereas the information obtained by the ECG-gated blood-
pool technique and by analysis of myocardial wallmotion
reflects only the consequences of impaired myocardial function,
analysis of Tl^{201} scintigrams provided the possibility of
obtaining qualitative information about irregularities in
regional myocardial perfusion.

Recent cardiological studies indicate, however, that for
objective evaluation of myocardial ischemias and for characterization of cryptogenic cardiomyopathies with as yet unidenti-
fied metabolic etiology, quantitative, not qualitative, information about myocardial perfusion and metabolism is necessary
(8-15). This requirement stimulated an interest in the development of alternative myocardial agents which would provide the
possibility of quantitative assessment of some parameters of
myocardial metabolism.

It is evident that external monitoring of myocardial
metabolism in vivo can only be performed by use of radiopharmaceuticals which are incorporated directly into metabolic pathways in the myocardium. Therefore, much effort was invested
in developing suitable labelling procedures for such metabolic substrates. So far the most detailed results were obtained
with radioactively labelled free fatty acids (RLFFA). The
RFLLA's seem to be particularly useful for the detection of

metabolic alterations associated with ischemia and congestive cardiomyopathy, because

1. free fatty acids are the main physiological substrate for myocardial energy production (16-22,39);
2. the metabolism of free fatty acids requires aerobic conditions 16-21) and
3. the myocardial extraction of long chain fatty acids is drastically reduced under conditions of hypoxia and normal perfusion (8-13).

In the last decade various fatty acids were labelled in the ω- and α-position with Br^{77}, Cl^{34m}, I^{123} and C^{11}, and tested in the mice (see fig 1) (23-27). These studies revealed that for metabolic studies in vivo the most suitable radio-pharmaceuticals are C^{11} labelled palmitic acid (CPA) and heptadecanoic acid labelled with I^{123} in the ω-position (IHA). Both of these compounds showed high uptake and similar kinetics. Significantly lower uptakes were obtained using ω-chloro- and ω-bromo-fatty acids as well as α-halofatty acids. The smaller uptake of ω-chloro- and ω-bromo-fatty acids may be explained by the stronger binding to serum proteins. The low uptake of α-halofatty acids seems to be due to steric and inductive effects that inhibit the esterification of fatty acids with co-enzyme A and carnithine. Due to this inhibition the ability of the cell to extract effectively the α-halofatty acids from blood is reduced, and the passage of fatty acids through the mitochondrial membrane decelerated.

The utility of C^{11} palmitate for imaging the myocardium with positron emission tomography (PET) was demonstrated first by Hofman et al (16) and Weiss et al (12,13). Their studies suggested efficient extraction of this labelled long-chain fatty acid by myocardium. Because the compound disappeared rapidly from blood, high quality cross-sectional images could be obtained (fig 2).

In dogs with experimentally induced myocardial infarction, cross-sectional images of the myocardium clearly depicted infarcted segments as regions with reduced C^{11} activity. The size of the defect on the cross-sectional images corresponded

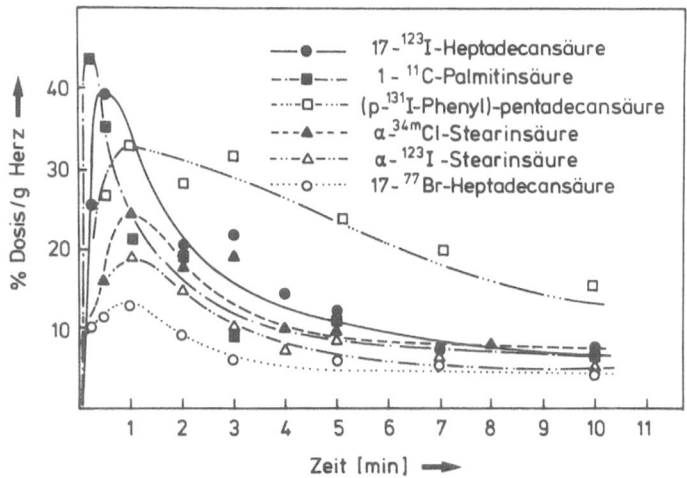

Fig. 1. The time course of radioactivity in mouse heart muscle after i.v. injection of 17-^{77}Br-, 17-^{123}I-heptadecanoic acid, 15 (p-^{131}I-phenyl) pentadecanoic acid (1-^{11}C) palmitic acid, α-^{34m}Cl, α-^{123}I-stearic acid; (200 μl of a 6% HSA solution containing 100 mCi). Average deviations are within ± 22% of indicated values.

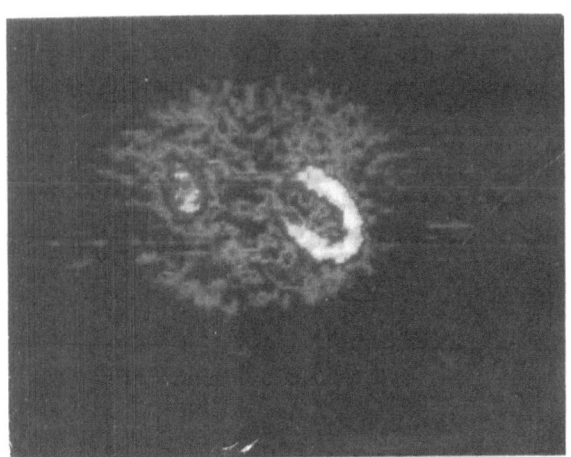

Fig. 2. Image of the myocardium registered by positron-emission trans-axial tomography at the level of A-V valves after i.v. injection of 2 mCi 1-^{11}C-palmitic acid.

to the histological and biochemical extent of the experimental
infarct and permitted accurate and reliable measurements of
infarct size by PET and C^{11} palmitate (28). These observations
also applied to man, where the extent of reduced C^{11} palmitate
uptake agreed with the biochemical estimate of infarct size as
obtained from the integral of serial CK concentrations.
Defects in regional C^{11} palmitate uptake may represent both
ischemia and necrosis (8-12,28).

Schelbert (28) demonstrated in dog experiments that the
clearance of C^{11} palmitate from myocardium is characterized
by two components. The rate of clearance of C^{11} activity from
myocardium during the initial phase closely correlated with
cardiac work and contractility as defined by the heart rate
blood-pressure development. Under ischemic conditions, the
rate of clearance was markedly prolonged.

The analysis of time-activity curves registered after CPA
(fig 3) and IHA application in normal persons revealed that
also the human myocardium activity release from the heart is
characterized by two components. In the case of CPA the rapid
elimination phase was characterized by an average half time of
6.5 ± 1.0 min. For the slow phase a half time of 160 ± 103
min was observed. The amount of activity being released in
the rapid phase to that in the slow phase can vary significantly. The ratio's (Q) of these two values for CPA^{11} ranged
between 1.8 to 5.4. The corresponding analysis of the data
obtained by the use of IHA^{123} indicated an average half time
of the rapid phase of 9 ± 3 min and for the second slow phase
of 45 ± 27 min. The ratio's (Q) for IHA^{123} ranged between
0.7 to 7.

In patients suffering from coronary artery disease, in
areas of accumulation defects not only normal, but also significantly prolonged or significantly shortened CPA/IHA elimination were observed (39). This data indicates that the ischemia
induced alteration of CPA/IHA accumulation is not necessarily
accompanied by alteration of fatty acid turnover rates. Consequently, for the evaluation of coronary artery disease, not
only an analysis of regional IHA accumulation but also a

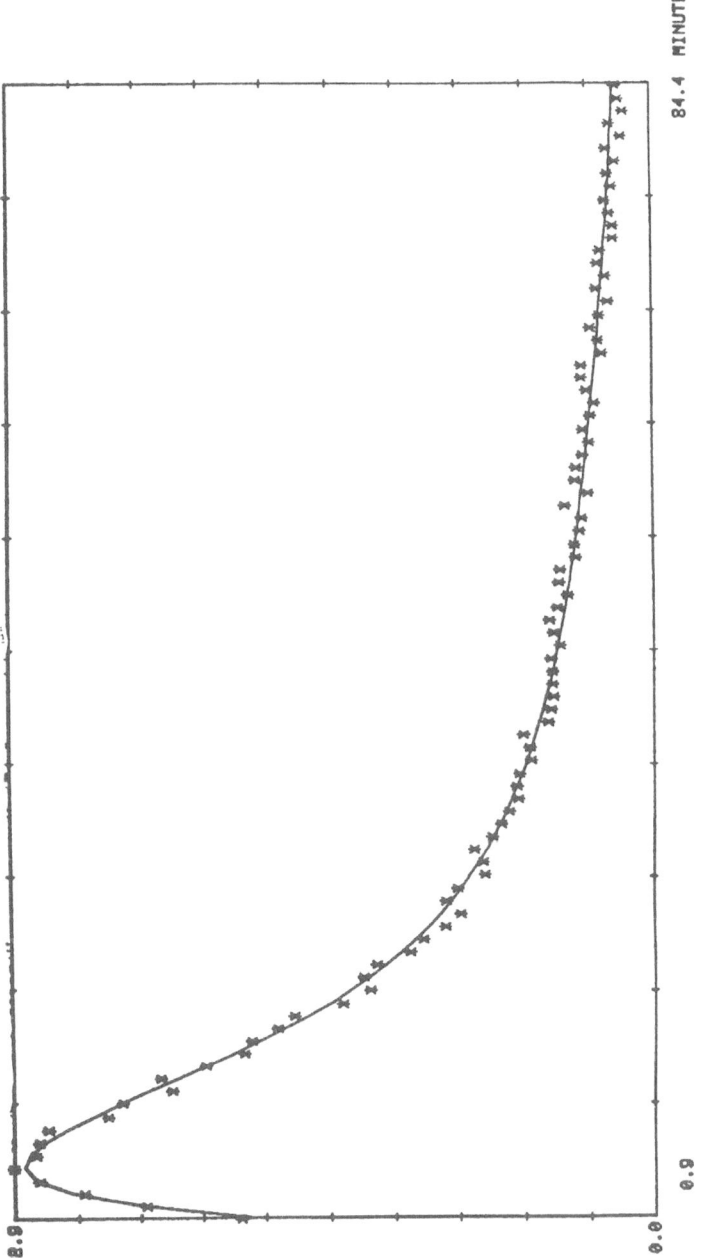

Fig. 3. Typical time activity curve registered over left ventricular myocardium after i.v. injection of
11c-palmitic acid. This curve was corrected for the activity in the blood.

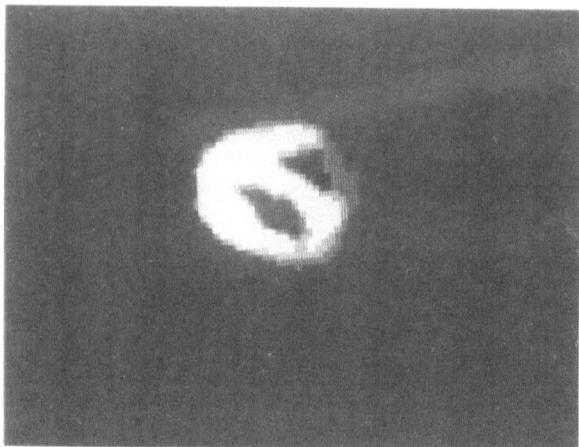

Emission image

Fig. 4. ECG-gated diastolic image of the myocardium registered by positron emission transaxial tomography, at the level of A-V valves, after intravenous injection of 2 mCi (p-^{75}Br-phenyl) pentadecanoic acid in a normal subject. The section is viewed from a cephalic-to-caudial orientation. Both ventricles which are clearly delineated are characterized by a homogenous distribution of activity in myocardium. The transmission image (see next page), obtained with the use of ^{68}Ge as a positron source at the same level, was sued to indicate the location of the heart within the thorax and to obtain attenuation factors, prior to i.v. injection of (p^{75}Br-phenyl) pentadecanoic acid.

detailed knowledge of regional IHA elimination rates are required.

High uptake, but different elimination kinetics were observed for (p-Br^{75}-phenyl) pentadecanoic acid (BPPA) (29). The uptake was approximately the same as that observed for IHA and C^{11}-palmitate, but the elimination rate was significantly lower. This indicates that, even if the halogenated phenyl residue in the ω-position does not affect the extraction process of BPPA, it inhibits the metabolic acceptance of this indicator. Due to the high accumulation and low elimination rate the BPPA, however, seems to be an excellent agent for myocardial imaging.

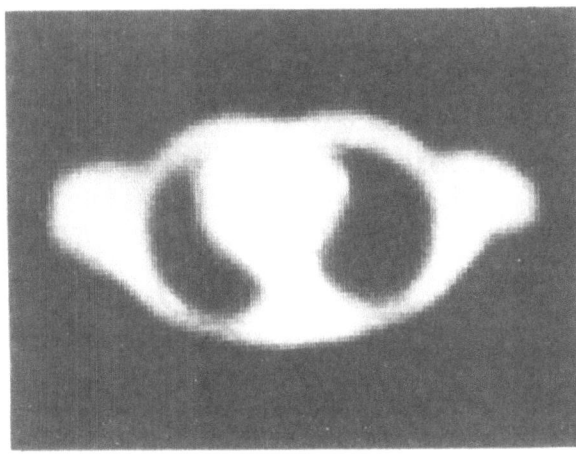

Transmission image

Fig. 4. (see legend previous page)

In fig 4 the ECG gated tomographic image detected at the level of A-V valves in a normal subject, 5 min after i.v. administration of 1.5 mCi BPPA is demonstrated. The collection period was 6 min and the activity was observed to be homogeneously distributed in both right and left ventricles. The characteristic horseshoe pattern of activity distribution observed at the level of A-V valves, is due to the fact that at this level the posterior portion of the heart comprises the atrial rather than ventricular myocardium.

In order to obtain more information which would contribute to the interpretation of these results as well as to obtain more knowledge about the pharmacokinetics of the radioactively labelled fatty acids, it was necessary to carry out additional animal experiments. For this IHA and (p-I[131]-phenyl) penta-decanoic acid (IPPA) were injected into mice, and the animals were sacrificed at different time intervals following applica-tion of the indicator (30,31).

The data obtained suggested an efficient extraction of

362

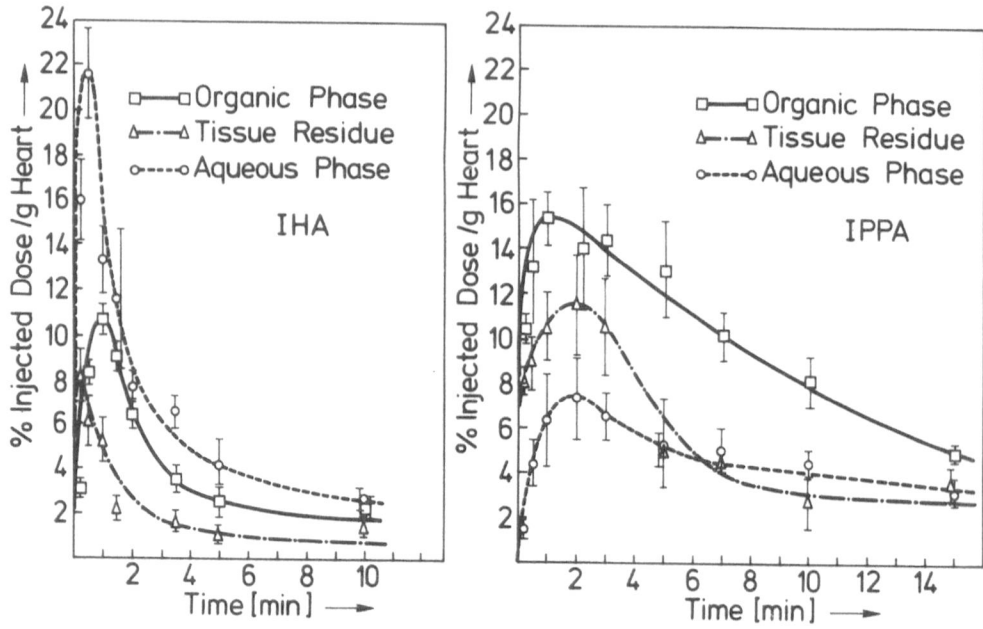

Fig. 5. Time course of radioactivity detected in different fractions
extracted from the homogenates of the heart muscle of mice, after injection of ω-131I-heptadecanoic acid (IHA) (fig. 5a) and (p-131I-phenyl)
pentadecanoic acid (IPPA) (fig. 5b). In general, 1.0-1.5 μCi IPPA or
IHA were dissolved in 0.2 ml 4% human serum albumin, sterilized by milli-
pore filtration and i.v. injected into mice (females, NMRI strain).
Mice were sacrificed at several time intervals up to 15 min and the
activity in the heart was determined. Subsequently, the hearts were
homogenized in 2.0 chloroform/methanol (2/1) and 0.65 ml 0.02 NH_2SO_4,
and 0.65 ml 40% aqueous solution of urea were added. The solution was
centrifuged (5000 RPM) for 15 min., the organic and aqueous phases, as
well as the tissue residue separated (22,23) and the activity in all
fractions was determined.

IHA and IPPA by the myocardium (36.3% and 32.5% dose per g
heart). Maximal accumulation of both compounds was very close
to that observed for CPA. This means that neither the phenyl
residue in IPPA nor the iodine in the ω-position of IHA
represents the steric hindrance of the enzymatic activity
involved in the extraction and accumulation of radioactively
labelled fatty acids (RLFA) in myocardium.

The half time of the elimination of IPPA activity from
the myocardium (3.5 min) was significantly higher than that
observed for IHA and CPA (2.4 min); from that we concluded

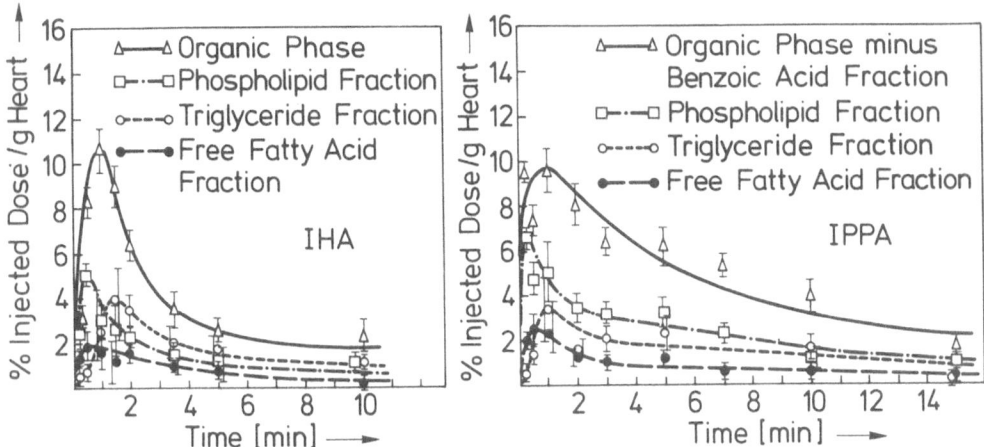

Fig. 6. Time course of radioactivity ($\bar{x} \pm S_x$; n = 5 animals/time interval) in various fractions separated from the organic phase by means of
thin layer chromatography (TLC) (Silica-gel 6QF-254 AL foil; 200x200x0.2
mm; N-heptane-diethyl-ether-acetic acid (90:10:1) was used as a solvent.
As standards in TLC, the inactive IPPA and IHA (for free fatty acids)
peanut oil DAB 7 (for triglycerides), lecithin (for phospholipids), and
paraiodobenzoic acid (for iodo-benzoic acid) were used. The recovery of
I^{131}-activity separated on TLC was 85.6 ± 5% (30,31).

that the phenyl residue in IPPA might interfere with enzymes
involved in the fatty acid catabolic pathway, whereas iodine
in ω-position (HA) does not alter the biological behaviour of
this compound. This conclusion is supported by results obtained by fractionation of myocardial tissue (30,31,32). The
elimination of IPPA activity from organic and aqueous phases
as well as from the tissue residue was significantly lower
than the IHA elimination rate (fig 5).

Thin layer chromatography (fig 6) of the organic phase
revealed that immediately after application of IHA, a considerable amount of activity can be detected in fractions co-migrating with phospholipids (PL) and free fatty acids (FFA). After
some delay, activity also appears in the fraction co-migrating
with triglycerides (TG). These data support the hypothesis of

Stein et al (33,34) that in myocardial cells a triglyceride
pool exists, which has a high turnover and which may serve as
an easily accessible store for fatty acids used for myocardial
energy production.

Since RLFA elimination from such a pool represents one of
the components determining the externally detected IHA elimination rate, it must be concluded that changes in the TG, PL,
and FA pools, as well as ischemic dependent alterations in the
enzyme systems involved in the activation of fatty acids from
these pools, might be the reason for the observed variation in
IHA elimination rates.

With regard to IPPA, the amount of activity in PL was
significantly higher, and the amount of activity in TG was
significantly lower than those observed for IHA. The elimination
of activity from both PL and TG fractions was found to be
slower for IPPA compared to IHA. These observations suggest
that the enzymes involved in the utilization of myocardial
fatty acid, phospholipid and triglyceride pools possess a
high steric specificity.

The detection of I^{131}-benzoic acid (30-32), the main
catabolic product of IPPA β-oxidation, in myocardial cells
immediately after application of IPPA leads to the conclusion
that not all of the fatty acids extracted by the myocardium
are first incorporated into PL and TG fractions; fatty acids
partially seem to be directly catabolized via the carnithine
shuttle in the β-oxidation pathway. This means that not only
changes in TG and PL pools but also the ischemia dependent
changes of the carnithine shuttle system as well as the changes
in β-oxidation rates themselves known to occur under conditions
of ischemia, must be considered as possible reasons for alteration of IHA elimination rates. The possibility that repeated
transient ischemia may result in reversible changes in the
carnithine shuttle system, was demonstrated in animal experiments carried out by Idell-Wenger et al (35) indicating a
significant reduction of carnithine availability in cytosol
under conditions of repeated transient ischemia.

Even though we are aware that at the moment a full interpretation of our in vivo observations is not possible, we feel that the data presented so far are sufficient to demonstrate that in ischemic myocardium, significant alterations in free fatty acid metabolic pathway exist which may be traced by using RLFA as an indicator.

However, not only the RLFA, but also radioactively labelled glucose and its structural analogs, were shown to be promising agents, for measuring regional myocardial metabolism in vivo by the means of PET. This approach was initiated by Stratmann et al (36) and Wolf et al (37), who in 1973 developed a procedure for C^{11}-labelling of glucose. This initial effort was, however, limited by a low extraction of this compound from coronary circulation and by relatively high accumulations of C^{11} glucose in many other organs, including the lung.

Based on the finding that glucose transport across the cell membrane is a passive carrier-facilitated process, Gallagher et al (38) concluded that accumulation of glucose within a tissue against the concentration gradient can not occur, and consequently that for the monitoring of myocardial glucose metabolism, not glucose itself, but some analog is desirable. Such a compound should be transported, phosphorylated, and thus trapped intracellularly in the same way as glucose, but it should not undergo subsequent metabolic steps. A radio-pharmaceutical which fulfills these requirements is F^{18}-2-fluoro-2-deoxyglucose (FDG). FDG (the fluorinating reagent was developed at Brookhaven National Laboratory) is trapped in myocardial cells as $FDG-6-PO_4$ since enzymatic conversion to $glucose-1-PO_4$ and $fructose-6-PO_4$ is inhibited by 2-deoxy-analog of glucose. Moreover, the cellular membrane permeability of $FDG-6-PO_4$, as well as the activity of glucose-6-phosphatase for conversion of $FDG-6-PO_4$ back to FDG are very low.

The results obtained with FDG demonstrate that this compound exhibits a number of important characteristics for myocardial imaging. It is rapidly taken up by the myocardium, has a long term tissue retention, and has a rapid blood-clearance. The FDG images provide high contrast between myocardium, blood, lung, and liver. The analysis of FDG accumulation rates seems to provide quantitative information about myocardial metabolic rates for exogenous glucose in vivo.

It is well established that the heart uses FFA as its prefered energy substrate, depending on plasma, FFA concentrations. The experiments obtained so far suggest, however, that in ischemia glycogen stores are depleted and that the exogeneous glucose may represent the significant source for glycolysis. Hence, FDG accumulation in this situation may in fact reflect the glycolytic flux. Schelbert (28) concluded from his measurements that the phosphorylation of FDG to FDG-6-phosphate in the previously infarcted segment indicates the presence of still metabolically active and hence viable myocardium and that the normal regulatory mechanisms for FFA and glucose utilization are no longer in effect in ischemic myocardium.

Even if the FDG provides the information about the glucose metabolic rate it does not allow the evaluation of glucose influx rate and thus, the analysis of the activity of hexose carrier system. As demonstrated in animal experiments, however, this information might be of basic importance for the assessment of the early changes occuring by ischemic insult.

In order to obtain this information we developed a new method which permits the external assessment of the transmembrane sugar transport and local perfusion (40-42). For this we used positron emission tomography and C^{11}-labelled methyl-D-glucose (CMG) or 3-fluor-deoxyglucose (3FDG) as indicator. Both -CMG - and 3FDG - are transported across the cell membrane by the same carrier as glucose, but they are not phosphorylated and further metabolized. They return to the circulating blood.

The CMG- or 3FDG-techniques, used in our studies for the analysis of the rate constants for glucose influx and efflux from the myocardial tissue, are based on the concomitant evaluation of CMG/3FDG blood and CMG/3FDG tissue concentrations.

In order to register the time changes of the local tissue CMG/3FDG concentration the dynamic positron emission tomography was used.

For this 5-6 mCi of CMG or 3FDG were injected into an antecubital vein of the patient and transaxial activity distribution in the chest in one selected slice was register- ed with ECAT II Scanner at 1 min intervals for a total period of 30 min.

The images were reconstructed using the measured attenua- tion correction. Subsequently the entire study was corrected for the activity in the blood. For this first 1 min image representing predominantly the activity distribution in the blood was used as internal standard. In images thus obtained different regions of interest were selected and time activity curves created.

The time activity curves registered over myocardium correct- ed for activity in blood were considered as a measure for the heart tissue CMG/3FDG concentration. As an estimate for the capillary CMG/3FDG concentration either the data obtained by the arterial blood-sampling or the time activity curves registered over the left ventricular cavity can be used.

In all studies the glucose plasma concentration was deter- mined just before indicator application and immediately after the completion of the examination.

Both CMG and 3FDG were found to be effectively accumulated in normal myocardium. A typical image of myocardium obtained after application of 5 mCi of CMG is demonstrated in fig 7. This image is corrected for the activity in the blood. The left ventricle as well as right ventricle can be easily re- cognized. Typical time activity curves registered in a normal individual over the left ventricular cavity, left ventricular myocardium and over subendocardial and subepicardial regions are shown in fig 8.

The time activity curve registered over left ventricular cavity showed usually initially rapid decrease of activity, which probably reflects mixing of indicator in the blood-pool and its equilibrium with tissue. This is followed by a phase of very slow indicator elimination indicating a high retention of non-metabolisable indicator in the blood.

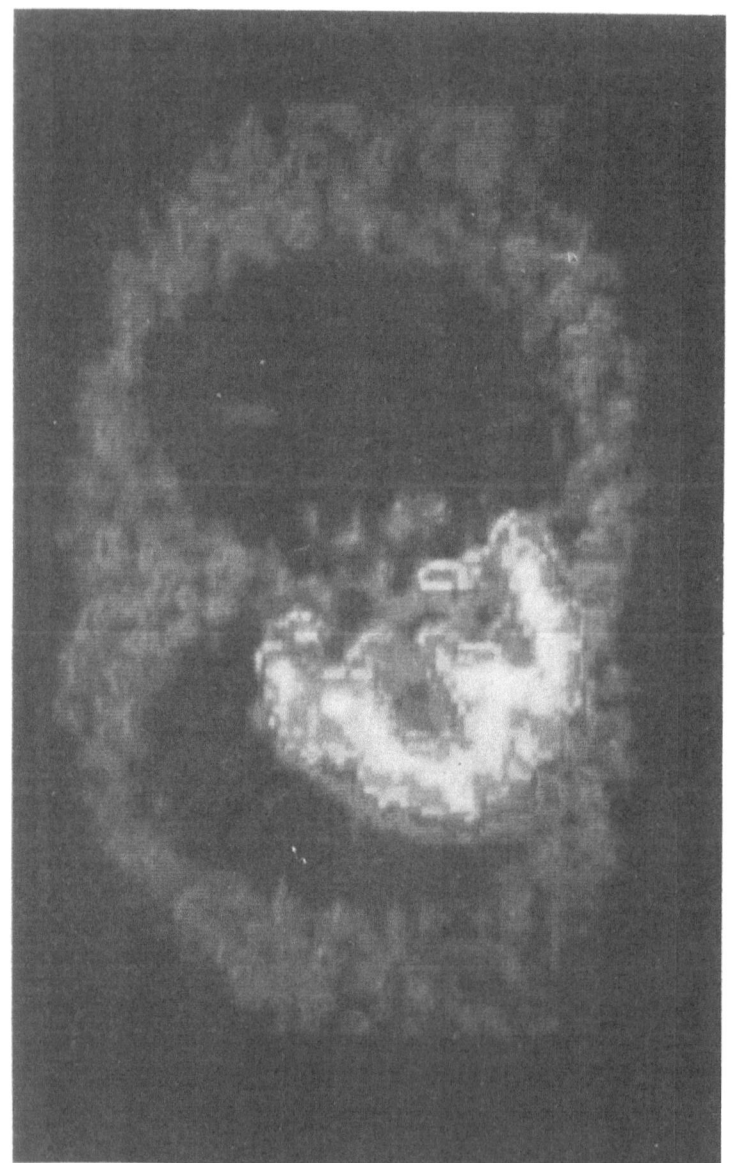

Fig. 7. Image of the myocardium registered by positron-emission-transaxial tomography at the level of A-V valves after i.v. injection of 5 mCi of CMG. The image is corrected for the activity in the blood. For better orientation the transmission image is superimposed in the same image.

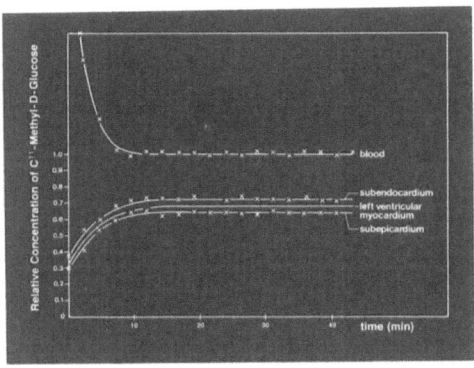

Fig. 8. Typical time activity curves registered in a normal person over the left ventricular cavity, left-ventricular myocardium and over sub-endocardial and subepicardial regions after i.v. application of 5 mCi of CMG.

The time activity curves registered over myocardium exhibited a rapid accumulation phase and a very slow elimination phase. The activity in equilibrium was in myocardium approximately 60-70% of the blood-activity.

In order to evaluate this data we considered the following model (fig 9): in plasma CMG or 3FDG completes with glucose for a common carrier for transport into a primary precursor pool in heart tissue. Since CMG/3FDG is not phosphorylated it accumulates in the myocardial tissue and proportional to its concentration in heart tissue it escapes back to circulation. Therefore, the rate of CMG accumulation in the heart tissue dc_T/dt is equal to the difference between the rate of CMG inflow and CMG outflow. According to experimental data of Betz and Gilboe (43-45) the rate of glucose inflow is proportional not only to the rate constant k_1 characterizing the catalytic activity of the carrier system but also to the total amount of the CMG being available for the transport at unit of the time.

The amount of CMG being available in unit of time is given by the product of blood CMG concentration, c_B, local flow-rate per gram of tissue (f). The proportionality constant which

370

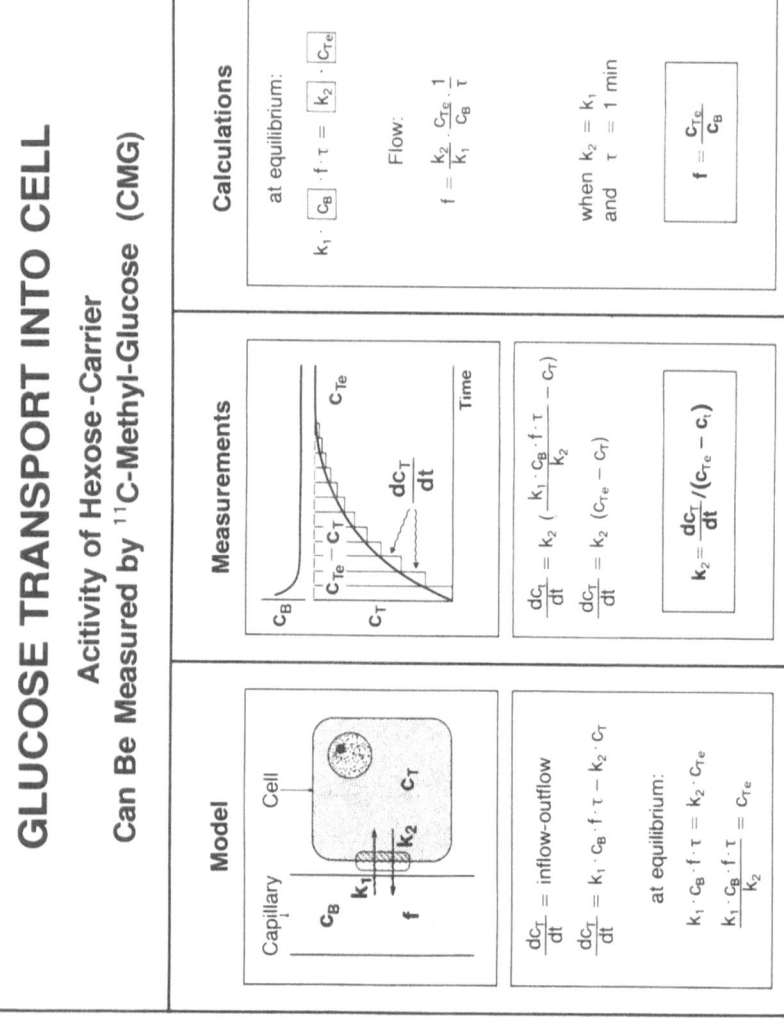

Fig. 9. Schematic description of the model and procedures used by the evaluation of CMG data.

has the dimension min is labelled in fig 9 as τ.

The CMG efflux is given by the product of k_2 and CMG tissue concentration, c_T; k_2 is the rate constant characterizing the catalytic activity of carrier system for CMG efflux.

At equilibrium when

$$\frac{dc_T}{dt} = 0$$

the inflow equals the outflow and

$$k_1 \cdot c_B \cdot f \cdot \tau = k_2 \cdot c_{Te}$$

where c_{Te} is the CMG concentration in tissue at equilibrium.

As shown at the bottom of fig 9, this equation demonstrates that the "tissue concentration at equilibrium" c_{Te} is directly proportional to k_1, c_B, and f and indirectly proportional to k_2.

If it is assumed that initial mixing of the indicator in the blood can be neglected, the rate equation for CMG accumulation in tissue may be rearranged as indicated in the first line in the middle of fig 9.

By comparing the first term in the parenthesis in this equation with expression for CMG tissue concentration at equilibrium c_{Te} it can be seen that we are dealing with the same values. Therefore, it can be concluded that the rate of CMG accumulation in heart tissue is given by the product of k_2 and difference between c_{Te} and c_T.

This equation demonstrates that rate constant for CMG efflux k_2 may be determined by the analysis of the rate of CMG approach to equilibrium.

On the right side of fig 9 are first summarized the conclusions drawn so far from our model. It says that at equilibrium the inflow equals outflow. This means that the product of k_1, c_B, f and τ equals to the product of k_2 and c_{Te}.

In this relationship the values of c_B and c_{Te} can be determined by the analysis of the activities in ROI's left ventricular cavity and heart tissue.

The value of k_2 is determined by the analysis of the rate of the approach of CMG tissue concentration to the equilibrium. If this equation, characterizing the activity distribution at equilibrium, is rearranged as indicated below, it becomes evident that the local perfusion rate per gram tissue is given by the product of the ratio's k_2/k_1, c_{Te}/c_B and $1/\tau$.

Since the glucose transport across the cell membrane is generally assumed to be comparable with reversible enzyme catalysed reaction the rate constants characterizing the carrier activity for glucose influx and glucose efflux k_1 and k_2 can be expected to be the same (41,42).

Under these conditions the local perfusion rate is equal to the ratio of the CMG activities in tissue and blood under equilibrium conditions.

Using the approach described so far, the myocardial perfusion rate was determined to be 68 ml per min and 100 g of tissue. In order to study the regional differences in perfusion rate we subdivided the left ventricular myocardium in halfs and selected subendocardial and subepicardial regions. In subendocardial region a local perfusion rate was found to be 73 ml/min and 100 g of tissue. For subepicardial region a value of 65 ml/min and 100 g of tissue was recorded. These values are in close agreement with observations reported by Lichtlen, Maseri and Kirk (46,47) by the use of standard methods.

The analysis of the slope of the approach of CMG concentration to the plateau value demonstrated that glucose influx rate in normal myocardium is about 0.35 μmol/min g. The studies done on patients with old myocardial infarction have demonstrated that the infarcted areas can be easily recognized as accumulation defects in CMG images.

The CMG scintigraphy in a patient with narrowing of the right coronary artery, in which Tl-scintigraphy under rest conditions was normal, revealed large accumulation defects in the postero-lateral wall (see fig 10). When compared with normal CMG image the damages appear to be more pronounced in subendocardial regions.

In agreement with Tl[201]-scintigraphy the quantitative

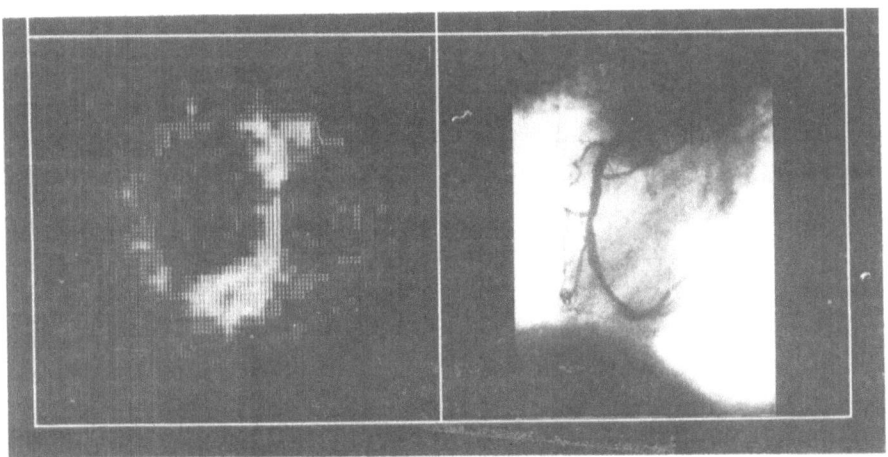

Fig. 10. The ECG gated image of the myocardium registered by PET at mid-ventricular level after i.v. application of CMG in a 49-year old patient with 50% and 30% narrowing of the right coronary artery.

analysis of CMG data has demonstrated that the local perfusion rate in these areas was normal, at rest. The local glucose transport rate was, however, significantly reduced.

This finding, which is in agreement with the results obtained by ω-I^{123} heptadecanoic acid scintigraphy in the same patient, indicates that repeated exposure of myocardial tissue to transient ischemia might produce an damage of the glucose transport system.

We conclude from the data that, for the diagnostic evaluation of ultimate heart damage, simultaneous quantitative assessment of both local perfusion rate and local glucose transport rate is of basic importante. There is some evidence that the CMG technique is an excellent tool which provides this possibility.

In addition to metabolic studies positron-emission tomography provides at the present time several methods which permit accurate measurements of regional myocardial bloodflow in units of ml/min/100 g. For example, Wisenberg et al developed a method for the determination of the local perfusion rate by the use of microspheres labelled with Ga^{68} (28). For the labelling of the microspheres, another generator-produced isotope-Copper-62 may be also used (48).

Schelbert et al (28) used for the determination of myocarddial blood-flow N^{13}-ammonia. At control flow of 80 ml/min/100 g, the extraction fraction of N^{13}-ammonia during a single capillary transit in myocardium was shown to be 90%. It decreases as flow increases. Over the physiological flow range, however, the myocardial net extraction or tissue concentrations were almost linearly related to myocardial blood-flow.

Other approaches for the measurement of regional myocardial blood-flow have included highly extractable indicators such as O^{15}-labelled water or C^{11}-labelled alcohols (28). Their potential for quantification of flow has recently been pointed out by Hack et al (49).

Also potassium-38 (50) and rubidium-82 (51) seems to be suitable indicators for detection of myocardial perfusion. Rubidium-82 is a potassium analog, which may be eluted from generator system so that it eliminates the need for on-site-cyclotron production. Its 2-min physical half-life minimizes the radiation dose to the patient. This indicator poses, however, some difficulties in practical use and data acquisition.

It is evident that the development of labelled metabolic substrates for myocardial studies in vivo has only begun. The examples mentioned so far demonstrated that use of radioactively labelled metabolic substrates indeed can provide an unique possibility of assessing metabolic alterations in disease heart, without the need for direct biochemical analysis of the myocardium. The in vivo measurement of metabolic rates has become a reality.

REFERENCES

1. Adam WE, Sigel H, Geffers H, et al, Analyse der regionalen Wand-
   bewegungen des linken Ventrikels bei koronarer Herzerkrankung durch
   ein nichtinvasives Verfahren (Radionuclid-Kinematographie).
   Z. Kardiol. 66:545, 1977.

2. Adam WE, Tarkowska A, Bitter F, et al, Equilibrium (gated) radionuclide ventriculography. In: Cardiac Medicine. Holman B, Abrams HL,
   Zeitler E, (eds), Springer Verlag, Berlin, Heidelberg, New York, p 21,
   1979.

3. Stauch M, Sigel H, Geffers H, et al, Radionuklid-Ventriculographie.
   II. Klinische Ergebnisse: Parameter der globalen Ventrikelfunktion.
   Nucl. Med. 17:211, 1978.

4. Strauss HW, Pitt B, In: Principles of cardiovascular nuclear medicine.
   Holman LB, Sonnenblick EH, Lesch M, (eds), p 161, 1977/1978.

5. Lebowitz E, Greene MW, Fairchild R, et al, Thallium-201 for medical
   use. I. J. nucl. Med. 16:151, 1975.

6. Ritchie JL, Albro PC, Caldwell JH, et al, Thallium-201 myocardial
   image a comparison of the redistribution and rest images. J. nucl.
   Med. 20:477, 1979.

7. Verani MS, Marcus ML, Razzak MA, et al, Sensitivity and specificity
   of Thallium-201 perfusion scintigrams under exercise in the diagnosis
   of coronary artery disease. J. nucl. Med. 19:733, 1978.

8. Sobel BE, Advanc. Cardiol. 26:15, 1979.

9. Sobel BE, Weiss ES, Welch MJ, et al, Detection of remote myocardial
   infarction in patients with positron emission transaxial tomography
   and intravenous ^{11}C-palmitate. Circulation 55:853, 1977.

10. Sobel BE, Assuming the current needs of cardiology. J. nucl. Med.
    20:589, 1979 (abstract).

11. Weiss ES, Hoffman EJ, Phelps ME, et al, External detection of altered
    metabolism of ^{11}C-labelled substrates in ischemic myocardium. Clin.
    Res. 23:383A, 1975 (abstract).

12. Weiss ES, Hoffman EJ, Phelps ME, et al, External detection and
    visualization of myocardial ischemia with ^{11}C-substrates in vitro and
    in vivo. Circ. Res. 39:24, 1976.

13. Weiss ES, Ahmed SA, Welch MJ, et al, Quantification of infarction in
    cross sections of canine myocardium in vivo with positron emission
    transaxial tomography and ^{11}C-palmitate. Circulation 55:66, 1977.

14. Vyska K, Freundlieb C, Höck A, et al, Myocardial imaging and measure-
    ment of myocardial fatty acid metabolism using ω-123I-heptadecanoic
    acid. In: Advances in clinical cardiology. Vol. 1: Quantification of
    myocardial ischemia. Kreuzer H, Parmley WW, Rentrop P, Heiss HW,
    Witzstrock G, (eds), New York, p 422, 1980.

15. Feinendegen LE, Vyska K, Freundlieb C, et al, Non-invasive analysis
    of metabolic reactions in body tissues, the case of myocardial fatty
    acids. Eur. J. Nucl. Med. 6:191, 1981.

16. Hoffman EJ, Phelps ME, Weiss ES, et al, Transaxial tomographic imaging
    of canine myocardium with 11C-palmitic acid. Nucl. Med. 18:57, 1977.

376

17. Rothlin ME, Bing RJ, Extraction and release of individual free fatty acids by the heart and fat depots. J. clin. Invest. 40:1380, 1961.

18. Miller HI, Gold M, Spitzer JJ, Removal and mobilization of individual free fatty acids in dogs. Amer J. Physiol. 202:370, 1962.

19. Ballard FB, Danfarth WH, Neagle S, et al, Myocardial metabolism of fatty acids. J. clin. Invest. 39:717, 1960.

20. Evans JR, Importance of fatty acid in myocardial metabolism. Circulat. Res. (suppl. II), 15:96, 1964.

21. Evans JR, Opie LH, Shipp JC, Metabolism of palmitic acid in perfused rat heart. Amer. J. Physiol. 205:766, 1963.

22. Evans JR, Gunton RW, Balcer RG, et al, Use of radioiodinated fatty acids for photoscans of the heart. Circulat. Res. 16:1, 1965.

23. Kupfernagel C, Qualitätskontrolle und Pharmacokinetik 14C-, 18F-, 34mCl-, 77Br- und 125I-markierter Fettsäuren. Berichte der Kernforschungsanlage Jülich nr. 1551, ISSN 0366-0885, p 1, 1979.

24. Machulla HJ, Stöcklin G, Kupfernagel C, et al, Comparative evaluation of fatty acids labelled with C-11, Cl-34m, Br-77, and I-123 for metabolic studies of the myocardium. Concise communication. J. nucl. Med. 19:298, 1978.

25. Machulla HJ, Marsmann M, Dutschka K, Biochemical concept and synthesis of a radioiodinated phenylfatty acid for in vivo metabolic studies for the myocardiun. Eur. J. Nucl. Med. 5:171, 1980.

26. Stöcklin G, Recent radiochemical developments in production and application of radiodiagnostics for cardiology. Sec.Int. Congr. of the World Fed. of Nucl. Med. and Biology. Sept. 17-21, 1978.

27. Stöcklin G, Coenen HH, Harmond HF, et al, ω-(p-bromo-phenyl-) pentadecanoic acid, a new potential agent for myocardial imaging. J. nucl. Med. 21:58, 1980 (abstract).

28. Schelbert HR, Henze E, Phelps ME, Emission tomography of the heart. Sem. Nucl. Med. 10:255, 1980.

29. Vyska K, Höck A, Freundlieb C, et al, Regional myocardial metabolism of free fatty acids. In: Microcirculation of the heart. Tillmanns H, Kübler W, Zebe H, (eds), Springer-Verlag, Berlin, Heidelberg, New York, p 216, 1982.

30. Daus HJ, Reske SN, Vyska K, et al, Pharmacokinetics of ω-(p-131I-phenyl)-pentadecanoic acid in heart. Proc. 18th Int. Annual Meeting of Eur. Soc. of Nucl. Med. Nürnberg, Sept. 9-12, 1980. Schattauer-Verlag, Stuttgart, New York.

31. Daus HJ, Massmann P, Dutschka K, et al, Radioaktive Isotope in Klinik und Forschung. 14. Gasteiner Int. Symp. Höfer R, Bergmann H, (eds), Teil I. Egerman, Wien, p 369, 1980.

32. Vyska K, Höck A, Freundlieb C, et al, Stoffwechseluntersuchungen am Herzen mit 123J-Fettsäuren und 11C-Methylglucose. Nukl. Med. 20:148, 1981.

33. Stein O, Stein Y, Metabolism of fatty acids in the isolated heart. Biochim. biophys. Acta 70:517, 1963.

34. Stein O, Stein Y, Lipid synthesis, intracellular transport and storage. III. Electromicroscopic autoradiographic study of the rat

heart perfused with tritiated oleic acid. J. Cell Biology 36:63, 1968.

35. Idell-Wenger JA, Grutyohann IW, Neely JR, Co-enzyme A and carnithine distribution in normal and ischemic hearts. J. biol. Chem. 25:3310, 1978.

36. Stratmann M, Welch MJ, Int. J. appl. Radiat. Isot. 24:234, 1973.

37. Wolf AP, Christman DR, Fowler JS, et al, In: Radiopharmaceuticals and labeled compounds. Vol. 1, IAEA, Vienna, p 345, 1973.

38. Callagher BM, Ansaa A, Atkins H, et al, Radiopharmaceuticals. XXVII. 18F-labeled-2-deoxy-2-fluoro-D-glucose as a radiopharmaceutical for measuring regional myocardial glucose metabolism in vivo: tissue distribution and imaging studies in animals. J. nucl. Med. 18:990, 1977.

39. Freundlieb C, Höck A, Vyska K, et al, Myocardial imaging and metabolic studies with (17-123I)-iodoheptadecanoic acid. J. nucl. Med. 21:1043, 1980.

40. Vyska K, Freundlieb C, Höck A, et al, Analysis of LPR and LUGTR in brain and heart in man by means of CMG and dPET. In: Radioaktive Isotope in Klinik und Forschung. Höfer R, Bergmann H, (eds), 15:129, 1982.

41. Vyska K, Kloster G, Feinendegen LE, et al, Regional perfusion and glucose uptake determination with 11C-methyl-glucose and dynamic positron emission tomography. In: Positron emission tomography of the brain. Heiss WD, Phelps ME, (eds), Springer-Verlag, Berlin, Heidelberg, New York, p 169, 1983.

42. Vyska K, Profant M, Schuier F, et al, The use of 11C-methyl-D-glucose for assessment of glucose transport in the human brain: Theory and application. In: Lecture notes in biomathematics. Tracer kinetics and physiologic modeling. Theory to practice. Proc. Sem. St. Louis, June 1983. Lambrecht RM, Rescigno A, (eds) Springer-Verlag, Berlin, Heidelberg, New York, p 411, 1983.

43. Betz IA, Gilboe DD, Kinetics of cerebral glucose transport in vivo. Inhibition by 3-0-methyl-glucose. Brain Res. Rev. 65:368, 1974.

44. Betz IA, Gilboe DD, Yudilevich DL, et al, Kinetics of unidirectional glucose transport into the isolated dog brain. Amer. J. Physiol. 225:586, 1973.

45. Betz AL, Gilboe DD, Drewes LB, Effects of anoxia on net uptake and unidirectional transport of glucose into the isolated dog brain. Brain Res. Rev. 67:307, 1974.

46. Lichtlen PR, Engels HJ, In: Cardiac Nuclear Medicine. Holman BL, Abrams HL, Zeitler E, (eds), Springer Verlag, Berlin, Heidelberg, New York, p 63, 1979.

47. Kirk ES, Hirzel HO, Critical role of coronary collateral blood flow in the pathophysiology of myocardial infarction. In: Coronary heart disease. Kaltenbach M, Lichtlen P, Balcon R, Bussmann WD, (eds), Thieme Verlag, Stuttgart, p 11, 1978.

48. Robinson JD, Copper-62: A short-lived generator produced positron emitting radionuclide for radiopharmaceuticals. J. nucl. Med. 17:559, 1976 (abstract).

49. Hack SN, Eichling JO, Bergmann SR, et al, Quantitative myocardial flow extraction data using gated ECT. J. nucl. Med. 21:16, 1979 (abstract).

50. Lambrecht RM, Hara T, Gallagher BM, et al, Cyclotron isotopes and radiopharmaceuticals. XXVIII. Production of potassium-38 for myocardial perfusion studies. Int. J. appl. Radiat. Isot. 29:667, 1979.

51. Grant PM, Erdal BR, O'Brien HA, A ^{82}Sr-^{82}Rb isotope generator for use in nuclear medicine. J. nucl. Med. 16:300, 1975.

VI. IMPACT OF RADIONUCLIDE TECHNIQUES
ON CLINICAL CARDIOLOGY

IMPACT OF RADIONUCLIDE TECHNIQUES ON CLINICAL CARDIOLOGY

O. PACHINGER

INTRODUCTION

In recent years, considerable advances have been made in our ability to image the heart by means of radionuclide techniques. The utility of these procedures in clinical cardiology must be considered in relation to that of other diagnostic techniques: the basic clinical assessment, other non-invasive approaches such as echocardiography, digital subtraction angiography, nuclear magnetic resonance, and cardiac catheterization. The clinician must choose the technique which provides the most useful diagnostic information in a given cardio-vascular disorder.

This review will deal with the impact of currently available radionuclide techniques on the clinical evaluation of patients with different cardiovascular diseases.

Evaluation of the patient with suspected coronary artery disease

The assessment of the ambulatory patient with either chest pain or suspected coronary artery disease represents one of the major applications of nuclear cardiology studies (1-4). Radionuclide techniques, when combined with physiologic stress, specifically bicycle exercise, provide relevant diagnostic and functional insights into patients with coronary artery disease. Radionuclide techniques augment the diagnostic accuracy achieved with exercise electrocardiography alone.

The two major exercise radionuclide approaches to the diagnostic evaluation of patients with coronary disease are radionuclide angiography and Tl^{201} imaging. Since 1979, the sensitivity and specificity of these two procedures have been examined in many centres around the world. The sensitivity of exercise planar Tl^{201} myocardial imaging is approximately 85% (5,6) when visual interpretation is used and 90 to 92% when quantitative computer techniques (7) or tomographic imaging (8) is applied. The sensitivity of radionuclide ventriculography is also in the range of 85 to 95% (6,9). Although the diagnostic sensitivities of these two techniques are roughly comparable, the exercise Tl^{201} study has a higher specificity than the exercise ventricular performance study (6). This lower specificity is not surprising because many conditions other than coronary artery disease may cause an abnormal left ventricular functional response to exercise. Furthermore, the optimal definition of normal left ventricular reserve during exercise is in doubt. Although exercise-induced regional wall-motion abnormalities are specific for coronary artery disease, they occur less frequently than abnormal ejection fraction responses (9-11).

At this time, it is unclear which exercise radionuclide technique should be recommended for the initial diagnostic assessment of patients with suspected coronary artery disease. The ultimate decision should be based upon the available instrumentation, the experience of the laboratory and the clinical subset into which a given patient falls.

Although the degree of left ventricular dysfunction with exercise generally is related to the severity of coronary artery disease, exercise radionuclide angiocardiography has not proved useful in identifying individual coronary artery lesions. In this regard, quantitative exercise Tl^{201} perfusion imaging with kinetic evaluation may be preferable. In the future, the choice between routine exercise testing, quantitative or tomographic exercise Tl^{201} imaging, and exercise radionuclide angiocardiography in the evaluation of the patient may not be determined primarily by the respective sensitivities and specificities of the technique. The prognostic relevance of a test may be of far greater value. If prognostic stratification of patients based upon the number of size of Tl^{201} perfusion defects or on the extent of left ventricular reserve during exercise proves feasible than it may become a primary factor in optimal clinical strategy.

The predictive accuracy of any diagnostic test depends not only upon its sensitivity and specificity, but also upon the prevalence of the disease in the population under study. The results of a radionuclide exercise test provide a probability statement concerning artery disease based upon a continuum of risk (12). The maximal discriminating power of these methods occurs in patients whose pre-test estimate of disease prevelance is between 30 and 70%. Based upon this BAYESIAN analysis, the optimal diagnostic use would include patients with major coronary disease risk factors, atypical chest pain, asymptomatic ST-segment depression during exercise, chest pain but no ST-segment changes during exercise, asymptomatic arrhythmias, or a negative exercise stress test with a submaximal heart rate response. The ultimate role of either radionuclide exercise technique in screening for coronary artery disease in an asymptomatic population remains to be determined and must remain speculative.

In addition to dynamic exercise other form of stress tests can be applied using radionuclide techniques, isometric handgrip (13,14), rapid atrial stimulation and cold pressure test. Several groups have demonstrated that Tl^{201} imaging after intravenous dypiridamol administration offers an alternative to exercise scintigraphy for the detection of coronary artery disease (15-18). Candidates for dypiridamol test may include individuals who can not exercise because of a muscular skeletal handicap or those unable to achieve even modest levels of exercise due to poor motivation or non-cardiac symptoms. The diagnostic accuracy is comparable with that of bicycle exercise scintigraphy (19).

At the present time no other non-invasive technique can achieve a higher sensitivity than suggested by current radionuclide techniques. The discrepancy between the anatomic presence of disease and its functional significance precludes perfection for any technique that does not define anatomic presence of disease. Although future developments in radio-

pharmaceutical agents or other non-invasive technologies may
allow detection of early atherosclerotic plaques within the
coronary artery, progress in this area has been slow and the
rate of future success is uncertain. However, improved specificity for the detection of ischemic versus other forms of myocardial disease is likely to be achieved with some of the
other non-invasive techniques. For example, it is likely that
monitoring of metabolic function by positron emission tomography or flow by nuclear magnetic resonance technique, or
both, will allow separation of ischemic and non-ischemic
causes of the impairment in ventricular function during stress
(20).

Evaluation of the patient with known coronary artery disease
Functional significance of anatomic stenoses: Following
cardiac catheterization, the anatomic features of the disease
are well defined. In some cases, however, the degree and
extent of physiologic impairment of blood-flow and the question
of myocardial viability are not well determined, and further
functional evaluation may be helpful in deciding the course of
management. Not infrequently, the clinical angiographer is
faced with the dilemma of determining whether a particular
anatomic lesion is "significant", particularly with respect
to a borderline 50% lesion. Because Tl^{201} uptake by the myocardium is directly related to blood-flow at the capillary
level, exercise scintigraphy may be helpful in assessing the
presence of functionally significant disease. Indeed, no
other conventional non-invasive technique at the present time
can provide similar information regarding myocardial blood-
flow distribution. Quantitative Thallium analysis improves
the sensitivity in this respect (21,22).

Functional significance of collateral coronary vessels:
As with the borderline coronary artery narrowing, the functional significance of a collateral vessel is not well evaluated
by the anatomic angiographic technique. Rigo et al (23) evaluated the influence of coronary collateral vessels under
results of Thallium scintigraphy. In this study, perfusion

abnormalities were noted in the distribution of all coronary arteries that were occluded and did not have visible collateral vessels, whereas no perfusion defects were seen in 39% of the occluded arteries with angiographically visible collateral vessels. Tubau et al (24) evaluated collateral vessel and single vessel coronary artery disease and demonstrated that patients with large collateral vessels more frequently showed negative exercise Thallium results than did patients without collateral vessels. Thus, in some patients collateral vessels do appear to protect against the development of exercise induced ischemia.

Evaluation of myocardial viability: The coronary angiogram is more limited in the assessment of myocardial viability than it is in the assessment of the functional significance of coronary narrowing. Because Tl^{201} uptake and washout depend on cell membrane integrity, this technique has the potential for assessing the presence of viable myocardium. Based on experimental animal studies of transient ischemia and infarction (25-27) and current interpretation of stress-redistribution Tl^{201} scintigrams, myocardial segments showing initial defects after exercise with delayed redistribution represent ischemic but viable regions which usually revert to normal Tl^{201} uptake following successful coronary revascularization. It is not always true, however that persistant Thallium defects during sequential imaging represent fibrosis or irreversible damaged myocardium. Segments with persistant Thallium defects before surgical procedure may demonstrate normal uptake and washout postoperatively. Thus, by applying quantitative criteria to Tl^{201} scintigraphy, this method appears useful in assessing myocardial viability and hence the potential response to revascularization procedures.

Evaluation of surgical intervention: Results of bypass graft surgery have been evaluated with Thallium myocardial imaging and radionuclide ventriculography (28,29). The value of these techniques in this clinical setting depends on the completeness of revascularization and on the comparability with a preoperative scintigraphic finding. With successful

revascularization procedures, most myocardial regions with
reversible perfusion or wallmotion abnormalities preoperatively demonstrate normalization postoperatively (29). This
phenomenon occurs despite the patients exercising to a higher
heart rate blood-pressure product, which would be expected to
enhance detection of perfusion defects in the absence of
successful revascularization. In few of these findings, if the
original perfusion defect reappears postoperatively, it can be
assumed that either the bypass graft supplying the involved
segment has occluded or residual ungrafted disease is present.
If, on the other hand, a region is normal preoperatively and
become abnormal postoperatively at the same or a lower heart
rate blood-pressure product, the region is likely to be
associated with intraoperative damage, graft occlusion, or
progression of native disease in an ungrafted vessel. If no
change is seen in an normal region between pre- and postoperative studies, no accurate statement can be made with
respect to bypass graft patency in that region. Some bypass
grafts supply regions that were not identified as abnormal in
the preoperative study. In these segments, the absence of a
perfusion defect in the postoperative study does not confirm
the patency of the graft. The incidence of perioperative infarction in patients undergoing bypass graft surgery has been
accurately determined by pre- and postoperative infarct-avid-
imaging.

With the combined information (operative report, preoperative angiogram and postoperative radionuclide study) the
results of the surgical intervention can be predicted with
high degree of accuracy.

Evaluation of percutaneous transluminal angioplasty.
During the past years the non-surgical percutaneous transluminal angioplasty procedure has become an established intervention in patients with coronary artery disease (31). Radionuclide techniques can be applied to the evaluation of this
therapeutic intervention since a successful balloon dilatation
must be reflected in a normalization of left ventricular
ejection fraction or wallmotion or Tl[201] distribution (32,33).

With these techniques one can also follow these patients and
detect a recurrance (34,35); we have recently shown that using
a quantitative circumferential profile analysis the predictive
accuracy of the results of balloon dilatation can be increased
from 76% to 94% (36). A redistribution index in the dilated
coronary vessel correlated well with changes of pressure
gradient and changes of luminal diameter after the dilatation.

Evaluation of thrombolytic therapy. Various radionuclide
approaches have been used to assess clinical reperfusion in
patients with acute myocardial infarction undergoing intracoronary or intravenous thrombolytic therapy with streptokinase (37-40). The clinical evaluation of these therapeutic
procedure is still highly controversial. In the majority of
patients this intervention does result in myocardial damage
and its success can only be judged by a reduction of infarct
size (42). In the clinical setting this is a very difficult
task to quantify. However, on the other hand it will be highly
decisive for this intervention whether one can prove that a
significant amount of ischemic myocardium has been protected
from necrosis. For this evaluation radionuclide techniques
appear to be better suitable than conventional electrocardiographic enzymatic and other parameters of left ventricular
hemodynamics. We have evaluated results of intercoronary
thrombolytic therapy with Tl^{201} perfusion scintigraphic and
metabolic studies using I^{123} labelled fatty acids in the
distribution of the recanalized coronary vessel (39,40). We
found a discrepancy between establishing perfusion and restor-
ing metabolic function within the first 48 hours (39). Our
results indicate that restoration of coronary blood-flow might
be able to salvage viable myocardium. However, reperfusion
does not lead to an immediate restoration of metabolic dysfunction. Despite these preliminary exciting results, much
more work needs to be done to understand Tl^{201} kinetic
behaviour during several hours of occlusion followed by reflow. It is still not clear which mode of Tl^{201} administration,
whether intravenous or intracoronary, is superior in assessing the efficacy of thrombolytic therapy. At present, we can

say that demonstration of enhanced Thallium uptake in the reperfused zone after thrombolytic therapy indicates that reflow has been established and that some tissue is capable of extracting Tl^{201}. We can not state with certainty, however, that the postrecanalization images provide meaningful information relative to the degree of myocardial salvage following successful clot lysis. It is clear that positron emittors would be suitable to solve such complex issues since they could provide simultaneous information on metabolism and perfusion on the cellular level.

Determination of prognosis. One important application of radionuclide techniques is the determination of prognosis in patients with known coronary artery disease. High risk subsets of patients with angina pectoris and myocardial infarction have been identified by these techniques (30,43,44). Submaximal exercise Thallium myocardial imaging and radionuclide ventriculography before hospital discharge have been found to be more sensitive than the electrocardiogram in detecting areas of jeopardized myocardium and subsequent risk of cardiac events (45-47). Moreover, as suggested by Brown et al (46), the demonstration of a large quantity of myocardium at jeopardy for ischemia exercise scintigraphy may be more useful in predicting the risk of an adverse clinical outcome than conventional contrast angiography. Since left ventricular performance is a powerful indicator of prognosis its evaluation during the various phases of coronary disease, this measurement provides important clinical information (48,49). In data derived from the Seattle Heart Watch program, the left ventricular ejection fraction was one of the best predictors of subsequent mortality in patients who had sudden cardiac death, but who survived the event. Following acute myocardial infarction, the resting left ventricular ejection fraction has been identified as an important harbinger of early mortality and subsequent congestive heart failure with sudden death. The concept seems attractive that the functional consequences induced by exercise stress or by myocardial infarction may impinge more on prognosis than the mere number of stenotic vessels. This has been greatly facilitated by myocardial imaging with radionuclide techniques.

Use in acute myocardial infarction. The development of mobile gamma cameras facilitated their use at the bedside in the Coronary Care Unit. The advantage of a non-invasive method becomes especially important in the acute setting (50). Radionuclide ventriculography, myocardial and infarct scintigraphy provide a number of parameters which allow the evaluation of the consequences of myocardial infarction in a quantitative manner (51-53). We have evaluated in the past years 186 patients with acute myocardial infarction in the acute phase with these techniques and analysed their potential for the management of the patients (54). 69% of all patients with anterior myocardial infarction developed heart failure (Killip III and IV) during the evolution of their course. They had a one year mortality of 25%. More than half of the patients with posterior myocardial infarction has a non-complicated course associated with a significantly lower one year mortality (12%). We also could demonstrate that the clinical picture does not always reflect the accurate state of left ventricular performance; on the other hand for the determination of prognosis in the acute phase the objectively determined left ventricular ejection fraction was a very sensitive parameter (54-56). Radionuclide angiography in acute myocardial infarction does not enhance diagnostic evaluation rather than the consequences of infarction on global and regional pump function and, thus, provides information on short and long term prognosis (55-57).

In cardiogenic shock radionuclide techniques allow a differentiation between postinfarction aneurysm or global inoperable hypokinesia (58). This diagnostic information can influence the further management of these patients. Thallium scintigraphy has been employed to detect and to localize acute myocardial infarction. Thallium scintigraphy appears to have a greater sensitivity than pyrophosphate imaging. However, Thallium scintigraphy is less specific than pyrophosphate scanning because old myocardial infarction and ischemia produce a positive Thallium perfusion image. Consequently, Thallium scintigraphy does not allow differentiation between old and new myocardial infarction or unstable angina pectoris. In a practical sense, however, these limitations may not be serious because most cases of suspected acute infarction are readily diagnosed by the combination of a typical medical history, evolutionary electrocardiographic changes and a rise and fall of myocardial-specific MB creatinine kinase.

As such Thallium scintigraphy performed during the early phase of acute myocardial infarction might more properly be considered a test for estimating short term prognosis. Silverman et al (59) had recently shown that in patients with extensive regions hypoperfused myocardium at the time of admission for acute infarction, the probability of proceeding to cardiogenic shock is high, regardless of clinical classification at the time of admission.

Finally, rest- redistribution imaging may differentiate unstable from acute myocardial infarction. During the early phase of infarction scintigraphically detected perfusion abnormalities reflect both necrosis and ischemia.

Repeated Thallium imaging on several days after acute infarction has revealed a decrease of the size of defects which implies resolution of ischemia at the time of follow-up imaging. Several authors have demonstrated the impact of the initial Thallium defect on prognosis. Since Thallium scintigraphy and infarct avid imaging with pyrophosphate provide different pathophysiologic information they can be applied in a complementary way. Since infarct size is the most important determination for the patient's prognosis an exact quantification of this measure would be desirable and was an important aim of radionuclide techniques during the past years. From a clinician's standpoint a method would be ideal which could define normal, necrotic and ischemic zones immediately after the admission and which could detect changes by interventions. This has not been accomplished so far in the clinical setting. With the presently available radionuclide techniques the status of the myocardium can be characterized in a more physiological way than do ECG, enzymes and ventricular performance, however, up until today no exact quantification as a measure of gram of tissue has been accomplished. May be tomographic approaches and especially the use of positron emission tomography could provide an important inpetus for further progress.

Evaluation of the patients with valvular heart disease

Valvular heart disease is usually recognized by suggestive medical history, physical examination, electrocardiogram, or chest roentgenogram. Furthermore, these basic clinical tools may indicate the severity of the abnormality. Heart failure in patients with valve disease may result from mechanical factors or depression of ventricular contractile function. The differentiation of the contribution of each of these factors to cardiac insufficiency can be facilitated by nuclear imaging techniques.

The clinical importance of these applications in terms of management of the patient and prognosis, however, varies with the individual valvular lesion. Radionuclide angiography is less important in obvious clinical situations, but is more important in complex disorders or perplexing situations, particularly in patients with associated coronary artery disease or after valve operations. Echocardiography is generally the non-invasive procedure of choice when evaluating patients with valvular heart disease. Furthermore, echocardiography is less expensive than other techniques. High quality echocardiograms are sometimes difficult to obtain for technical reasons, however. Radionuclide angiography is helpful if the echocardiogram does not provide adequate information about ventricular function, particularly in patients with valvular regurgitation (60).

Radionuclide studies may be helpful in solving difficult clinical problems such as timing of the operation or estimation of operative risk (61-63). It is difficult to predict the surgical results in patients with preoperative diminished ventricular function (64,65). We have assessed the response of patients to afterload reduction and whether such pharma-

cological interventions might be useful in predicting the improvement that can be expected after valve replacement (61).
Although in the majority of patients a decrease in volume
overload by pharmacological afterload reduction could be observed, that was not accompanied by an increase of left ventricular ejection fraction to the same degree. Radionuclide angiography is able to confirm the presence of ventricular overload
and left ventricular dysfunction (60,63). Exact volume determination at rest and after intervention may identify patients
in whom earlier surgery should be considered as well as
patients who might benefit from valve replacement (66). At the
same time criteria for optimal timing of valve replacement in
patients with either asymptomatic aortic insufficienty or
aortic regurgitation associated with severe left ventricular
function are not yet precisely defined. The use of ejection
fraction response to exercise in asymptomatic patients with
aortic regurgitation as suggested by Borer (65) appears to be
inappropriate because of the complex entity of ejection
fraction in aortic regurgitation. The volume of regurgitation
decreases per beat with exercise because of a shorter diastole
and an exercise induced decrease in peripheral resistance. As
a results, the total stroke volume and the enddiastolic volume
decreases during exercise but the forward stroke volume actual-
ly increases. Because the ejection fraction reflects the total
stroke volume and does not separate regurgitant from forward
stroke volume, it is possible to have both a fall in ejection
fraction and an increasing forward stroke volume during exercise. Therefore, the ejection fraction response to exercise
in patients with aortic regurgitation is likely to be different from that in normal patients. Furthermore, no study has
so far demonstrated the prognostic value of the exercise
response of the ejection fraction in this patient population.

Because many patients with valvular heart disease are
older adults, it is not unusual to find associated coronary
artery disease (67). Radionuclide approaches are suggested to
detect coronary artery disease in these patients, partly to
avoid catheterization, if the clinical diagnosis of the val-

vular disease is apparent. However, both exercise Thallium and exercise radionuclide angiographic studies appeared to be unreliable in detecting or excluding coronary artery disease in association with significant aortic steonis (68). Cardiac catheterization is the only means of determining the presence of coronary disease in these patients. On the other hand, in patients with the combination of aortic stenosis, coronary artery disease, heart failure and a depressed left ventricular ejection fraction, Thallium imaging at rest may be helpful in defining the amount of viable myocardium present, as opposed to the amount of scar tissue from previous infarction. Therefore, radionuclide studies may be useful in this setting to assess to overall impact of the coronary disease on the patient's left ventricular myocardium.

Evaluation of the patients with myocardial disease
Nuclear techniques allow the determination of the functional type of cardiomyopathy as well as quantitative evaluation of right ventricular and left ventricular function (69-71). For example, patients with dilative cardiomyopathy usually demonstrate both right and left ventricular dilatation and dysfunction. Again, from a standpoint of cost-effectiveness, echocardiography is clearly superior in evaluating patients with primary myocardial disorder. In the late stage of the disease, definitive diagnosis can be established without heart catheterization (72). The ischemic type of cardiumyopathy still requires invasive evaluation, however, because occasionally potential surgical candidates are found in this group. A combined scintigraphic approach - gated blood-pool imaging and Tl^{201} imaging - is very useful in distinguishing dilated cardiomyopathy from severe coronary disease (58,63,74/.

Radionuclide imaging appears useful in following the progression of the disease and in evaluating the efficacy of therapeutic interventions (73). However, it is no substitute for the echocardiographic approach but complement the diagnostic armamentarium if echocardiographic studies are not satisfactory.

Future directions

The clinical impact of radionuclide techniques on the
evaluation of patients with various forms of heart diseases
have been and will continue to be great. New imaging techniques, advances in computer technology and improvement and
development of new radiopharmaceuticals will undoubtedly open
new areas for clinical investigations. Positron emission
computed tomography might offer an improved understanding of
global and regional myocardial pathophysiology in various
diseased states; its clinical utility will be defined within
the next year. It is possible that advantages in digital left
ventriculography, quantitative echocardiography, nuclear
magnetic resonance imaging and other non-invasive techniques
will replace some of the currently applied radionuclide techniques. It is undeniable that the ability of the clinician to
diagnose disease, to assess the effect of therapeutic interventions and to determine prognosis with radionuclide imaging
techniques has been gratifying. The information provided with
currently available techniques - their insight into pathophysiology, diagnosis, therapy and prognosis, are an important
impetus for the further progress. The potential to relate
these techniques to prognosis is an exciting new area in
nuclear cardiology.

LITERATURE

1. Berger HJ, Gottschalk A, Zaret BL, Radionuclide assessment of left and right ventricular performance. Radiol. Clin. North Amer. 18:441, 1980.

2. Bodenheimer MM, Banka VS, Helfant RH, Nuclear cardiology. I. Radionuclide angiographic assessment of left ventricular contraction: uses, limitations and future directions. Amer. J. Cardiol. 45:661, 1980.

3. Okada RD, et al, Exercise radionuclide imaging approaches to coronary artery disease. Amer. J. Cardiol. 46:1188, 1980.

4. Strauss HW, et al, Of linens and laces : the 8th anniversary of the gated blood-pool scan. Sem. Nucl. Med. 9:296, 1979.

5. Bailey IK, Griffith LSC, Rouleau J, Strauss WH, Pitt B, Thallium 201 myocardial perfusion imaging at rest and exercise: Comparative sensitivity to electrocardiography in coronary artery disease. Circulation 55:79, 1977.

6. Okada RD, Boucher CA, Strauss HW, Pohost GW, Exercise radionuclide imaging approaches to coronary artery diseases. Amer. J. Cardiol. 46:1188, 1980.

7. Berger BC, Watson DD, Taylor GJ, et al, Quantitative Thallium 201 exercise scintigraphy for detection of coronary artery disease. J. nucl. Med. 22:585 1981.

8. Rizi HR, Kline RC, Thrall JH, et al, Thallium 201 myocardial scintigraphy: A critical comparison of seven-pinhole tomography and conventional planar imaging. J. nucl. Med. 22:493, 1981.

9. Brady TL, Lo K, Thrall JH, Walton JA, Brymer JF, Pitt B, Exercise radionuclide ejection fraction: Correlation with exercise contrast ventriculography. Radiology 132:703, 1979.

10. Brady TL, et al, Exercise radionuclide ejection fraction: Correlation with exercise contrast ventriculography. Radiology 132:703, 1979.

11. Brady TL, et al, Exercise radionuclide ventriculography: Practical considerations and sensitivity of coronary artery disease detection. Radiology 132:697, 1979.

12. Epstein SE, Implications of probability analysis on the strategy used for noninvasive detection of coronary artery disease. Role of simple or combined use of exercise electrocardiographic testing, radionuclide cineangiography and myocardial perfusion imaging. Amer. J. Cardiol. 46:419, 1980.

13. Bodenheimer MM, Banka VS, Fooshee CM, Gillespie JA, Helfant RH, Detection of coronary heart disease using radionuclide determined regional ejection fraction at rest and during handgrip exercise: Correlation with coronary arteriography. Circulation 58:640, 1978.

14. Peter CA, Jones RH, Effects of isometric handgrip and dynamic exercise on left ventricular function. J. nucl. Med. 21:1131, 1980.

15. Albro PC, et al, Non-invasive assessment of coronary stenoses by myocardial imaging during pharmacologic coronary vasodilation. III. Clinical trials. Amer. J. Cardiol. 42:751, 1978.

16. DeAmbroggi L, et al, Assessment of diagnostic value of dipyridamole testing in angina pectoris. Clin. Cardiol. 5:269, 1982.

17. Pachinger O, et al, Assessment of myocardial ischemia during pharmacologic vasodilatation. In: Quantification of myocardial ischemia. Kreuzer H, Parmley WN, Rentrop P, Heiss HW, (eds), Witzstrock Publish House, Inc, New York, pp 82-91, 1980.

18. Leppo J, et al, Serial thallium-201 myocardial imaging after dipyridamole infusion. Diagnostic utility in detecting coronary stenoses and relationship to regional wallmotion. Circulation 66:649, 1982.

19. Tavazzi L, et al, Dipyridamole test in angina pectoris. Diagnostic value and pathophysiologic implications. Cardiology 69:34, 1982.

20. Pitt B, et al, Impact of radionuclide techniques on evaluation of patients with ischemic heart disease. J. Amer. Coll. Cardiol. 1:63, 1983.

21. Berger BC, et al, Quantitative thallium-201 exercise scintigraphy for detection of coronary artery disease. J. nucl. Med. 22:585, 1981.

22. Maddahi J, et al, Improved non-invasive assessment of coronary artery disease by quantitative analysis of regional stress myocardial distribution and washout of thallium-201. Circulation 64:924, 1981.

23. Rigo P, et al, Influence of coronary collateral vessels on the results of thallium-201 myocardial stress imaging. Amer. J. Cardiol. 44:452, 1979.

24. Tubau JF, et al, Influence of coronary collaterals on 14 lead ECG and thallium-201 exercise test results. Circulation 60:266 (suppl. II), 1979.

25. Beller GA, Pohost GM, Mechanism of thallium-201 redistribution after transient myocardial ischemia. Circulation 56:171, 1977.

26. Beller GA, Watson DD, Pohost GM, Kinetics of thallium distribution and redistribution: Clinical applications in sequential myocardial imaging. In: Cardiovascular nuclear medicine. Strauss HW, Pitt B, (eds), Mosby CV, St. Louis, 1979.

27. Beller GA, et al, Time course of thallium-201 redistribution after transient myocardial ischemia. Circulation 61:791, 1980.

28. Ritchie JL, Narahara KA, Trobaugh GB, Williams DL, Hamilton GW, Thallium-201 myocardial imaging before and after coronary revascularization: Assessment of regional myocardial blood flow and graft patency. Circulation 56:830, 1977.

29. Gibson RS, et al, Prospective assessment of regional myocardial perfusion before and after coronary revascularization surgery by quantitative thallium-201 scintigraphy. J. Amer. Coll. Cardiol. 1:804, 1983.

30. Olson H, Lyons K, Aronow W, Waters H, Identification of high risk unstable angina patients for mortality and myocardial infarction (abstr.) Circulation 55:173 (suppl. III), 1977.

31. Grüntzig AR, Senning A, Siegenthaller WE, Non-operative dilatation of coronary artery stenosis percutaneous transluminal coronary angioplasty. New Engl. J. Med. 301:61, 1979.

32. Hör G, Kanemoto N, Kaltenbach M, Standke R, Maul FD, Klepzig H, jr, Transluminale Angioplastik: Erfolgskontrolle mit Verfahren der Nuklearmedizin nach nichtoperativer Dilatation kritischer Koronararterienstenosen. Herz 5:168, 1980.

33. Hirzel HO, Grüntzig AR, Nuesch K, Thallium 201-imaging for the evaluation of myocardial perfusion after percutaneous transluminal angioplasty of coronary artery stenosis. Circulation 58:180, 1978.

34. Hirzel HO, Nuesch K, Grüntzig AR, Luetolf UM, Short- and longterm changes in myocardial perfusion after percutaneous transluminal coronary angioplasty assessed by thallium-201 exercise scintigraphy. Circulation 63:1001, 1981.

35. Cherrier F, Godenir JP, Amor M, Cuilliere M, Annouf S, Danchin N, Bertrand A, Interet des methodes isotopiques pour l'indication et l'evaluation des resultats de l'angioplastie transluminale coronaire. In: Non invasive methods in ischemic heart disease. Faivre G, Bertrand A, Cherrier F, Amor M, Neimann J, (eds), Specia, Nancy, pp 399-409, 1982.

36. Pachinger O, Sochor H, Ogris E, Probst P, Klicpera M, Kaindl F, Evaluation of transluminal coronary angioplasty by quantitative 201-thallium scintigraphy. J. nucl. Med. 24:P17 (abstr.), 1983.

37. Maddahi J, et al, Myocardial salvage by intracoronary thrombolysis in evolving acute myocardial infarction. Evaluation using intracoronary injection of thallium-201. Amer. Heart J. 102:664, 1981.

38. Markis JE, et al, Myocardial salvage after intracoronary thrombolysis with streptokinase in acute myocardial infarction. Assessment by intracoronary thallium-201. New Engl. J. Med. 305:777, 1981.

39. Pachinger O, Sochor H, Probst P, Ogris E, Klicpera M, Kaindl F, Scintigraphic evaluation of myocardial viability after coronary reperfusion using intracoronary streptokinase. Eur. Heart J. 2:65, (suppl. A), 1981.

40. Pachinger O, Sochor H, Probst P, Klicpera M, Ogris E, Selektive Thrombolyse bei akutem Koronarverschlusz. Acta Med. Austr. 9:35, 1982.

41. Reduto LA, et al, Coronary artery reperfusion in acute myocardial infarction. Beneficial effects of intracoronary streptokinase on left ventricular salvage and performance. Amer. Heart J. 102:1168, 1981.

42. Schuler G, et al, Thrombolysis in acute myocardial infarction using intracoronary streptokinase assessment by thallium-201 scintigraphy. Circulation 66:658, 1982.

43. Olson H, Lyons K, Aronow W, Waters H, Identification of high risk unstable angina patients for mortality and myocardial infarction. Circulation 55:56 (suppl. III), III-173 (abstr.) 1977.

44. Corbett JR, Dehmer GJ, Lewis SE, et al, The prognostic value of submaximal exercise testing with radionuclide ventriculography before hospital discharge in patients with recent myocardial infarction. Circulation 64:535, 1981.

45. Turner JD, Schwartz KM, Logic JF, et al, The detection of residual jeopardized myocardium three weeks after myocardial infarction by exercise testing with thallium 201 myocardial scintigraphy. Circulation 61:729, 1980.

46. Brown K, et al, Prognostic value of exercise thallium-201 imaging in patients presenting for evaluation of chest pain. J. Amer. Coll. Cardiol. 1(4):994, 1983.

47. Nicod P, et al, Prognostic assessment after myocardial infarction. Comparison between coronary angiography and submaximal exercise testing with radionuclide ventriculography. Amer. J. Cardiol. 49:991, 1982.

48. Phillips P, et al, Prognostically critical coronary stenoses. Identification by radionuclide cineangiography. Amer. J. Cardiol. 49:991, 1982.

49. Rigo P, Murray M, Taylor DR, Weisfeldt M, Strauss HW, Pitt B, Hemodynamic and prognostic findings in patients with transmural and non-transmural infarction. Circulation 51:1064, 1975.

50. Pitt B, Thrall JH, Thallium 201 versus technetium 99m pyrophosphate myocardial in detection and evaluation of patients with acute myocardial infarction. Amer. J. Cardiol. 46:1215, 1980.

51. Tobinick E, Schelbert HR, Henning H, et al, Right ventricular ejection fraction in patients with acute anterior and inferior myocardial infarction assessed by radionuclide angiography. Circulation 57:1078, 1978.

52. Leitl GP, Buchanan JW, Wagner HN, Monitoring cardiac function with nuclear techniques. Amer. J. Cardiol. 46:1125, 1980.

53. Rigo P, Murray M, Strauss HW, Pitt B, et al, Scintiphotographic evaluation of patients with suspected left ventricular aneurysm. Circulation 50:985, 1974.

54. Pachinger O, Einsatz von Radionuklidmethoden in der kardiologischen Intensivstation. In: Verhandlungen der Deutschen Gesellschaft für Herz- und Kreislaufforschung. Band 59, Seite 99-106, 1983.

55. Shah KP, Pichler M, Berman DS, Singh BH, Swan HJC, Left ventricular ejection fraction determined by radionuclide ventriculography in early stages of first transmural myocardial infarction. Amer. J. Cardiol. 45:542, 1980.

56. Nichols AB, McKusick KA, Strauss HW, Dinsmore RE, Block PC, Pohost GM, Clinical utility of gated cardiac blood imaging in congestive left heart failure. Amer. J. Med. 65:785, 1978.

57. Pitt B, Thrall JH, Thallium-201 versus technetium-99m pyrophosphate myocardial in detection and evaluation of patients with acute myocardial infarction. Amer. J. Cardiol. 46:1215, 1980.

58. Bulkley DH, Hutchins GM, Daly I, Pitt D, Thallium-201 imaging and gated cardiac blood pool scans in patients with ischemic and idiopathic congestive cardiomyopathy. A clinical and pathologic study. Circulation 55:753, 1977.

59. Silverman KJ, et al, Value of early thallium-201 scintigraphy for preducting mortality in patients with acute myocardial infarction. Circulation 61:996, 1980.

60. Boucher CA, Okada RD, Pohost GM, Current status of radionuclide imaging in valvular heart disease. Amer. J. Cardiol. 46:1153, 1980.

61. Ogris E, Sochor H, Pachinger O, Probst P, Klicpera M, Assessment of left ventricular performance and regurgitant fraction in chronic aortic insufficiency before and after pharmacologic afterload reduction. In: Radioactieve isotope. Höfer R, Bergman H, (eds), Klin. Forsch. 15:15, 1982.

62. Klicpera M, Probst P, Pachinger O, Assessment of left ventricular reserve in patients with chronic aortic regurgitation using systemic vasodilation. Eur. Heart J. 2:96, 1981.

63. Rigo P, Alderson PO, Robertson RM, Becker LC, Wagner HN, Measurement of aortic and mitral regurgitation by gated cardiac blood pool scans. Circulation 60:306, 1979.

64. Clark DG, McAnulty JH, Rahimtoola SH, Valve replacement in aortic insufficiency with left ventricular dysfunction. Circulation 61:411, 1980.

65. Borer JS, Rosing DR, Kent KM, et al, Left ventricular function at rest and during exercise after aortic valve replacement in patients with aortic regurgitation. Amer. J. Cardiol. 44:1297, 1979.

66. Slutsky R, Karliner J, Ricci D, et al, Left ventricular volumes by gated equilibrium radionuclide angiography: A new method. Circulation 60:556, 1979.

67. Hancock EW, Aortic stenosis, angina pectoris, and coronary artery disease. Amer. Heart J. 93:382, 1977.

68. Bailey IK, et al, Thallium-201 myocardial perfusion imaging in aortic valve stenosis. Amer. J. Cardiol. 40:889, 1977.

69. Goldman MR, Boucher CA, Value of radionuclide imaging techniques in assessing cardiomyopathy. Amer. J. Cardiol. 46:1232, 1980.

70. Pachinger O, Ogris E, Sochor H. Probst P, Zasmeta H, Kaliman J, Klicpera M, Szintigraphische Aspekte bei Kardiomyopathien. Acta Med. Austr. 2:35, 1979.

71. Pachinger O, Ogris E, Probst P, Sochor H, Joskowicz G, Kaindl F, Radionuclide assessment of left and right ventricular performance in congestive cardiomyopathies. Trans. Eur. Soc. Cardiol. 1:38, 1978.

72. Pachinger O, Ogris E, Sochor H, Probst P, Zasmeta H, Kaindl F, Radionuclide assessment of cardiac performance and myocardial perfusion in congestive cardiomyopathies. Clin. Cardiol. 2:264, 1979.

73. Alexander J, Dainiak N, Berger HJ, et al, Serial assessment of doxorubic in cardiac toxicity with quantitative radionuclide angiocardiography. New Eng. J. Med. 300:278, 1979.

74. Pachinger O, Ogris E, Probst P, Sochor H, Joskowicz G, Kaindl F, Assessment of right ventricular performance in coronary artery disease and cardiomyopathies. In: Coronary heart diseases. Kaltenbach M, (ed), Thieme G, Stuttgart, pp 244-246, 1978.

AUTHOR INDEX

SUBJECT INDEX

404